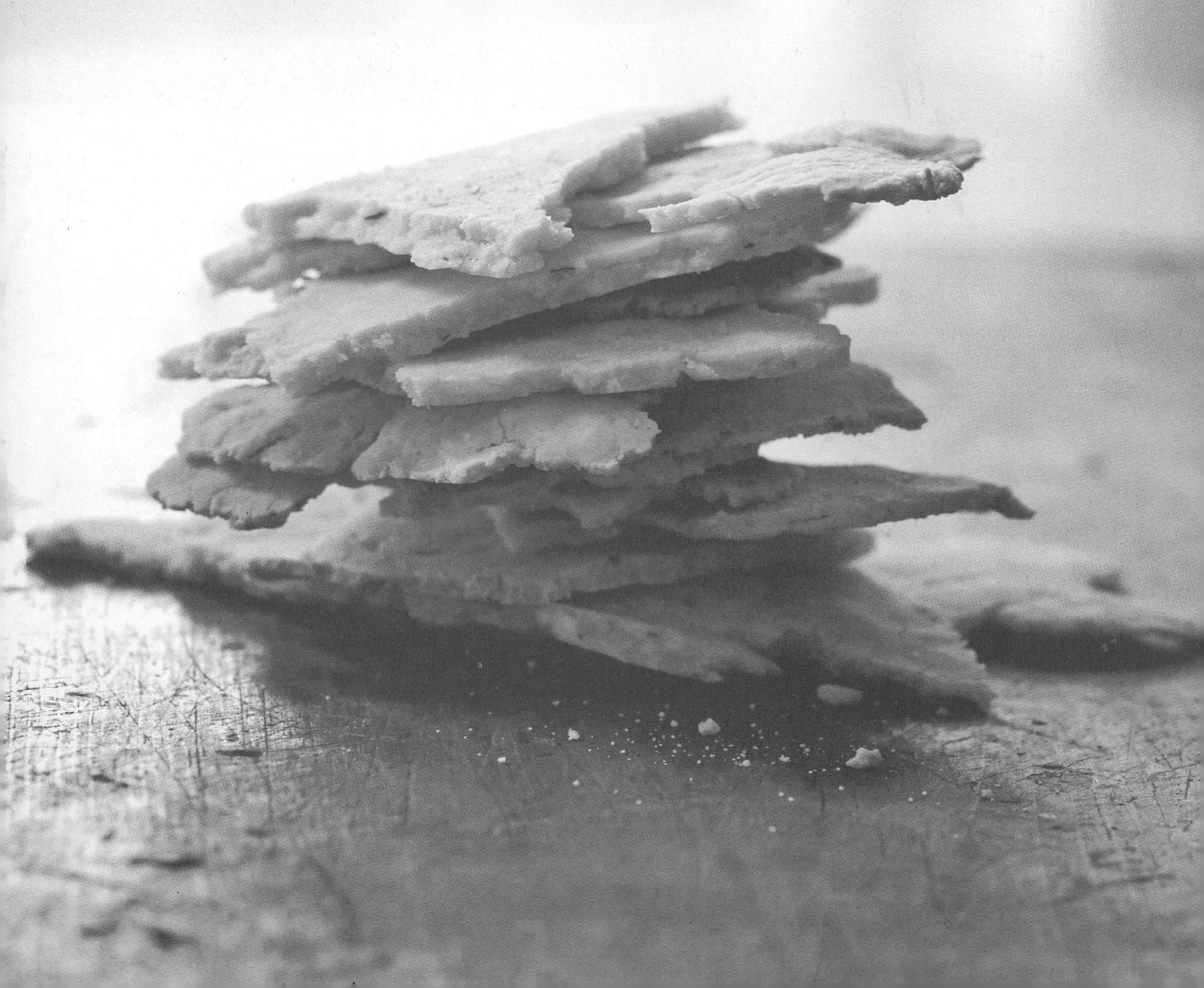

Gluten-Free Girl
AMERICAN CLASSICS
REINVENTED

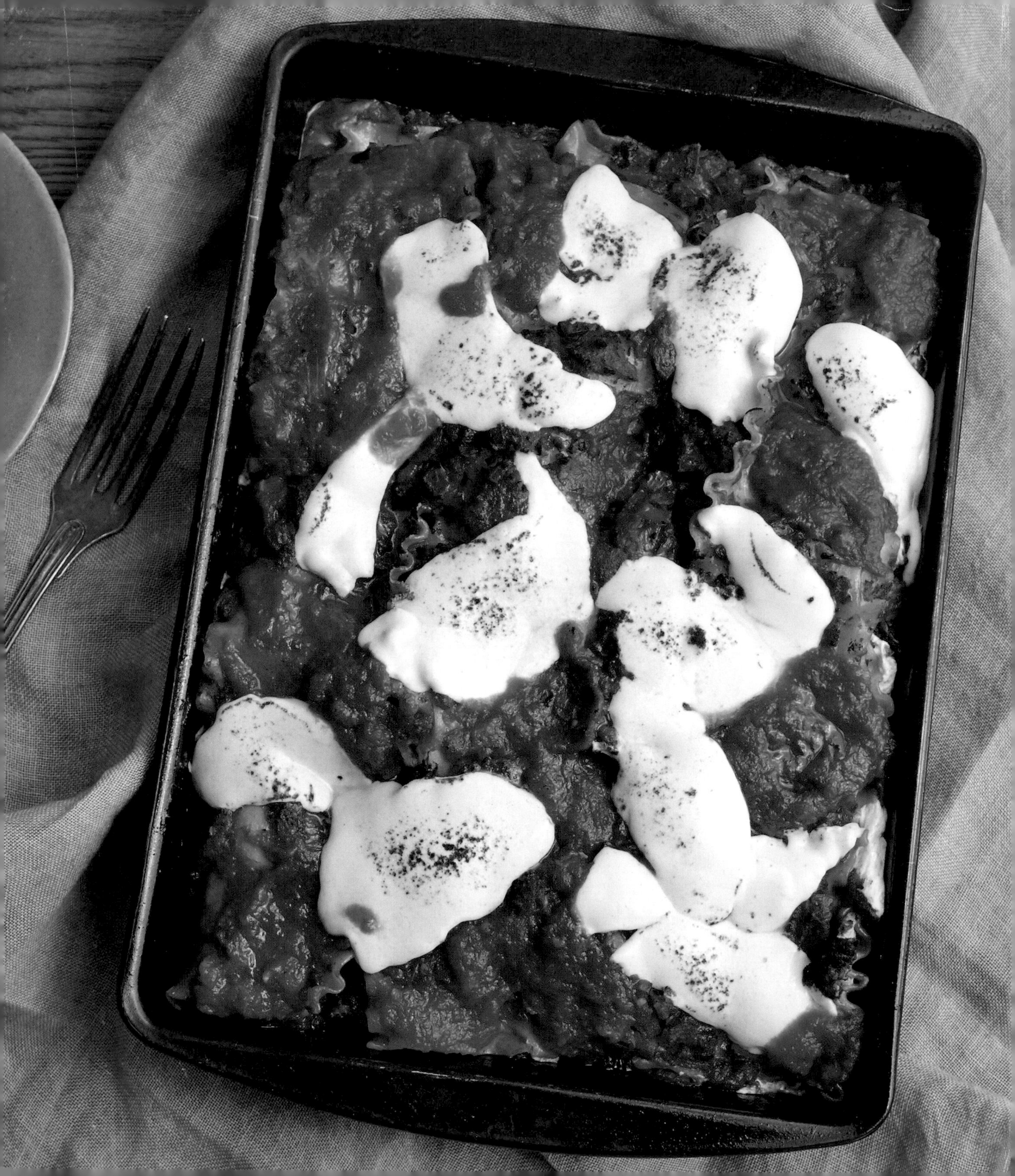

Gluten-Free Girl AMERICAN CLASSICS REINVENTED

Shauna James Ahern with Daniel Ahern

PHOTOGRAPHY BY LAUREN VOLO

HOUGHTON MIFFLIN HARCOURT
BOSTON NEW YORK 2015

Food styling by Mariana Velasquez

Prop styling by April Flores

www.hmhco.com

Library of Congress Cataloging-in-Publication Data

Ahern, Shauna James.

Gluten-Free Girl American classics reinvented / Shauna James Ahern and Daniel Ahern ;
photography by Lauren Volo.

pages cm

Includes index.

ISBN 978-0-544-21988-5 (paper over board) — ISBN 978-0-544-25691-0 (ebook)

1. Gluten-free diet —Recipes. 2. Cooking, American. I. Ahern, Daniel, date. II. Title.

RM237.86.A3378 2015

641.5973 —dc23

2015007133

Printed in China

Design by Gary Tooth / Empire Design Studio

C&C 10 9 8 7 6 5 4 3 2 1

for every person who needs to be gluten-free and still wants a slice of damned good pie

CONTENTS

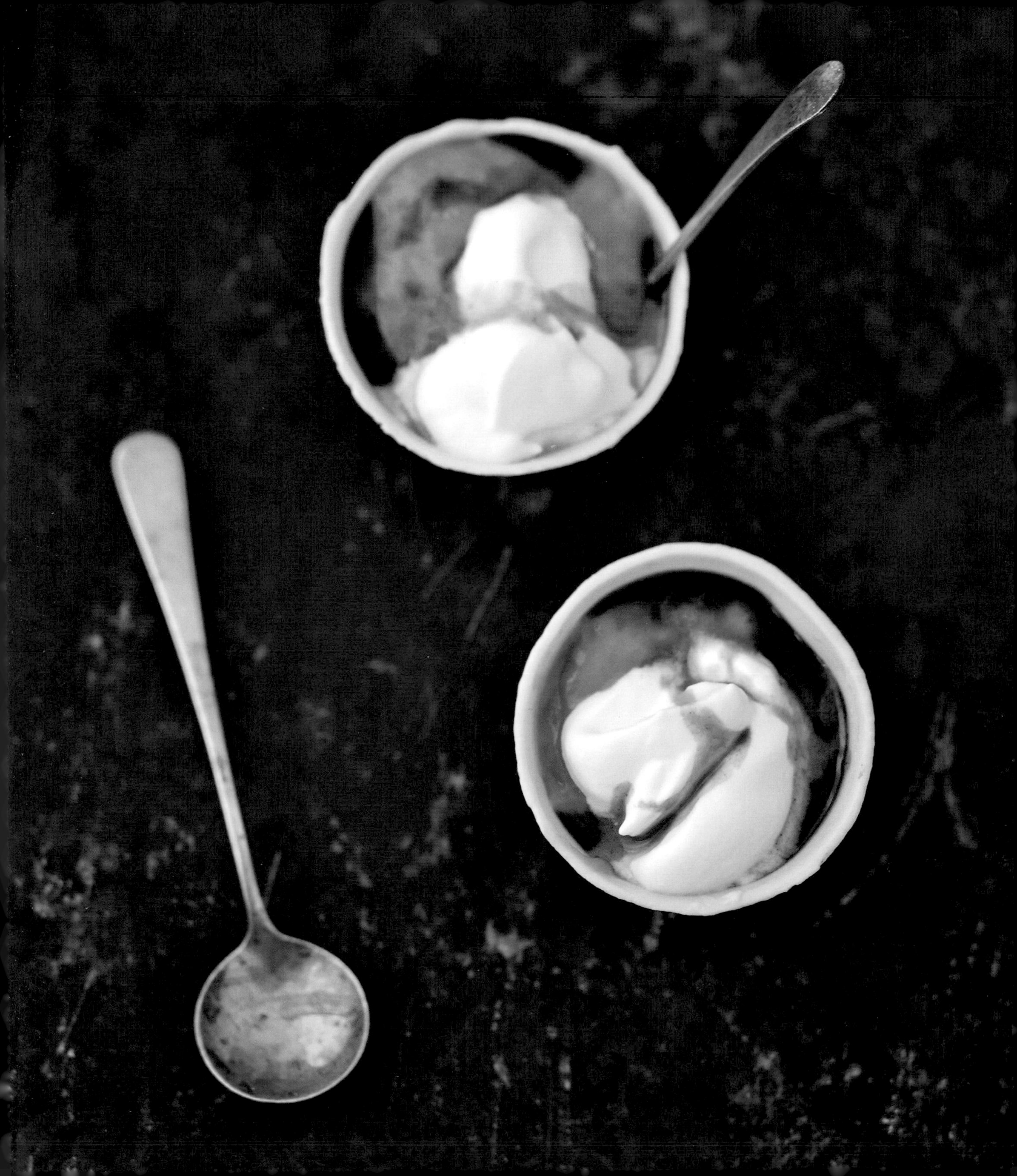

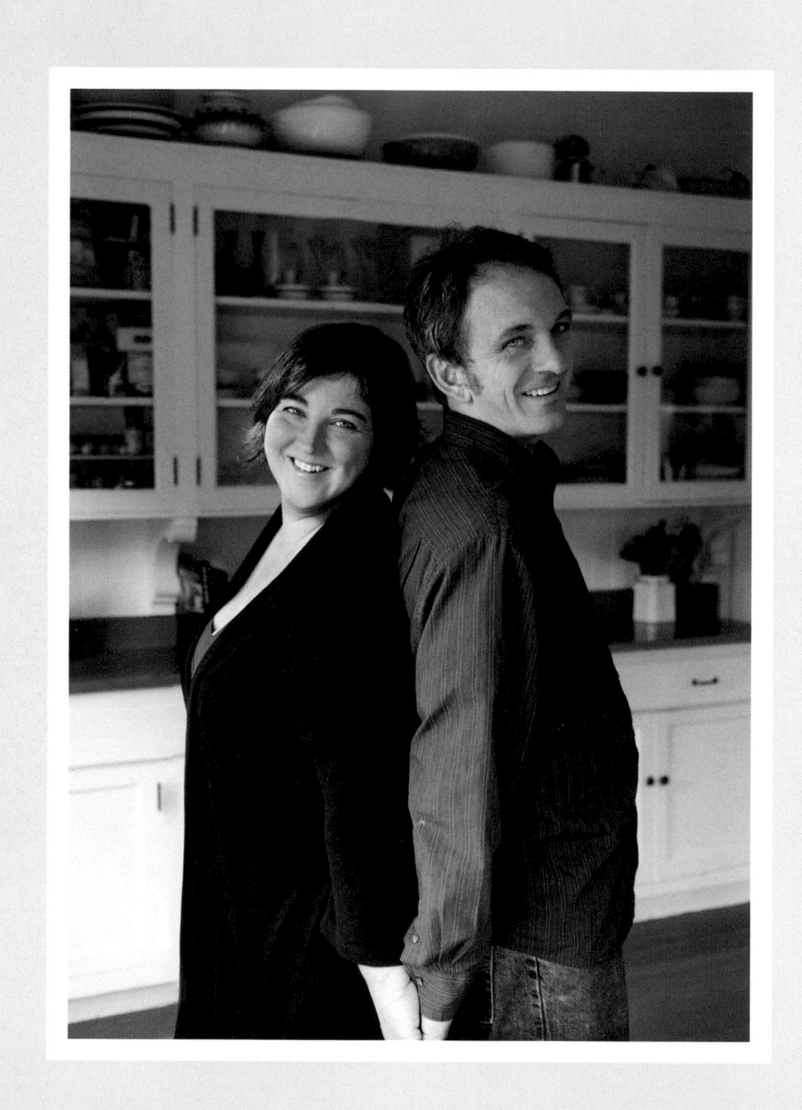

Acknowledgments

Thank you!

Thank you to every reader who sent us impassioned pleas and suggestions for recipes that *must* be made gluten-free, from shoofly pie to tater tot hot pot to red velvet cake. You missed your comfort foods and the ease of eating them at family gatherings and birthday parties. Thank you for trusting us to make these recipes right for you.

Thank you to every person who helped us arrange potlucks in community centers, church basements, and people's homes across New England and down the length of California. We loved sharing food and laughter with you.

Thank you to Jovial Foods, Bakery on Main, and Attune Foods for sponsoring our road trips as well as providing gluten-free pasta, granola, and cereal for everyone who attended our potlucks. We love your food and your companies.

Thank you to Lauren Volo for her clear, sumptuous photographs, April Flores for her meticulous choice of props, and Mariana Velasquez for her incredible food styling for the photo shoot for this book. You made this food truly beautiful.

Thank you to the entire team at Houghton Mifflin Harcourt for your hard work and close attention to detail, especially Jacqueline Beach, whose kind, gentle urgings to make the manuscript as clear as possible made this book much better.

Thank you to Justin Schwartz, as always, for insisting we pay close attention to every detail of every recipe and pushing us to write this book. We cannot imagine creating a cookbook without you editing it.

Thank you to Stacey Glick for being the best darned agent we could ever imagine. You're our constant cheerleader and guiding voice.

Thank you to Claire Moncrief for coming into our professional lives just when we needed you most. You provided us with direction and so many laughs those long days in the studio. Without you, we wouldn't have boxes of Gluten-Free Girl flour blends available for sale by the publication of this book.

Thank you to the 1563 people who backed our Kickstarter campaign to bring those flour blends to the market. The community came together to make magic happen and we are so grateful.

Thank you to our good friends who cheered us on, tested recipes, tasted dishes, and watched the kids when we were really in a crunch. Adrienne and Michael, Trish and Clint, Tracy and Kim, Anna and Michael, Tita and John, Gypsy and Steve, Andy and Dana, Richard and Mary, Alison and Scott, Sharon, and Sara and John—you are our community.

Thank you to our darling children, Lucy and Desmond. You are the light of our lives and the reason we work so hard. (Lu, this book is why Mama sometimes had to be on the computer at night when you came downstairs, supposed to be asleep, wanting me to read one more book. Let's make beignets again.)

Thank you, finally, to all the loyal and generous readers of *Gluten-Free Girl*. You've changed our lives in an extraordinary fashion.

Introduction

America, you have so much good food to offer.

From Key lime pie in Florida to Indian pudding in New England, broiled Kumamoto oysters with garlic-butter breadcrumbs in the Pacific Northwest, and Baja fish tacos in California, the four corners of this country are full of great food. But it's not just the coasts. It's smoky corn fritters from the Midwest; green chile breakfast pie from New Mexico; Philly cheesesteaks; gumbo from New Orleans; pecan pie; almond dim sum cookies; hot and sour soup; huckleberry pancakes from Montana; Kentucky hot browns; fried green tomatoes; and macadamia-encrusted mahi mahi from Hawaii. This country contains such a bounty of fresh produce, wild game, and ingredients from around the world that became standard American fare with the immigration of people across our borders, and a resilience that creates goodness from necessary change.

American food culture has received a bad rap for the past 75 years. With the rise of packaged and processed foods, and the way we've been persuaded by advertisers that our meals should be convenient and fast rather than homemade, so much of American food has come out of a box since the 1950s. But if you look at regional specialties and recipes that have been passed down from grandmother to uncle to someone cooking in an American kitchen in 2015, you'll see a spirit of making something good out of what is already in the pantry. You'll see beloved dishes like buttermilk chess pie and hush puppies and johnnycakes that have a history, a resonance from the 1800s to today, a story of what America used to be, still alive in this age. We are far more than the bill of goods we have been sold and the preservative-laden "food" we've been eating out of boxes. We can do better. We have before. We can do it again.

The America we see in popular media often seems divisive—full of arguments about politics and religion—or trivial—with endless conversations about celebrity gossip and sports—and sometimes annoying. But drive across this country, stopping in small family restaurants or people's homes or farmers' markets, and you'll find good people full of kindness and open minds around the table. Setting food down on the table opens the door to great conversations.

In the summer of 2003, I drove across America,

from New York to Oregon, with my best friend, Sharon. We were perfect traveling companions, having been best friends since 1982. We never failed for conversations on country roads where the radio reception faded. We stayed in tiny hotels every night, exhausted after traveling all day and laughing. We sang ABBA songs deep into the evening as we crossed Minnesota under starry skies. And mostly, we ate. Sharon and I ate everything that came our way. In New York, we shared two last slices of thin pizza at Sal and Carmine's, across the street from the apartment building we were leaving. In Indiana, we drove 60 miles off the highway to have chicken and noodles at an Amish restaurant, passing black carriages to reach the place. In Chicago, we ate great hot dogs after a run along Lake Michigan and deep-dish pizza in a restaurant where the walls were so festooned with signatures we could no longer see the white walls. The next day we ate Italian beef sandwiches at Al's #1 Italian Beef, the juices dripping onto the trunk of our white car. There were sandwiches alongside lakes, waffles for breakfast, and Indian fry bread in South Dakota. In Wyoming, Sharon turned the car around when she saw a tiny café selling homemade peach pie, even though we had already eaten a huge breakfast and lunch that day, plus snacks. We ended our trip in Ashland, Oregon, with a big breakfast of yogurt and hazelnut granola. After I flew home, I discovered that somehow I had lost eight pounds after that trip. We did try to go for walks and runs every day, but mostly I think it was the happiness and laughter. My metabolism seemed to have increased from joy. I have never been so in love with the country where I live as I was on that trip.

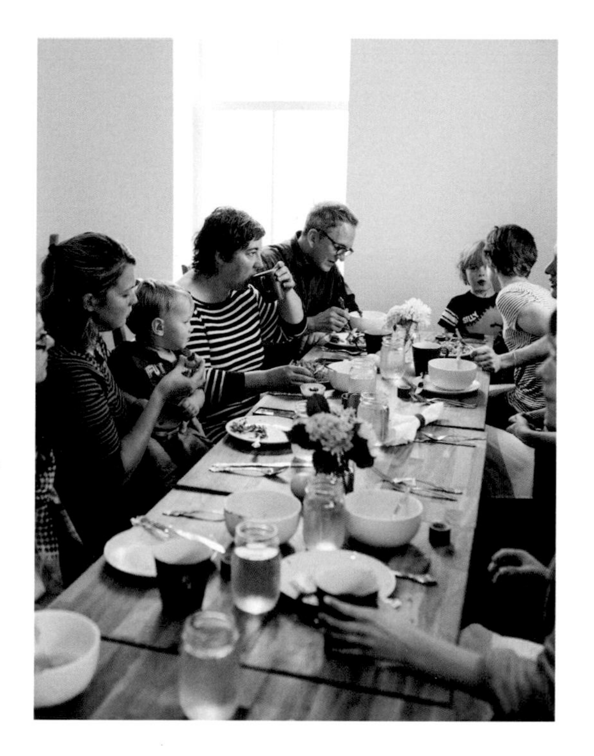

A few years later, however, I was deathly sick and no one could figure out why for months. By the time I was diagnosed with celiac sprue, the autoimmune disorder that causes the body to attack itself upon ingestion of gluten, I was thrilled to hear it. I didn't have cancer or anything fatal. And the only cure was removing gluten from my diet. Give me the disease where the cure is not chemotherapy or drugs or surgery, but eating really great food instead. Within weeks of giving up gluten entirely, I started to heal. Within a year of letting go of gluten, I had a popular food blog, a book deal, and my husband, who was a chef. Together, Danny and I started creating food that nourished us both, and then our daughter, along with the people who bought our cookbooks. Our first instinct is always to create food that is naturally gluten-free, foods everyone can share: fresh vegetables, succulent meat dishes, roasted potatoes or quinoa fritters, smoked salmon, big salads, soups full of flavor, and simple sweets made with honey and maple syrup. Most of the time, we're eating food that people don't think of as gluten-free. We just love good food.

But over time, and after the publication of our second cookbook, Danny and I began thinking of all the eating adventures in our lives. He grew up in Colorado, cooked in Seattle and New York, helped open a restaurant in Oklahoma, and loved his brief time in New Orleans. In each of those places, it was food that began the memories he shared with me. I grew up outside Los Angeles, moved to Seattle, lived in New York City (for a brief time, Danny and I lived twelve blocks from each other and never met), traveled fairly extensively, and even lived in London twice, giving me the chance to look at my country from the outside. Of course I remember the Huntington Library, orca whales off ferry rides, Central Park, and the Tate Gallery. But memories of those places wouldn't be complete without corn dogs at Disneyland, blackberry pie, knishes from Zabar's, and the time I grew excited to see a frozen Mexican TV dinner at Harrods when I was particularly homesick. And we talked continuously about the letters we received from people who read our site, letters asking how to convert their grandmother's Texas sheet cake recipe into gluten-free, or how to make a great pie dough for cherry pie in July, or how to make cream of mushroom soup for much-loved Midwestern casseroles. As much as we love kale and sausage breakfasts, noodles made of zucchini, and ribs right off the grill, we both under-stood the desire for foods that originally contained gluten.

Every Sunday, for the four years I lived in New York, I walked with my best friend, Sharon, up Broadway to Absolute Bagels. We always ordered the same: one plain bagel with cream cheese and lox, one sesame bagel with lox cream cheese. (The second one was cheaper.) We walked home, talking, the bagels calling to us from the bag. But we waited until we reached our apartment, made a pot of tea, spread the Sunday *New York Times* before us, and sat down at the kitchen table together. We spent all morning and well into the afternoon there, slowly eating our chewy bagels, the best in New York City, happy to be together. I find, often, when I miss a food with gluten, it's not the actual food I miss. It's the experience of sharing it with someone else.

Danny and I wanted to create food that resonates with you, bringing memories of Sunday morning breakfasts with family or cakes on special occasions or a decadent dessert for birthdays. But we also wanted to make food that is great on its own. We never aim for food that will make people say, "Hey, I can't even tell there's no gluten in there." We both smile widely if people say, "Man, that's good. Can I have some more?" You don't need gluten to make great food.

We both love a challenge. Danny's decades of chef experiences means he approaches recipes with enthusiasm and a deep curiosity to play with the food, rather than fear that it will never work. I am full of the geekery required to play with

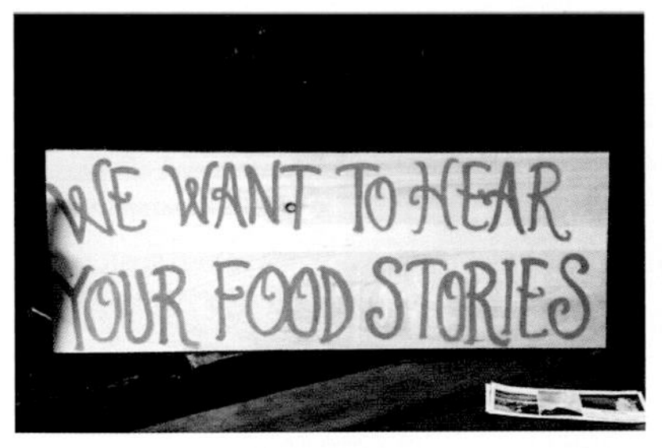

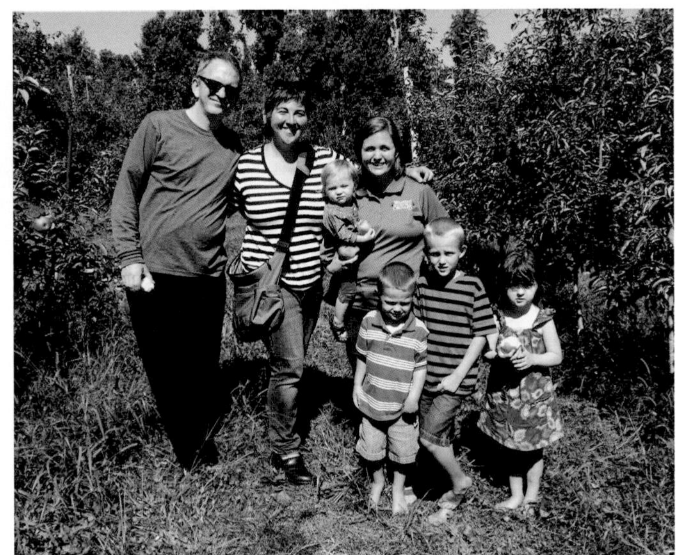

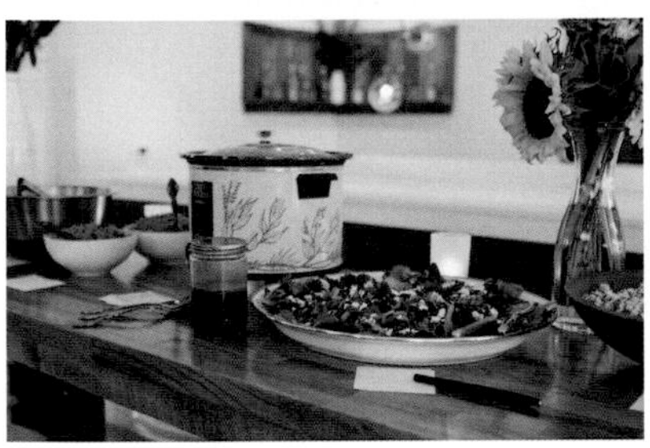

gluten-free flours, combine them, and see which ones work best for a pizza dough. (There were many failed attempts before we created the recipe you will find in this cookbook.) We decided to tackle this project: the most-requested American comfort foods, great without gluten.

We asked questions of everyone we met. For months, we asked fans of our website what they wanted to eat. If you are from the South, what do you miss? From the Rocky Mountain states? From New England? From the Southwest? What can we make for you? There was no shortage of opinions. We compiled long lists of everything people said—the hundreds and hundreds of fervent requests—and began compiling a recipe list. We researched online—thank you to everyone who has written down a much-loved recipe from relatives before you—and cracked open the battered covers of old cookbooks from Junior Leagues and PTAs and Fannie Farmer and all the regional cookbooks that we could find. We have a huge cookbook collection, but it grew enormously over the past two years. Some readers sent us their family recipes to adapt. Others just urged us on, sending good wishes and inspiration.

The best research we did happened on the road. Danny and Lucy and I climbed into a rented minivan one September and drove from New York City to Amish country, up to Vermont and over to Maine, through Rhode Island, and to the Berkshires, driving back to New York City full of stories and good food. Everywhere we went, we attended potlucks thrown by locals (we spent months arranging these, along with the companies who make good gluten-free foods who sponsored the trips for us), and ate great food, gluten-free. We ate in church basements and a beautiful barn in the Green Mountains of Vermont, in people's homes and restaurants, at picnics in the park and tiny community halls. We visited farms every day, everywhere we went, because nothing would end up on our plates without the work of farmers. And we listened to the stories of all the people we met. Listening to other people's food stories is one of

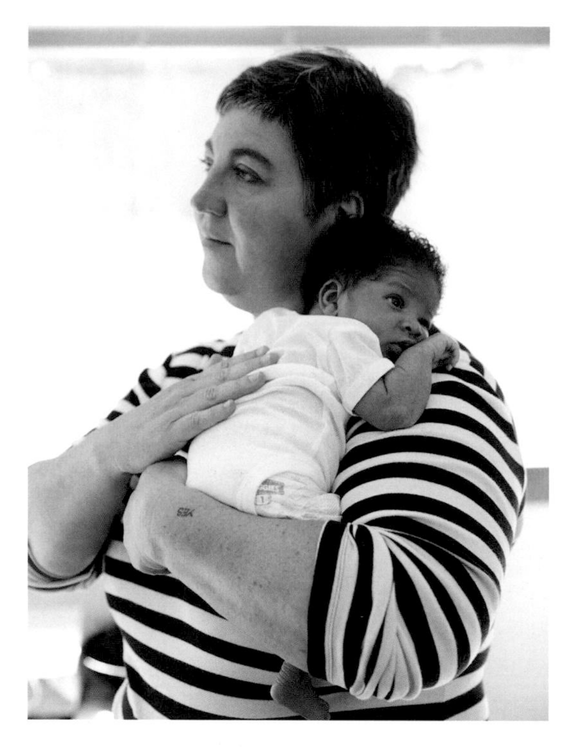

my favorite activities in the world. Later, we drove again, from Sacramento to San Francisco to the fertile area outside of Fresno to the coast of California, all the way down to Los Angeles. We were astonished again by the hard work of farmers, the stories of families gathered together over food, and the new memories we helped people make at every potluck. These visits were just as joyful as the trip across the country in a rented car with Sharon had been, but this time there was no gluten. I ate equally well on all those trips. (We planned a potluck trip through the Midwest and another one in the South, but our darling son, Desmond, arrived, after three years of trying to adopt, so that put the kibosh on long road trips for a while. We're hoping we can come see you with the publication of this book.)

And then we returned home to cook and bake. We made three or four dishes a day, writing it all down, playing, discussing, tweaking, and eating. Luckily, we have a lot of friends who want to eat our food, or we would have been swimming in casseroles and pie. We crossed some recipes off the list after we made them—I'm sorry, but funnel cake with or without gluten is too greasy-gross for my taste—and added others. In each chapter we planned, we gave ourselves a little space to play, making up a new dish based on the flavors of an area, rather than merely re-creating a dish. I think you'll like the Reuben Sandwich Soup (page 140) and the California Roll Sushi Salad (page 161) especially well.

We liked sharing the process along the way with folks on the Internet. This is the new America, after all. Whenever we posted a photograph of a first draft of sourdough bread or the Cuban pork sandwiches on Instagram, there were loud cries of excitement and want. ("Recipe, please?!") We felt bad about making you wait for so long to hold this book in your hands. But after more than two years of researching, writing, traveling, testing, tweaking, writing some more, feeding people, editing, photographing, pondering, and mostly eating a lot of really great food, we're ready to share with you.

Here it is, finally. *American Classics Reinvented.*

A few notes about ingredients and techniques

When you make gluten-free food and baked goods, the first question everyone asks is pretty simple to guess: how do you make [insert name of food here] without gluten?

It's much easier than you might expect. In fact, we've done most of the hard work for you.

First, realize that we have, as a society, overprivileged gluten in our food culture, specifically wheat. For thousands of years, bakers have been reaching for wheat flour primarily because it was the one most widely available to us. But there are plenty of places in this country where people found it hard to grow wheat in their climate and so relied on corn or buckwheat instead. This explains the popularity of buckwheat crepes in northern Maine or johnnycakes in New England and the South. It's only recently that we began demanding a common food culture of wheat, and that demand grew louder when we started living on processed food. As well, there has been a birth of new grains and flours available in the United States, such as teff, sorghum, millet, almond flour, and starches such as potato starch and sweet rice flour. In the past decade or so, pastry chefs and bakers have started playing with other flours in their work, not as a substitute for wheat, but as a powerful way to build flavor and create structure in baked goods. Kim Boyce's wonderful cookbook, *Good to the Grain*, inspired countless bakers to start playing with whole grains of all kinds. Alice Medrich's cookbook *Flavor Flours* honors flours such as corn flour, coconut flour, and sorghum flour, not as good enough for gluten-free baking, but as incredible flours every baker should use. (In fact, that book was not marketed as a gluten-free book at all, but simply as a book for adventurous bakers.) Bakers everywhere are starting to realize this: gluten-free does not have to be the ugly stepsister of baking to the Cinderella of wheat.

In fact, many baked goods are better without gluten. Read that sentence again. I mean it. The only reason we traditionally use gluten in pancakes, muffins, quick breads, and pie dough is because we always have. Think about the properties of gluten. It adds bulk to a recipe. Gluten-free flours do that just as well. It binds ingredients in a recipe. Most gluten-free flours do that well too. The only place where gluten is really necessary is in breads, flatbreads, pizza doughs, and any baked good that requires elasticity or particularly strong dough. There's no reason to use gluten in crepes, fried fish or chicken, casseroles, waffles, banana bread, or soups. We just need flours for those.

Gluten-Free Flour Blends

So let's talk about flours.

There are more gluten-free flours in the world than gluten flours. Did you know that? Most of them might feel unfamiliar—have you tried banana flour or kaniwa flour?—but that doesn't mean they're not useful. Think about it—at some point in U.S. history, olive oil felt like a really exotic foreign ingredient. And that was only 50 years ago. So embrace the change and start playing with the flours available to you.

We have been playing with flours for years. I have probably made at least 120 different flour mixes in the past nine years, combining flours for protein levels, flavor combinations, fats, and availability in most stores. Some of them have been disastrous. (Do NOT mix coconut flour and buckwheat together. Bleh.) Some of them have worked better than others. Some of them have worked brilliantly, but suggesting those particular combinations of flours would require that you order pounds of expensive flours online. That wasn't going to work.

After our daughter was born, and particularly now that our son is here too, I understand why so many of our readers asked if we could come up with blends for our recipes instead of listing six different flours for each baked good. And, after all that playing and baking, we have two mixes we adore, flour mixes we have not only used in creating this book but also that we keep in big containers in our kitchen and use to make everything we bake for our family. Throughout the book, you'll see that we have suggested one or the other flour mix for particular recipes, based on their properties. However, we have formulated every recipe in this cookbook to work with either mix. If you find you cannot eat grains, you can still make almost every recipe in this cookbook with our Grain-Free Flour Mix.

ALL-PURPOSE GLUTEN-FREE FLOUR BLEND

Makes 1000 grams (1 kilogram)

This flour blend works well in every recipe in this book. It's the all-purpose flour of gluten-free. Because it's 40 percent whole-grain millet flour, it contains enough protein to create structure in baked goods. The sweet rice flour is special, so super-starchy that it binds other ingredients together in the recipe, somewhat like gluten does. And the potato starch lends a certain lightness and moisture to baked goods and foods. Together, these three flours are our super-flours, our favorite all-purpose gluten-free flour blend.

400 grams millet flour

300 grams sweet rice flour

300 grams potato starch

Put the flours and starch in the bowl of a food processor or stand mixer with the paddle attachment. Whirl them together until they are one color. You now have a flour blend. Store it in a large jar or container. You can now make any recipe in this book.

Why is this recipe in grams? Huh?

This question comes up immediately. (Several times readers of our website have asked why our recipes aren't in American! To which I've always been tempted to say, "Grams and science are American too.") So let me answer it immediately. Each gluten-free flour has a different density and weight than every other flour. Teff flour is far heavier than potato starch, for example. If you try to substitute a cup of one for another, you're going to be mighty frustrated with the results. Danny and I want your baked goods to work. Baking by weight means the measurements will be accurate. This is the reason pastry chefs and professional bakers make all their recipes by weighing their ingredients. You won't see measuring cups in a bakery.

A kitchen scale costs about $30. You're going to spend that much on flours in recipes that don't work if you try to do them in cups. Trust us. No one who has made the switch to baking by weight has ever regretted it. (Plus, when you bake by weight, you simply zero out the scale and use the same bowl for the next ingredient. Fewer dishes!)

But I can't eat rice flour. How am I going to make your flour mix?

You won't make our flour mix. You'll use your flour mix. Many people who cannot tolerate gluten have other food allergies or intolerances besides that. If I use sweet rice flour in our recipes, and you can't tolerate rice, you can replace it with the same weight of tapioca flour or arrowroot in this formula. It might not produce the exact same result, but it will be good.

So here's all you have to remember: 40 percent whole-grain flour; 60 percent starches or white flours.

If you can't eat millet, or can't find it (but it is found online, easily), you could use to replace it: brown rice flour, sorghum flour, buckwheat flour, teff flour, or quinoa flour.

If you can't eat sweet rice flour or potato starch, you could use to replace either: tapioca flour, cornstarch, or arrowroot flour. Just use the same weights and you've made your own flour mix.

Also, once you have used this flour mix to make the recipes in this book and you have enjoyed the results, you can convert your own family recipes by using this simple trick: every 1 cup of all-purpose bleached white flour = 140 grams of this flour mix. That's about all you have to do.

GRAIN-FREE FLOUR MIX

Makes 1000 grams (1 kilogram)

What if I can't eat grains like millet or sweet rice?

Some folks who are gluten-free find that they do better without grains at all. There's no need to fear you will never eat banana bread again. We have a grain-free mix for you too.

300 grams raw buckwheat flour

200 grams almond flour

100 grams finely ground flaxseed meal

200 grams potato starch

200 grams arrowroot flour

Put the flours and starch in the bowl of a food processor or stand mixer with the paddle attachment. Whirl them together until they are one color. You now have a flour blend. Store it in a large jar or container. You can now make any recipe in this book.

Let us explain.

Almond flour is a wonder. It's full of good fats and high in protein. Many people create baked goods using only almond flour. But we find that baked goods with almond flour are a little too dense for our taste. When we first combined almond flour and raw buckwheat flour, we fell in love. The flavor of these two together is warm and nutty, familiar and new at the same time. However, we have to make clear that we want you to buy raw buckwheat flour, rather than traditional buckwheat flour. Most buckwheat flours on the market are toasted buckwheat flour, which has a very distinct taste, a little too bitter for us. Raw buckwheat flour is simply raw buckwheat groats ground down into a flour. That flour is nutty and warm and so good. Buckwheat is sort of a magic flour, fairly close to wheat in many ways. (But it's not wheat or even a grain. It's a seed from the rhubarb family.) Ground flaxseed meal adds a warm nutty flavor to complement the buckwheat and acts as a great binder for baked goods. The potato starch and arrowroot flour here add lightness and some moisture to the mix. You can use this grain-free flour mix in almost every recipe in the book.

Do I need any other flours for this book?

We highly recommend you start your sourdough starter with teff flour, which is also phenomenal in any baked good with chocolate. We use tapioca flour in our bagel recipe, to add a hint of chewiness. To sum up, you'll need millet flour, sweet rice flour, and potato starch, plus almond flour, buckwheat flour, and arrowroot flour, plus teff and tapioca. Or, you could choose one mix like the AP and do everything with three flours.

And if you don't want to buy and mix all these flours yourself, by the time of publication of this book, you can buy them from us directly, through our website. Go to www.glutenfreegirl.com/flours to order some today.

PSYLLIUM HUSK

In some of the bready recipes in this book, the doughs that rely more on gluten than muffins or cookies would, we use a teaspoon or two of psyllium husks. These husks are high in dietary fiber, have no real taste, and absorb water like you wouldn't believe. With these properties, a bit of psyllium husks can replicate some of the properties of gluten in doughs. Since I don't do well with xanthan or guar gum—they give me digestive upset as though I have eaten gluten, and I'm certainly not the only one—and psyllium is widely available in every grocery store, we use psyllium in our recipes. You might wish to play with ground flaxseed or chia seeds, or if you can tolerate the gums, use xanthan instead. Feel free to play, but we've seen the best results with psyllium.

Other Ingredients

Most of the ingredients we use are available in the grocery store. That's intentional. We want you to be able to cook and bake easily. But here are a few words about the food choices we have made.

FATS

You'll see it when you flip through the pages of this book: we believe in butter. We also use good-quality lard. We don't use the kind sold in grocery stores, since that is full of trans fats to make it shelf stable. We use lard that has been rendered from the fat around the kidneys of the pig, which is called leaf lard. That kind of lard is sold at farmers' markets and good butchers. (We actually render our own lard from the fat sold to us by local farmers.) These two fats are what American cooks used for hundreds of years. Around the 1970s, most Americans grew afraid of these fats, a fear instigated by the medical community and most of the media, which insisted that saturated fats cause heart disease and other chronic conditions such as diabetes. Guess what? They were wrong. Trans fats and hydrogenated fats are bad for our hearts, which means the margarine so many of us grew up eating was far worse for us than butter. Our doctor, who is one of the most respected doctors in Seattle, has told us that he believes the low-fat, no-fat craze of the past forty years has been the worst thing to happen to American health. And in fact, heart attacks and chronic diseases have risen dramatically since Americans started staying away from fat and lard. Did you know that pure lard is one of the healthiest fats you can eat, along with olive oil and coconut oil? Find out for yourself what works for your body, because each of us is different. But in our kitchen, we use butter, lard, coconut oil, and olive oil for 95 percent of our cooking.

When we are frying foods, we sometimes use other fats. We have a fried foods chapter in this book for a good reason. Fried foods were the most requested recipes of all the recipes we received. When we were in Maine on our potluck road trip, at the Common Ground Country Fair, we saw a booth that made us laugh out loud. On the side, it simply said HOT FRIED DOUGH. "That's America," we said, laughing. But we understand why. Hot fried dough can be delightful, if done right. And if you fry foods at the right temperature, with a good frying oil, frying does not have to be unhealthy or greasy. There's a place for fried chicken (we've converted Edna Lewis's recipe, using lard, butter, and country ham as the fat) and beignets in a good, healthy diet. I'm willing to say that if we expand the notion of "healthy diet" to mean eating with great variety and joy, a diet without the occasional fried pickle or apple cider doughnut is not much of a healthy diet. That's what we believe.

When you are making recipes from the fried foods chapter, you'll see that we have not specified the fry oil for the recipe. We'll let you make your own choice. For shallow frying, we tend to use lard, coconut oil, or olive oil. Or some combination of them, with butter added for the flavor. (If you have to be dairy-free, you can clarify the butter, which gives it a higher smoke point, making it better for frying anyway.) For a dish like hush puppies or doughnuts, we use a frying oil like peanut oil (for a strong savory taste) or rice bran oil (for a more neutral flavor, which works well for those doughnuts). Again, we'll let you decide what you can afford and what you want to use. Remember that you can reuse fry oil again and again, like restaurants do. Keep using the fry oil until you can't see the bottom of the pan when you pour in the oil, or the oil starts to smoke upon heating. We keep one jar of fry oil for savory foods and another for sweet foods in our kitchen.

SWEETENERS

When we first began creating this book, we thought about making it a gluten-free, grain-free, dairy-free, and sugar-free book. However, we let that go pretty quickly. Our intention in creating this book is to make the very best gluten-free versions of the foods so many folks requested of us. We've made many of the recipes dairy-free, or we've given you suggestions for how to make a recipe dairy-free, when that's possible. (See the Feel Like Playing? box at the end of every recipe.) We've given you a grain-free flour mix, if you need to be grain-free. And many recipes use honey or maple syrup because they taste better than sugar in those recipes.

However, we decided in the end that sugar was necessary in some of these recipes. Sugar helps to create structure in baked goods like cookies and cakes. Switching away from sugar meant losing loft and a certain flavor. But even more than that, we feel like having sugar occasionally isn't so bad. Honey, maple syrup, coconut sugar, and organic cane sugar—they're all sweeteners and the body reads them pretty much the same way.

Most of the foods in this book, particularly the sweet baked goods, are splurge foods. We don't have any right to tell you what to eat, and we won't. But seriously, don't do what we had to do to make this book by our deadline. Don't eat cake every day for a week. (Ugh, that was actually an awful week.) And after much experimenting with restrictive eating and low-fat foods, I've come to realize that my body does much better if I consciously choose and fully savor what I eat. We have fruit for dessert most evenings of the week. We have something like cake or pie or coffee milk custards once a week or so, mostly on the weekends after we have been running around or playing outside with the kids all day. And doing that—instead of restricting sweet things entirely—has allowed us to have great conversations with our daughter about sugar and the idea of "sometimes treats" far better than if they were never in the house.

In other words, eat these foods in moderation and enjoy them fully.

When we do use sugar, we use organic cane sugar instead of bleached white sugar. We prefer the taste and texture of organic cane sugar to bleached white sugar. These recipes here have been formulated with organic cane sugar. We also use coconut sugar, which has a deep caramel taste and comes from the sap of a coconut tree, in place of traditional brown sugar. But of course, you can use whatever works for you.

SALT

We use kosher salt for all savory foods and fine sea salt for baked goods. If you use the same amount of fine sea salt in place of the kosher salt, your food will be saltier.

WATCH OUT FOR THESE INGREDIENTS

When you have to be gluten-free, you learn to avoid commercially produced breads, pizzas, and beers pretty quickly. But there are ingredients you might not suspect to have gluten that can still make you sick. For example? Soy sauce. The few times I have ingested gluten by mistake mostly came from a well-meaning person giving me food that had been seasoned with soy sauce. Soy sauce is fermented with wheat. Even that small amount could make me (and you) sick. Gluten-free tamari actually tastes better! But you have to be vigilant with foods made by other people. Fish sauce, which we use at times in this book, often has wheat in it. Don't let go of it, however! Fish sauce adds such a wonderful umami depth to flavors in food that we always use it in our meat loaf. Our favorite brand, Red Boat, does not contain wheat. Even boxed chicken or beef stock can sometimes contain wheat. And make sure before eating them that cornmeal or other grains are produced in a gluten-free facility. In essence, check all your ingredients carefully before using them in these recipes.

Finally, we want you to know that this is not a "5-ingredients-or-less and we promise it will only take 20 minutes to make!" kind of book. These are recipes worth taking the time to make. If we're going to make the recipes we miss from our childhoods, the ones our grandmothers and grandfathers made, in the tradition of their grandmothers and grandfathers, we need to slow down. Great sourdough bread takes five full days to make a starter (and sometimes more like two weeks) and two full days of rising and waiting and proofing before baking. Believe me, that bread is worth the wait.

Those of us who cannot eat gluten can heal by avoiding gluten for the rest of our lives. But just because something is gluten-free doesn't mean it's going to help heal us. Cookies from a box with a long list of preservatives, additives, and food dyes are just as bad for us as the gluten boxed cookies with the same list. Make your own gingersnaps. Get the kids involved. Set aside some time to enjoy this. You'll all enjoy it more and you are in charge of what goes into your food. The first cheesecake with the gingersnap crust you make with your kids, from scratch, is going to be far more memorable than the one you bought in the freezer section of the store.

However, we're pretty sure you already know this. After all, you're buying a cookbook, not a grocery list. So, set aside some time, gather good food around you, and let's start cooking, America.

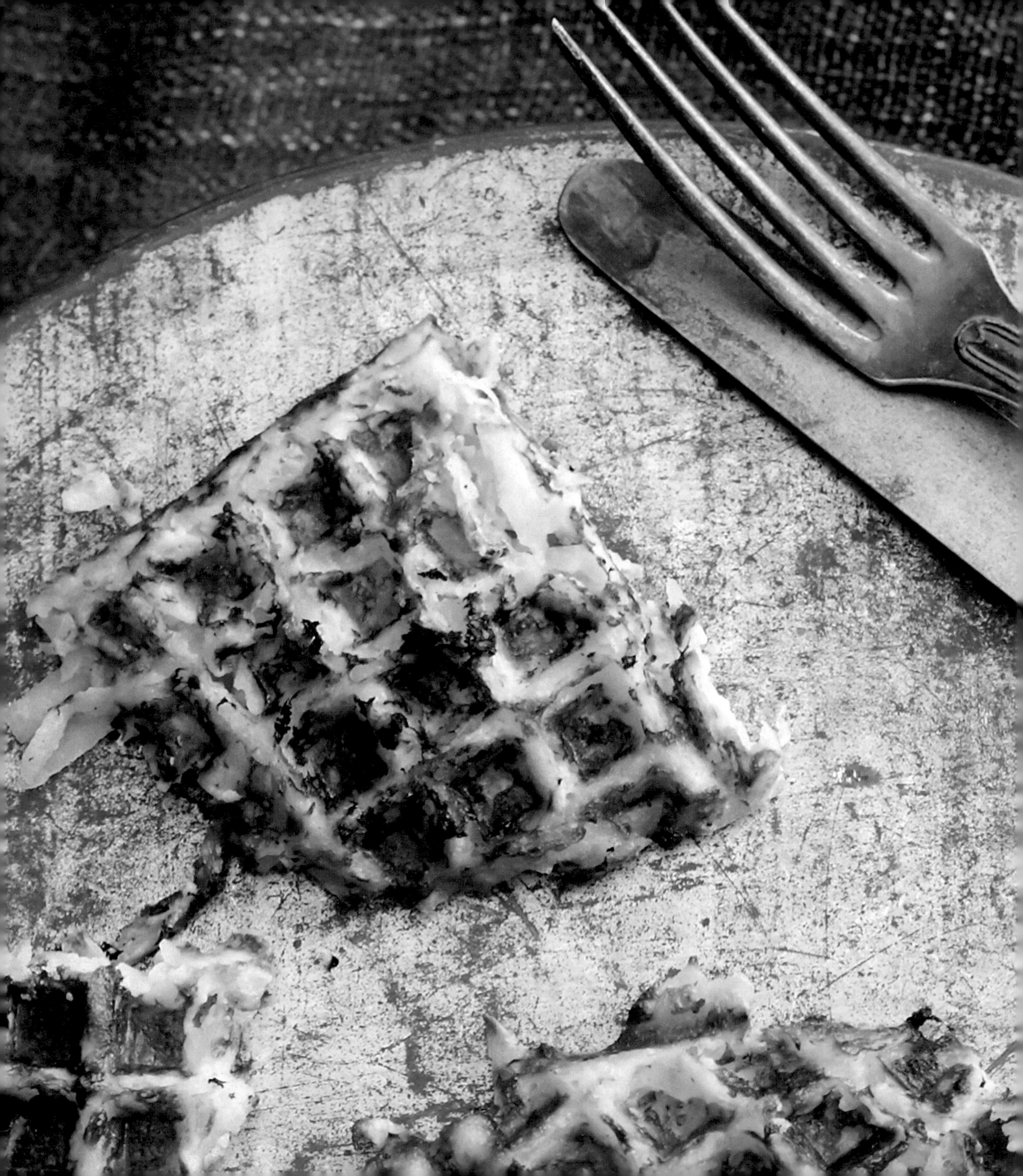

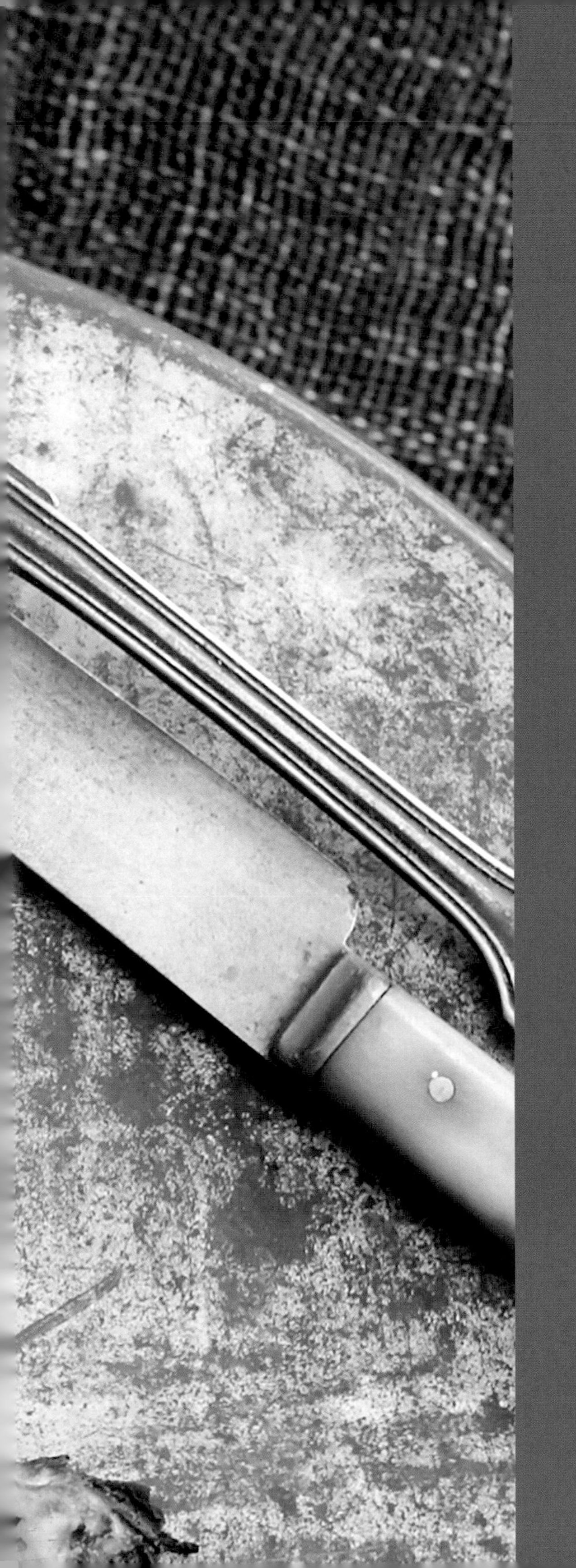

BREAKFAST

SMOKED SALMON EGGS BENEDICT

Feeds 4

The traditional eggs Benedict—toasted English muffin topped with ham, then poached eggs, then a hollandaise made with clarified butter—seems to have originated in New York City at the restaurant Delmonico's. Now, it's ubiquitous across the United States, in diners and good brunch places alike, particularly popular as a hangover cure. This version of eggs Benedict was inspired by the smoked salmon we make from wild Alaskan salmon every summer. The dairy-free hollandaise relies on olive oil, a technique Danny first encountered at a restaurant in Vancouver, Canada. So really, this dish comes from all over the place. And it could be on your table soon.

FOR THE HOLLANDAISE SAUCE

4 large egg yolks

1 cup extra-virgin olive oil

1 tablespoon fresh lemon juice

Dash Tabasco sauce

Kosher salt and freshly ground black pepper

FOR THE EGGS BENEDICT

2 teaspoons white vinegar

8 large eggs, at room temperature

4 gluten-free English Muffins (page 64), split open and toasted

8 ounces smoked salmon

Make the hollandaise. Set a medium pot over high heat. Fill it three-quarters of the way with water. When the water is boiling, put a metal bowl on top of it. Grab the side with a dry towel so you don't burn yourself. Add the egg yolks and 1 tablespoon of water. Whisk them together continuously until they have tripled in volume. Do not walk away from this or you will have scrambled eggs. If the eggs look anything like they are starting to cook and curd up, take the bowl off the boiling water. Put the towel on the counter and the bowl on top of it. Slowly drizzle in the oil, whisking vigorously, until all the oil is added. If the sauce looks at all like it is starting to separate, stop adding the oil and whisk until it is emulsified. If the sauce is starting to thicken up too much before the oil is added, add a tablespoon of water and continue whisking. Once all the oil is added, and the consistency is like a slightly thin mayonnaise, season with the lemon juice, Tabasco, and salt and pepper. Put the bowl back on the pot of water, with the heat off, on the back of the stove.

Poach the eggs. Set a large pot over high heat. Fill it with water and bring it to a boil. When the water is boiling, turn the heat down to low so the water simmers very slowly. Add the vinegar and stir it up. Crack each egg into its own ramekin or bowl. Use a large spoon to stir the water in one direction and make a little whirlpool. Carefully, drop one egg into the middle of the whirlpool. Quickly, add one more. Immediately turn off the heat and let the eggs sit in the water. For soft-poached eggs, pull the eggs out of the water with

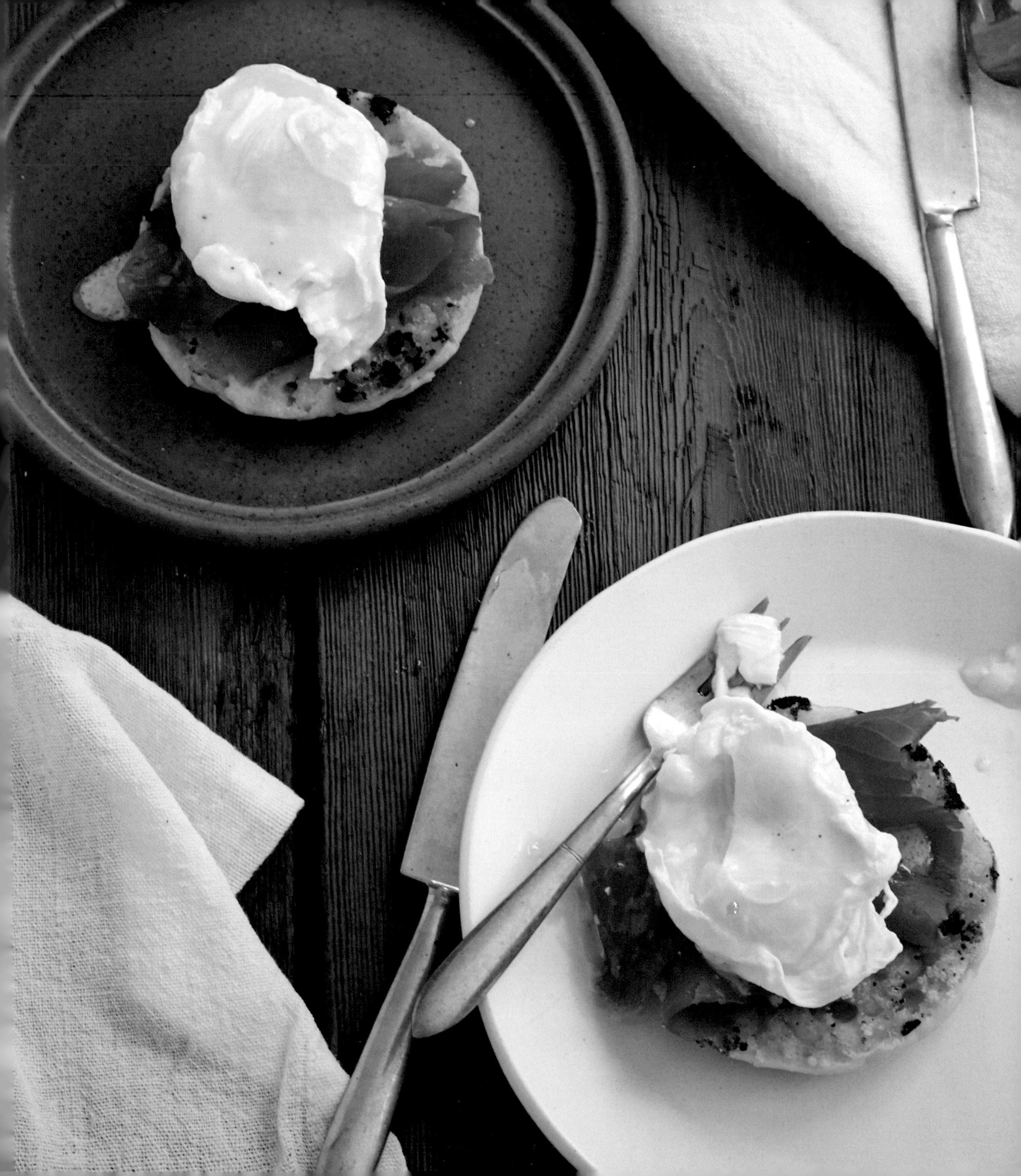

a slotted spoon after 2 minutes. For harder eggs, wait for 5 minutes. Move the eggs to a plate. Reheat the water and continue the same process with the remaining eggs. (If you have a big pot and you feel confident poaching eggs, you can poach 4 at a time.)

Assemble the eggs Benedict. Put two halves of the toasted English muffins onto a plate. Put some smoked salmon on each, then a poached egg on each, then ladle some hollandaise luxuriously on the top. Serve immediately.

Feel like playing?

If you really prefer the taste of hollandaise sauce made with clarified butter, use 8 ounces of it in this recipe, instead of the olive oil.

HUCKLEBERRY PANCAKES

Makes about 8 pancakes

Pancakes? You can make those anywhere in this country. Huckleberry pancakes? Well, you can make them where huckleberries grow freely, such as the Pacific Northwest or Montana. Or if you don't have access to fresh huckleberries, try to find them frozen. These tiny dark berries have a stronger flavor than blueberries that's pretty persuasive. Of course, you could use this recipe to make any kind of fruit-filled pancakes you wish.

250 grams Grain-Free Flour Mix (page 19)

1½ teaspoons baking powder

1 teaspoon kosher salt

1 cup low-fat buttermilk

2 large eggs, at room temperature

4 tablespoons (55 grams) unsalted butter, melted and cooled

2 cups fresh or frozen huckleberries

Fat for greasing the pan (we like bacon grease)

Combine the dry ingredients. In a large bowl, whisk together the flour mix, baking powder, and salt. Make a well in the center.

Combine the wet ingredients. In another bowl, whisk together the buttermilk, eggs, and melted better.

Make the batter. Pour the wet ingredients into the well of the dry ingredients. Stir the batter together well. Let the batter sit for 30 minutes before making the pancakes. If you like thick pancakes like we do, you have your batter. If you like thinner pancakes, stir in a couple of tablespoons of water or milk here. Stir in 1 cup of the huckleberries just before cooking.

Make the pancakes. Set a large cast-iron skillet over medium heat. (We also like a nonstick pan, if you use them.) Grease the pan with the fat of your choice. Pour about ¼ cup of batter into the greased pan for a pancake. Put two more pancakes in the pan. When bubbles have started to form and pop on the top of the pancakes, flip them. Cook for about 1 minute more. Put the pancakes on a plate. Continue cooking until you have cooked all the pancakes. Top with the remaining huckleberries.

Feel like playing?

Melted coconut oil works well in place of the butter here. And you can use any nondairy milk you wish. It doesn't affect the texture of the pancakes much.

HAZELNUT BANANA BREAD

Feeds 8

A long, leisurely breakfast is a wonderful way to start the day. However, most of us in this country don't seem to have the time for a full-course meal. And when you're on the run, a good quick bread can be a boon.

We make this banana bread with our grain-free flour blend. Bananas and buckwheat are complementary flavors, as are maple syrup, cinnamon, and coconut. Throw them all in together and bake them in a loaf pan? You have a warm, nutty banana bread that is ever so slightly sweet. Without the refined sugars, this banana bread tastes more of bananas and nuts than sweetness. Unlike so many quick breads, this one does not have a small suggestion of the flavors inside, hiding behind a scrim of sugar. It tastes of banana and hazelnuts and maple syrup. The fact that it's gluten-free, grain-free, dairy-free, and refined sugar–free? Well, that's nice for the people who need those things. But for you? This is a darned fine banana bread.

Fat for greasing the pan

210 grams Grain-Free Flour Mix (page 19)

1 teaspoon baking soda

½ teaspoon kosher salt

¼ teaspoon ground cinnamon

2 large eggs

½ cup maple syrup

About ⅓ cup (80 grams) coconut oil, melted

1 teaspoon vanilla extract

3 ripe bananas, mashed

About 1 cup (75 grams) chopped hazelnuts

Prepare to bake. Preheat the oven to 375°F. Grease a 5 x 9-inch loaf pan with the fat of your choice.

Mix the dry ingredients. In a bowl, whisk together the flour mix, baking soda, salt, and cinnamon.

Combine the wet ingredients. In another bowl, stir together the eggs, maple syrup, oil, and vanilla. Add the mashed banana and whisk until everything is combined well.

Make the batter. Add the dry ingredients, stirring as you go, a bit at a time to the wet ingredients. When all the flour has disappeared into the batter, and you can't find any more hiding at the bottom of the bowl, add the hazelnuts and stir.

Bake the banana bread. Pour the banana bread batter into the greased pan. Bake until the banana bread is springy to the touch, the edges are pulling away from the pan, and the top is browned, 45 to 60 minutes.

Cool the banana bread in the pan for 15 minutes, then move it to a wire rack. Turn the bread upside down so the bottom doesn't grow too moist.

Feel like playing?

You could use this recipe as a template for any banana bread you might like to make. Play with any nuts in place of the hazelnuts. You could also try honey in place of the maple syrup. If you want to make French toast with the banana bread, wait until it's a little stale. Soak it in beaten eggs, a little milk, and some sugar. Dunk the banana bread in, then put it in a hot pan with butter. Delicious.

HASH BROWN WAFFLES

Feeds 4

Hash browns—some form of potato diced or sliced or grated, mixed with fat and onions, then fried into a cake—are thought to be an American form of the Swedish rösti. It's not clear how long they have been on the table in the United States. There's a recipe for them, involving salt pork fat, in the first Fannie Farmer book, from 1896. But it's clear that hash brown potatoes were around earlier than this, from this reference to a speech given in 1892: "Mrs. Rorer gave her audience a shock the other day while lecturing at the Health and Food Exhibition in New Haven, Conn., by prophesying dire disaster as a result of indulgence in 'hashed brown potatoes.' She had visited insane asylums, she said, and found that many of the inmates had been addicted to the use of potatoes fried after being boiled. Ergo, potatoes cooked in this way appear to produce insanity." I think we're probably safe from the insanity, other than the fact that we're crazy about hash browns, many of which sold at restaurants are made with gluten flour. And our daughter is crazy about waffles. We combine the two for a hearty savory breakfast. (These puff up beautifully when you make them in a Belgian waffle maker.)

5 large russet potatoes, peeled and grated

Kosher salt

1 large yellow onion, peeled and grated

⅓ cup thick whole milk plain yogurt

1 tablespoon chopped fresh rosemary

½ teaspoon garlic powder

½ teaspoon onion powder

2 large eggs, at room temperature

3 tablespoons (45 grams) unsalted butter, melted (or you could use coconut oil)

Season the potatoes. Put the grated potatoes into a large bowl. Season them with a liberal pinch of salt, toss them to coat, and let the potatoes sit for 10 minutes. Wring the potatoes dry in a dish towel or paper towels until they are entirely dry. Put them back into the large bowl.

Make the potato mixture. Add the onion, yogurt, rosemary, garlic powder, and onion powder to the potatoes. Toss them all together to coat, then add the eggs and stir well. The potatoes should be well coated, a little wet but not sopping wet.

Make the waffles. Turn on the waffle iron. If you have a temperature setting on your waffle iron, set it on 80 percent heat. If not, then let the waffle iron grow hot to the touch but not ready to smoke. Brush the waffle iron with some of the butter. Spread one-quarter of the potato mixture evenly over the waffle iron, then close it. Let it cook until the edges of the waffle are crisp and middle of the waffle is fairly firm to the touch, 15 to 20 minutes. Take the waffle out of the iron and cook the remaining hash brown waffles the same way.

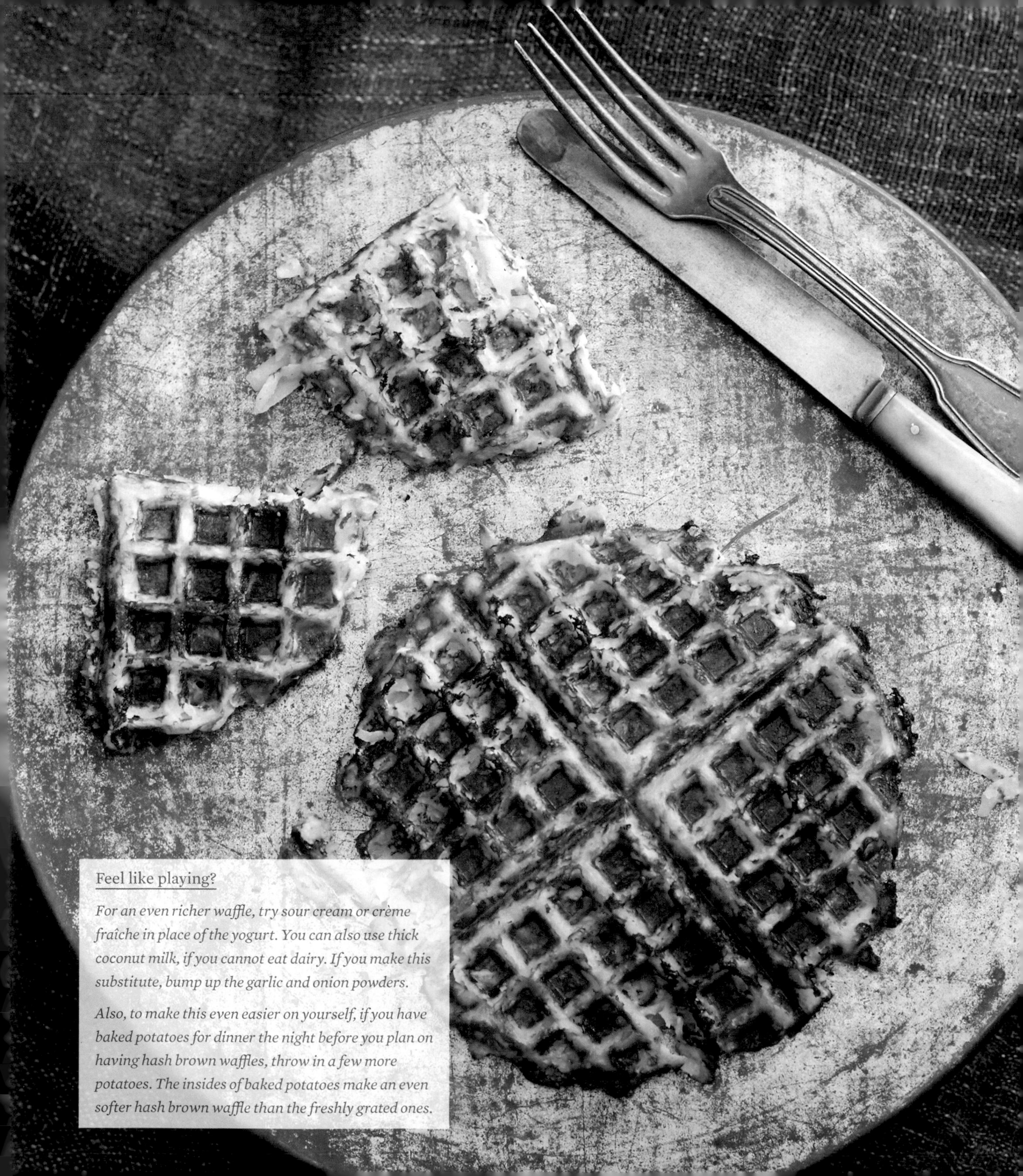

Feel like playing?

For an even richer waffle, try sour cream or crème fraîche in place of the yogurt. You can also use thick coconut milk, if you cannot eat dairy. If you make this substitute, bump up the garlic and onion powders.

Also, to make this even easier on yourself, if you have baked potatoes for dinner the night before you plan on having hash brown waffles, throw in a few more potatoes. The insides of baked potatoes make an even softer hash brown waffle than the freshly grated ones.

DUTCH BABY

Feeds 4

These sweet puffed-up pancakes, full of eggs and butter, are a wonderful lazy Sunday breakfast. Gluten-free, they may not rise as high as the versions with gluten, but Dutch babies deflate as soon as they come out of the oven anyway. By the way, this isn't a dish from Holland. Instead, it's based on a German pancake called apfelpfannkuchen. *Legend has it that the daughter of the owner of a Seattle restaurant called Manca's simply couldn't pronounce the word* Deutsch, *which means "German." She changed it to* Dutch, *and it stuck. That's a fairly typical American story, sadly. But there's nothing sad about eating this custardy pancake dish for breakfast.*

6 tablespoons (90 grams) unsalted butter

4 large eggs, at room temperature

100 grams All-Purpose Gluten-Free Flour Blend (page 17)

½ cup milk (use any nondairy milk you prefer)

½ teaspoon fine sea salt

1 lemon, juiced

Powdered sugar for sprinkling

Prepare to bake. Preheat the oven to 425°F. Set a large cast-iron skillet over low heat. Melt the butter.

Make the batter. Add the eggs, flour blend, milk, and salt to a blender. Whirl them up.

Bake the Dutch baby. Pour the batter into the melted butter in the hot skillet. Immediately put it in the oven. Bake until the Dutch baby is puffed up and browned, about 25 minutes.

Serve. Remove the Dutch baby from the oven. Show it to your family and guests fast because it will deflate immediately. Sprinkle on the lemon juice, followed by the powdered sugar. Slice the Dutch baby into wedges and serve immediately.

Feel like playing?

You can easily use any milk you like here. We like to macerate strawberries in honey and balsamic vinegar, when they are in season, and put them on top of the Dutch baby too.

JOHNNYCAKES

Makes about a dozen johnnycakes

These bare-bones corn cakes have been a staple of the American diet for a long time. Made only with easy-to-find pantry staples, these little savory cakes traveled well. (The original name might have been journey cakes, which somehow switched to johnnycakes. Or maybe it's jonnycakes. They're also known as hoecakes in the South.) Native Americans in what's now called the Northeast were growing corn before people immigrated to the United States from Europe. The new inhabitants of the area took to corn and corn cakes immediately. (The first written reference to hoecakes is in the Oxford English Dictionary *in 1745.) Later, these cakes traveled with settlers as they moved farther west. I noticed references to them in the* Little House on the Prairie *books when I read them to our daughter, Lucy. Rhode Island residents claim that the johnnycake originated in that fierce, small state, and I don't doubt them. Some Rhode Islanders like thick cakes and others like crisp, lacy ones like pancakes. This recipe works for the pancake-like johnnycake. And, they're naturally gluten-free! If you haven't made johnnycakes before, we want to make it easy for you to try.*

¾ cup whole milk

1 cup white or yellow cornmeal (make sure it's gluten-free)

⅓ cup water

1 teaspoon kosher salt

2 teaspoons unsalted butter, for greasing the pan

Scald the milk. Set a small pot over medium heat. Pour in the milk. When it is steaming and simmering, almost about to boil, pull it off the heat.

Make the johnnycake batter. In a large bowl, combine the cornmeal, milk, water, and salt. Whisk them together well.

Make the johnnycakes. Grease a large cast-iron skillet with the butter and set over medium-high heat. Before the skillet smokes, stir the batter again, then add 1 tablespoon of the johnnycake batter to the hot skillet and spread it out to make a 3-inch cake. Fill the pan spaciously. (You'll probably get 6 to a pan.) Cook until the johnnycakes are browned on the bottom, about 3 minutes. Flip the johnnycakes and cook for an additional 1 to 2 minutes. Remove the johnnycakes to a plate and cook the remaining batter. Serve immediately.

Note: Some folks from Rhode Island insist the only cornmeal to use in a johnnycake comes from Kenyon's Grist Mill. I wish I could. Kenyon's says on its website that they use the same millstone to grind both wheat and corn products. Gray's Grist Mill in Massachusetts, only 100 feet shy of the Rhode Island border, mills only Narragansett white flint corn, but they do have wheat in their facility to make a pancake mix. Most often, we use Italian cornmeal, used to make polenta, for our johnnycakes, cornmeal we know has been made in a mill that only grinds corn. If you are not celiac and thus not as sensitive as I am to cross-contamination with gluten, feel free to seek out Kenyon's cornmeal!

Feel like playing?

You could use any kind of milk here that works for you. I love topping these with cheese or caramelized onions to make them savory, but you may prefer maple syrup. You could also make a quick cranberry syrup to fit with the Northeast theme: add 1 cup of sugar and 1 cup of water to a large pot over medium-high heat. Bring the sugar and water to a boil, then lower to a simmer, until they form a thick syrup. Put 1 cup of fresh cranberries into the syrup and cook them until they start to break down. Turn off the heat and let the cranberries sit in the syrup for 30 minutes. Strain out the cranberries if you want a pourable syrup or leave them in and mash them up for a chunky compote.

BUCKWHEAT CREPES

Feeds 4

Danny teases me that I get crushes on grains and flours. It's true. Teff, millet, and oats—I've gone through love affairs with all of them. But buckwheat is my enduring love (as a flour, of course). The raw groats make for a nutty-flavored flour with some of the same qualities as wheat. I don't know why everyone is not in love with buckwheat. In the northern part of Maine, Americans who are descendants of French colonists still prize buckwheat highly. These crepes are a wonderfully easy way to start the day with a savory breakfast. (Thank you to David Lebovitz, my favorite Parisian resident, for the inspiration for this recipe.)

2 cups whole milk (or you can use your favorite nondairy milk)

175 grams Grain-Free Flour Mix (page 19)

3 large eggs, at room temperature

3 tablespoons (42 grams) unsalted butter, melted

½ teaspoon fine sea salt

Fat for greasing the pan

Make the batter. Add all the ingredients to a blender. Blend until smooth. Pour the batter into a bowl, cover with plastic wrap, and chill. For best results, chill the batter overnight.

Prepare to make the crepes. The next morning, remove the batter from the refrigerator. Let it sit on the counter and come to room temperature, about 45 minutes. Stir up the batter. It should have the consistency of heavy cream or well-stirred coconut milk. If the batter is thicker than this at room temperature, add 1 or 2 tablespoons of milk.

Cook the crepes. Set a large nonstick pan over medium-high heat. When the pan has come to heat, add a tiny amount of fat—less than a teaspoon—to the pan and wipe it over the entire surface of the pan.

Pour about ¼ cup of the batter in the middle of the pan, then lift the pan off the heat to swirl the batter around to cover the entire surface of the pan. You should have just enough time to coat the pan evenly with batter before it starts cooking. Let the crepe cook for 1 minute, then lift up an edge with a rubber spatula. Flip the crepe with the spatula. As you feel more experienced, you can simply use your fingers to grab the crepe and flip it. Cook for 30 seconds on the other side.

Serve the crepes. Slide the crepe off the pan and repeat the process with the remaining crepe batter until they are all cooked. Serve the crepes immediately.

CONTINUED

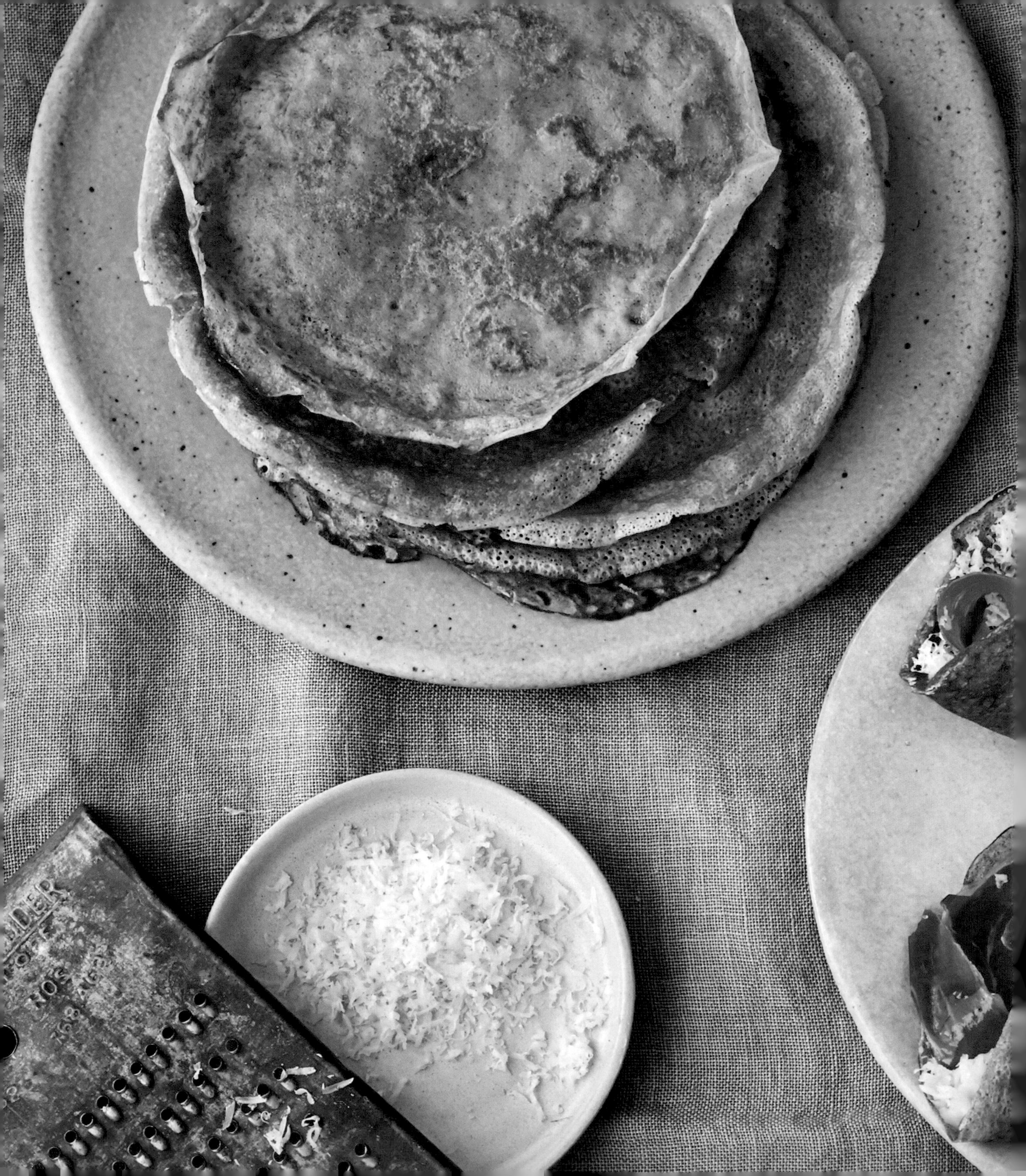

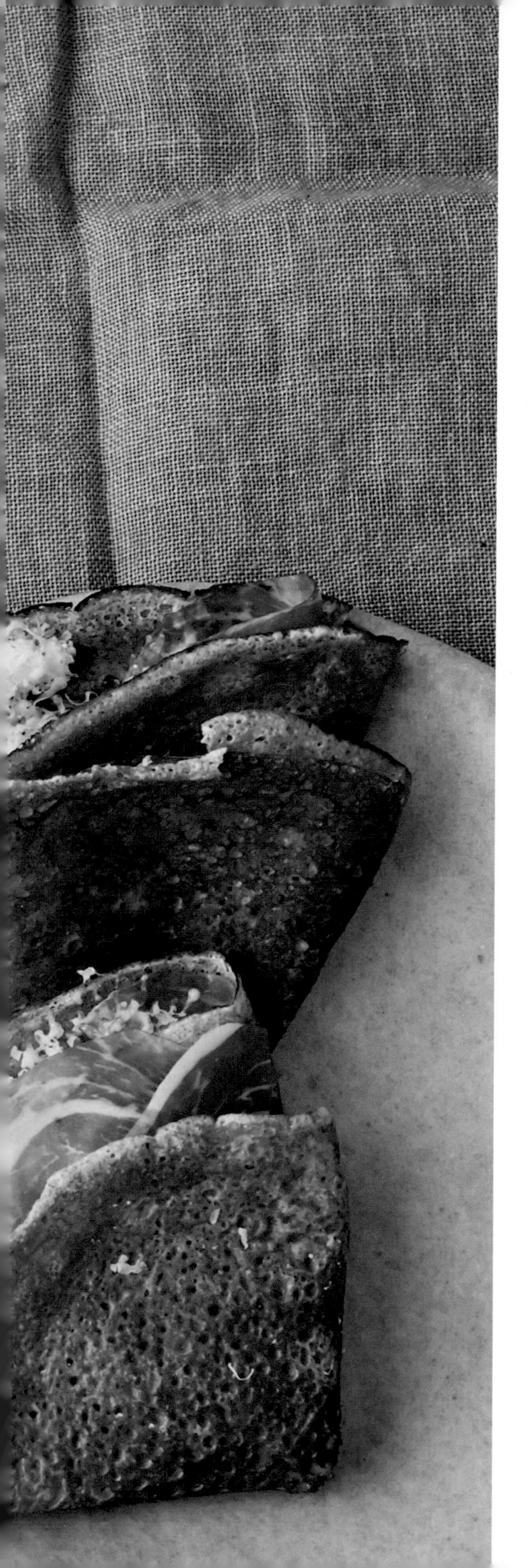

We like to fill ours with Gruyère and a little prosciutto. You might like sauerkraut and some scrambled egg. Really, a crepe is the perfect vehicle for your favorite food. If you want sweet crepes, add a couple of teaspoons of honey to the batter before you set it in the refrigerator.

Feel like playing?

If you have whole buckwheat groats, you can use those here in place of the flour. Put the whole groats in the blender with the other ingredients and let them sit in the blender overnight. In the morning, the groats will be so soft that you can blend up the batter on the spot.

ALMOND AND CHERRY GRANOLA

Feeds 6 to 12

Many of us mourned the loss of homemade granola when we found out we could no longer eat gluten. For decades, those with celiac were told to not eat oats. Oats in their pure form do not have the kind of gluten that damages celiacs. However, they are generally grown next to fields of wheat, transported in the same trucks as wheat, and processed in the same plants as wheat. Luckily, several years ago, certified gluten-free oats emerged onto the market, oats that had been grown in fields that had deliberately lain fallow for years to avoid any cross-contamination with wheat, and that are transported and processed with utmost care. (A small percentage of celiacs react to avenin, the protein in oats, with intestinal upset as well, so make sure you can handle oats before you start eating them regularly.) This granola recipe is only lightly adapted from our friend Megan Gordon's wonderful book, Whole-Grain Mornings. *Megan makes Marge Granola, a wonderful granola made with the best ingredients she can find. Because of our friendship, and her desire to feed everyone good granola, she now makes a gluten-free granola too. (You'll find it at www.margegranola.com.) I'm so happy to have good granola back.*

3 cups (300 grams) rolled oats (make absolutely sure they are certified gluten-free)

1¼ cups (190 grams) chopped almonds

½ cup raw sesame seeds

1 teaspoon fine sea salt

½ teaspoon ground ginger

¼ teaspoon ground cinnamon

½ cup maple syrup

½ cup coconut oil, melted

1 teaspoon vanilla extract

1 cup dried cherries

Prepare to bake. Preheat the oven to 325°F. Line a baking sheet with parchment paper.

Combine the dry ingredients. In a large bowl, stir together the oats, almonds, sesame seeds, salt, ginger, and cinnamon.

Combine the wet ingredients. In another bowl, whisk together the maple syrup, oil, and vanilla. Pour them over the oats mixture and stir well to evenly coat every ingredient. Use your hands for best results.

Bake the granola. Spread the granola onto the prepared baking sheet, making sure it's in one even layer. Bake for 15 minutes. Pull the baking sheet out of the oven and stir the granola, turning it all over. Bake for another 15 minutes and stir again. The granola might be done at this point. Granola hardens as it cools, growing crunchier than it is in the oven. Take care to not overbake. As soon as you pull the granola from the oven, add the dried cherries and stir up the granola.

Cool the granola completely before storing it in an airtight container.

Feel like playing?

Feel free to substitute any nuts for the almonds and any dried fruit for the cherries.

CINNAMON ROLLS WITH CREAM CHEESE FROSTING

Makes 16 cinnamon rolls

Common sense says we should have a healthier start to the day than cinnamon rolls. I hope you have that common sense most of the time. But sometimes, like Christmas morning or other family gatherings, we throw common sense aside and eat these cinnamon rolls for breakfast. There are 360 days a year for green salads and turkey burgers.

FOR THE CINNAMON ROLLS

300 grams All-Purpose Gluten-Free Flour Blend (page 17)

1 teaspoon brown sugar

1 tablespoon psyllium husks

1½ teaspoons fine sea salt

¾ teaspoon instant yeast

¼ cup (50 grams) organic cane sugar

1 teaspoon ground cinnamon

½ cup (125 grams) warm water

⅓ cup (100 grams) whole milk, at room temperature

FOR THE FILLING

8 tablespoons (115 grams) unsalted butter

1 tablespoon ground cinnamon

⅔ cup (140 grams) organic cane sugar

4 tablespoons (58 grams) unsalted butter, melted

1 batch Cream Cheese Frosting (page 268)

Make the dough. Put the flour, brown sugar, psyllium husks, salt, and yeast into the bowl of a stand mixer with the paddle attachment. Mix on medium speed until the dry ingredients are aerated. Add the sugar and cinnamon and mix until everything is incorporated. Scrape down the sides of the bowl with a rubber spatula and add the warm water and milk. If the dough feels dry, dribble in a bit more water. Keep the mixer running until the dough is fluffy and slumping off the paddle, about 5 minutes.

Cover the bowl with plastic wrap and let it sit in a warm space until the dough has hydrated and become kneadable, about 90 minutes.

Melt the butter. Set a large skillet over low heat and melt the butter.

Roll out the dough. Set half of the ball of dough onto a lightly greased piece of parchment paper. Lay another piece of paper on top of it. Going slowly, roll out the dough until it is about ½ inch thick and has reached the edges of the parchment paper. Peel off the top piece of paper.

Fill the rolls. Brush half of the melted butter over the top of the dough, leaving a 2-inch edge of dough with no butter on it all around the dough. Mix the sugar and cinnamon together and sprinkle a third of it over the butter. Grab the bottom of the parchment paper and pull it toward you a bit. The edge of the dough should flop over onto the filling. If not, give it a nudge with your fingers. Press it down onto the filling, then make another roll of the dough. Make a tight roll, using the parchment paper as your guide, moving slowly and patting the dough down gently as you go. If the filling oozes out as you reach the end, that's okay. That's a sign you're going to have good cinnamon rolls.

Cut the rolls. Grab a long piece of dental floss. Nudge the middle of the dental floss under the log of dough, about 2 inches from the end. Bring the two edges of the floss together to cross over the top. By doing this, you will slice a piece of the log. This makes for lovely, neat pieces instead of jagged hunks. Make your way down the log of dough with the dental floss. This should give about 8 pieces of dough.

Repeat the process with the remaining dough and filling.

Rise the rolls. Pour 2 tablespoons of the melted butter into the bottom of a pie pan, then repeat with the remaining 2 tablespoons of butter and another pie pan. (A glass-bottomed pie pan works best.) Sprinkle the remaining sugar on top of the melted butter. Put the sliced rolls into the buttered pans, filling side up, tightening the rolls if they have begun to unravel. Set them aside to rise for at least 1 hour. The rolls will fill out.

Prepare to bake. Preheat the oven to 350°F.

Bake the rolls. Bake the cinnamon rolls until they are firm to the touch when you press on both sides of one, but still with some give, about 25 minutes.

Allow the rolls to cool for 10 minutes, then invert them onto two plates.

Frost the rolls. Frost the rolls with the cream cheese frosting when they have come to room temperature.

Feel like playing?

You certainly don't have to splurge on cream cheese frosting every time. A simple powdered sugar and lemon juice glaze would work well, as would a bit of coconut cream and honey.

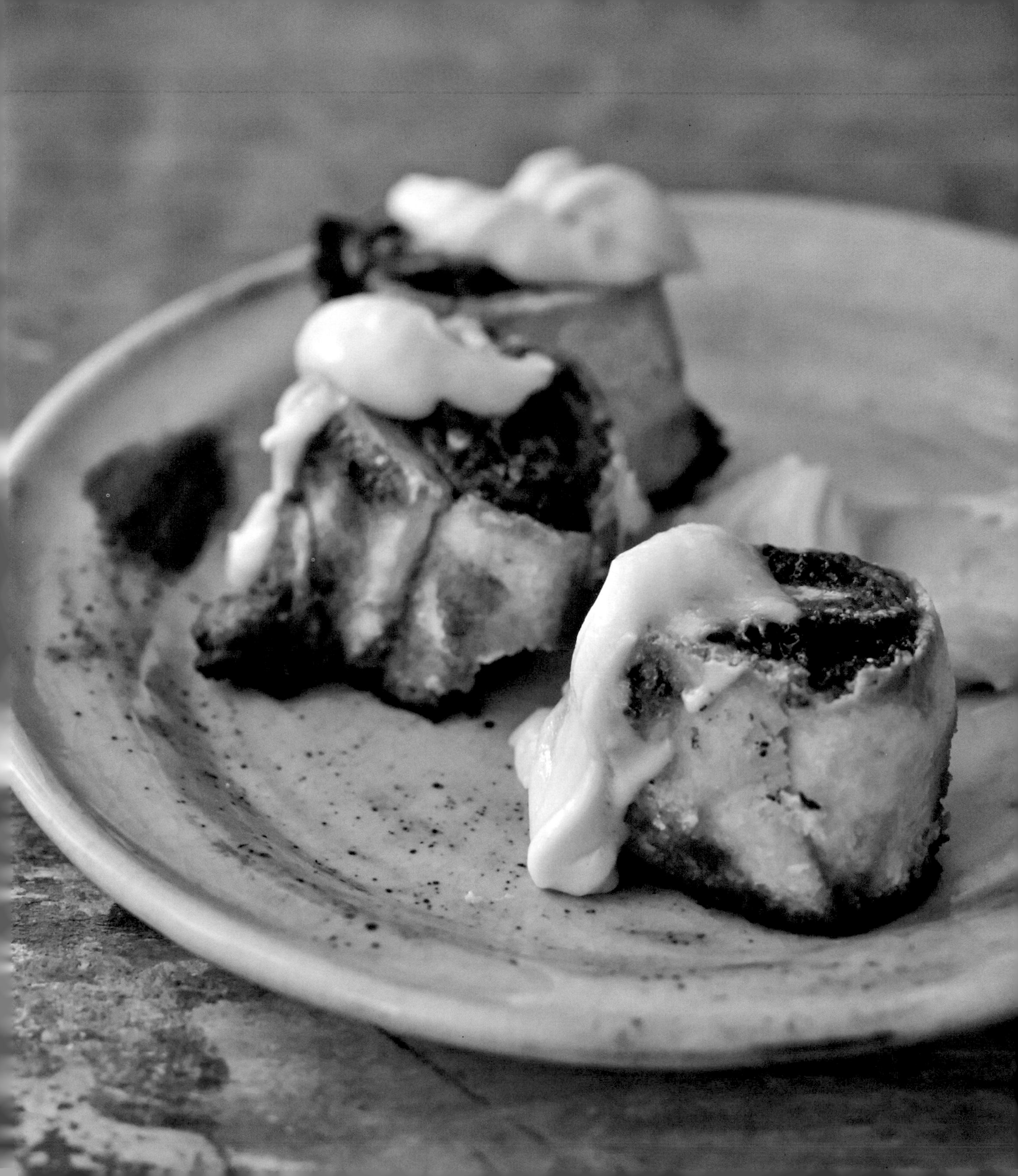

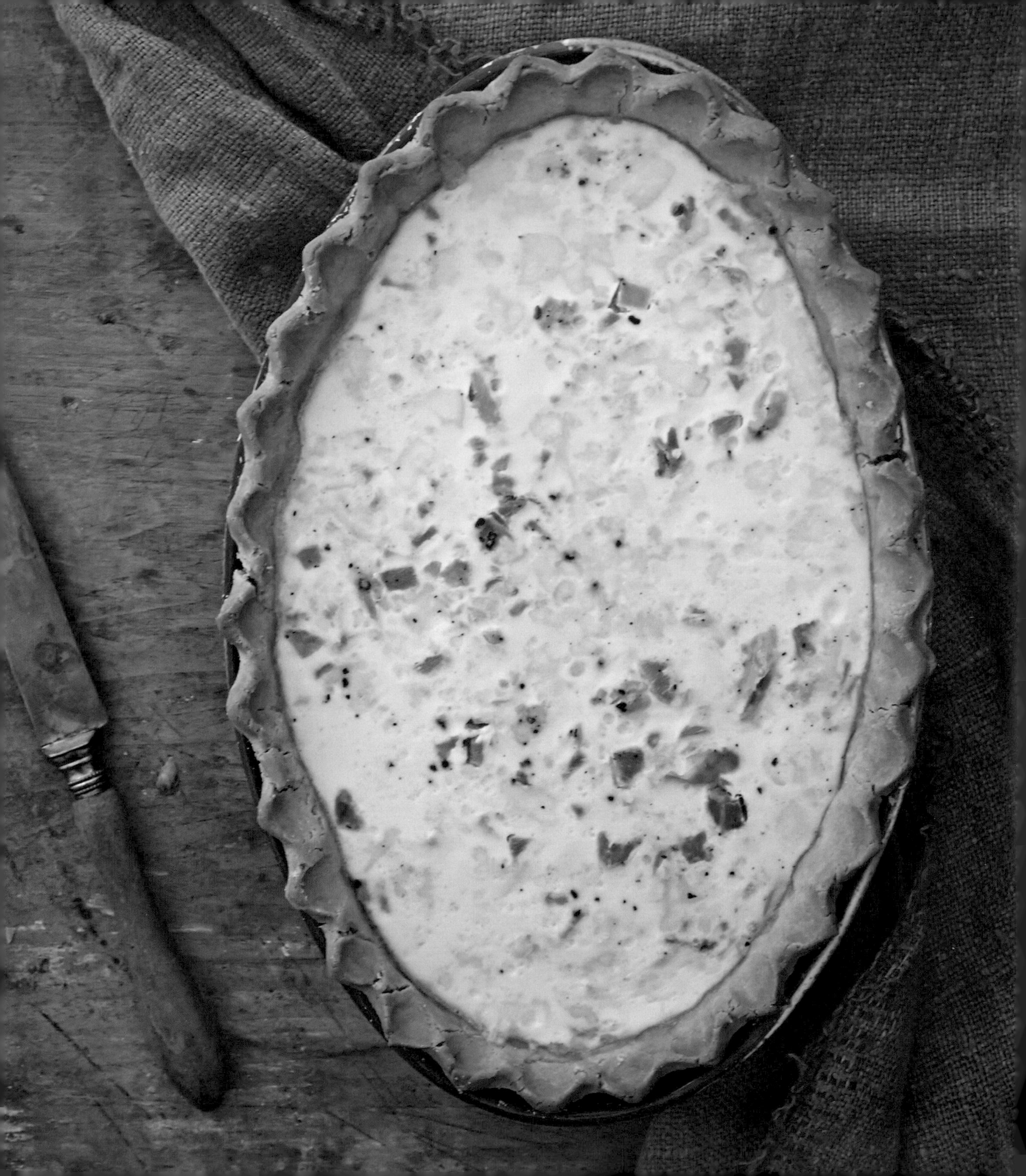

GREEN CHILE PIE

Feeds 6 to 8

When Danny and I decided that a savory breakfast pie with green chiles would be a great way to honor New Mexico and the Southwest, we went looking to see if anyone else had a recipe we liked that we could adapt to be gluten-free. Pretty quickly, we found one from Maya Angelou, in her gorgeous book Great Food All Day Long. *We looked no further. Ms. Angelou was not only a deeply inspiring woman, but also a woman who knew how to cook. We've made a few small changes here, and we've made it gluten-free. But when you make this pie—and you should—we ask you to raise a fork to Maya Angelou over breakfast.*

1 disk chilled Pie Dough (page 226)

6 ounces (1½ cups) freshly grated Monterey Jack cheese

2 ounces (½ cup) freshly grated Cheddar cheese

One 4-ounce can diced green chiles, drained

1 cup whole milk (or you can use your favorite nondairy milk)

4 large eggs, at room temperature

¼ teaspoon ground cumin

Kosher salt and freshly ground black pepper

2 ounces (½ cup) freshly grated cotija cheese

Prebake the piecrust. Preheat the oven to 350°F. Roll out the dough, put it in the pan, and crimp it (see page 227 for full instructions). Line the bottom of the dough with a lightly greased piece of aluminum foil. Pour dried beans on top of it. Bake the crust until it is barely golden brown, about 12 minutes. Remove the crust from the oven and let it cool to room temperature.

Prepare to bake. Turn down the heat to 325°F. Line a baking sheet with parchment paper.

Fill the pie. Sprinkle the Jack and Cheddar cheeses over the bottom of the crust. Scatter the chiles over the top of the cheeses.

In a bowl, whisk together the milk, eggs, cumin, and salt and pepper. Pour this over the cheese and chiles. Sprinkle the cotija cheese over the top of the pie.

Bake the pie. Bake the pie until the center of the pie is just set, 30 to 40 minutes.

Let the pie cool to room temperature before cutting into it. It's also delicious cold.

Feel like playing?

If you don't have access to cotija cheese, simply double up the Cheddar and sprinkle half of that over the top.

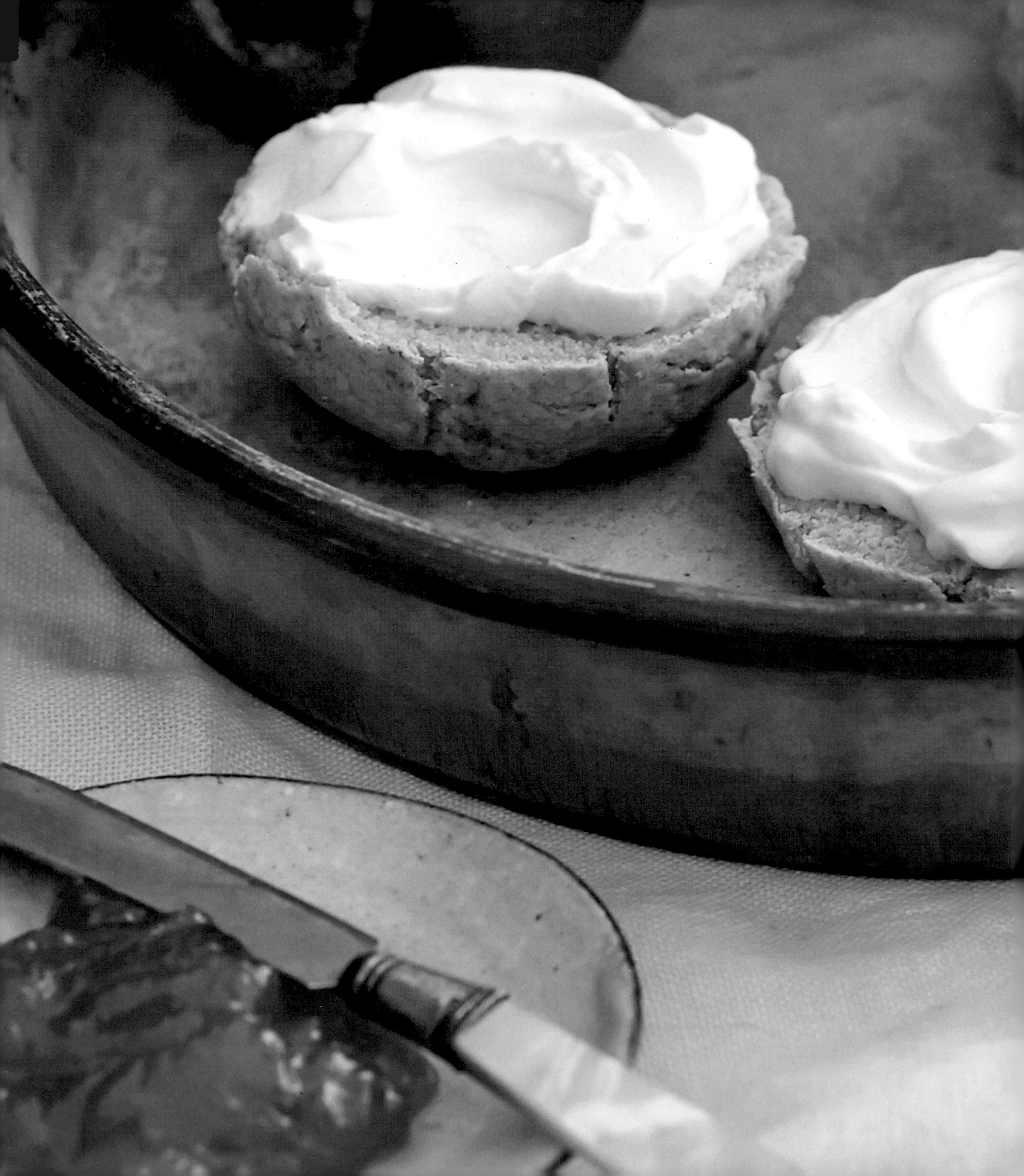

BREADS

SOURDOUGH STARTER

Sourdough is a fermented food, a living organism, good for the gut and utterly delicious in bread. When I was a kid, sandwiches on sourdough bread were always my favorite. The tang in the bread always made the ingredients inside far more interesting. And of course, when I visited San Francisco, I saw how proud that city's bakers were of their iconic sourdough bread.

But sourdough was not born in San Francisco. It's not just an American thing. Making a sourdough starter (or levain) is how humans made breads and baked goods for thousands of years. American women in the 1800s kept a starter going as a matter of course. (Reading *Little House on the Prairie* to our daughter, I noticed references to sponges and starters in nearly every other chapter. Women used to work far harder to make dinner for their families than we do now.) Yeast in packets, like the ones sold in grocery stores today, only came onto the market in the early twentieth century.

Yes, instant and active dry yeast help make a loaf of bread more quickly. But that loaf of bread won't be as good as one made slowly, with some of the starter you baby along in your own kitchen. We've included baked goods recipes in this book using commercial yeast, since that is what most people want to use. But when we bake for ourselves, we always use sourdough starter now. The breads are more flavorful, hold together better, have more spring, and behave more like traditional gluten breads do.

There's no need to be afraid of sourdough starter. Making a good gluten-free sourdough starter only requires attention, a little stirring, some dumping and whisking, and waiting. You can do this.

DAY ONE

Before noon, mix together 500 grams of teff flour and 500 grams of lukewarm water in a large container. (We use a sturdy rectangular restaurant container with a lid, made by Cambro. These are available online and at restaurant supply stores.)

Let the flour and water sit for 2 hours in a warm place, then cover the container and let it sit overnight.

DAY TWO

The next day, before noon, remove three-quarters of the mix. (You don't have to throw it out. See Notes.)

Add 500 grams of teff flour and 500 grams of lukewarm water. Stir them together well.

Let the flour and water sit for 2 hours in a warm place, then cover the container. By the end of the day, the mixture should have increased in volume. With a gluten sourdough starter, the mix will have doubled in volume. That won't happen without gluten, but you'll have some good activity going on.

Let the starter sit overnight.

DAY THREE

The next day, before noon, remove three-quarters of the mix.

Add 200 grams of teff flour, 300 grams of All-Purpose Gluten-Free Flour Blend (page 17), and 500 grams of lukewarm water. Stir them together well.

Let the flour and water sit for 2 hours in a warm place, then cover the container. By the end of the day, the mixture should look like a sour porridge and have a pungent smell.

DAY FOUR

Before noon, there should be bubbles all throughout the starter. The starter should look alive now. Remove three-quarters of the mix.

Add 500 grams of All-Purpose Gluten-Free Flour Blend and 500 grams of lukewarm water. Stir them together well.

Let the flour and water sit for 2 hours in a warm place, then cover the container. By the end of the day, the starter should be full of bubbles and smelling sour.

DAY FIVE

Before noon, the starter should feel gassy and goopy. Reach in with a wet hand and feel the starter. If you can pick up a handful of it and watch it drizzle slowly through your fingers, thicker than water and smelling of sour pungent wonderfulness, you're ready to bake.

NOTES:

Flours. Starting with teff is smart because that flour has the most wild yeast of any flour in the world. It sours easily, which is how injera bread is made in Ethiopia. We've had great success with sourdough starter made of only teff flour. However, if you want your sourdough starter to not be dark, you can start adding in lighter flours, as we have done here. We've made a mostly grain-free starter, using our Grain-Free Flour Mix (page 19), but it only works if we start with teff. By removing so much of the starter each day, the small amount of teff flour shouldn't bother those who feel better without grains. Feel free to use any combination of flours here that works best in your kitchen.

Removing the starter. Removing most of the starter each day strengthens the starter and is necessary to the process. However, there's no need to throw out the starter you remove each day. We use that not-quite-fully-matured starter to make pancakes, flatbreads, savory muffins and quick breads, and pizza dough. Simply replace any liquid in the recipe with the weight of starter you were going to throw away.

Consistency. If you look at pictures of some gluten sourdough starters, you might believe that your sourdough starter is too thin. Don't worry. Thick or runny really doesn't matter in terms of the consistency of the bread you bake. You just want a fully fermented starter.

How long it takes. Five days is the bare minimum required to make a healthy sourdough starter. That's how long it takes in our kitchen on fairly warm days, and we know what we're doing. If your starter takes 7 days of feeding the starter, removing the starter, and letting it all grow pungent and bubbly, that's fine. If you begin your starter in the middle of the winter, it might take as long as 2 weeks. Don't worry. Keep going.

What else do you need? Some folks add something to their starter to nudge along the growth of the yeast, such as grape skins, rhubarb pieces, or even yogurt. We haven't found that to be necessary. Flour and water are all it took to make a sourdough starter for thousands of years—it's pretty easy! But if you live in an especially cold place and you are worried, feel free to add your ingredient of choice.

What might go wrong. If you see a layer of water on the surface of your starter, you might be keeping it in a not-warm-enough place. If the water is clear, stir it in and keep going. If the water is dark and smells off, you've probably gone too long without feeding your starter and you've killed it. Throw it out (don't bake with that leftover starter) and begin again. It might take you a few times of trying to make a starter to get the hang of it. You'll get the hang of it.

SOURDOUGH BREAD

Makes 2 sourdough boules or 4 baguettes

Great bread takes a little work, a lot of time, a sourdough starter, and paying attention. This bread requires a few moments of your time for two days. Plan ahead and you could have great crusty bread with a dense, chewy crumb back in your life.

Morning of Day One

In the morning, remove all but 100 grams of the active sourdough starter you have built. Add 400 grams of water, 400 grams of All-Purpose Gluten-Free Flour Blend (page 17), and 100 grams of Grain-Free Flour Mix (page 19). Stir it all up well. Let the sourdough starter sit for 8 to 10 hours. This will be the strong starter you will use to make your bread.

Evening of Day One

350 grams lukewarm water

200 grams All-Purpose Gluten-Free Flour Blend (page 17)

200 grams Grain-Free Flour Mix (page 19)

In a large bowl, stir together the water, flour blend, and grain-free flour mix. Let this mixture sit for 30 minutes, then add:

120 grams of the sourdough starter you strengthened that morning

12 grams (2 tablespoons) psyllium husks

10 grams kosher salt

Mix these ingredients together well with a rubber spatula, folding and mixing to make sure that everything is well combined. It will look a little wetter than typical bread dough. Cover the bowl with plastic wrap and let it sit in a warm place.

Before going to bed, fold the dough over on itself once or twice. Let the dough sit overnight.

Morning of Day Two

Ease the dough onto a clean counter. (If the dough starts to stick, sprinkle on a little of the all-purpose flour blend.) Fold the dough onto itself once or twice, then cut the dough into 2 equal pieces with a bench scraper. Roll each piece of dough around and

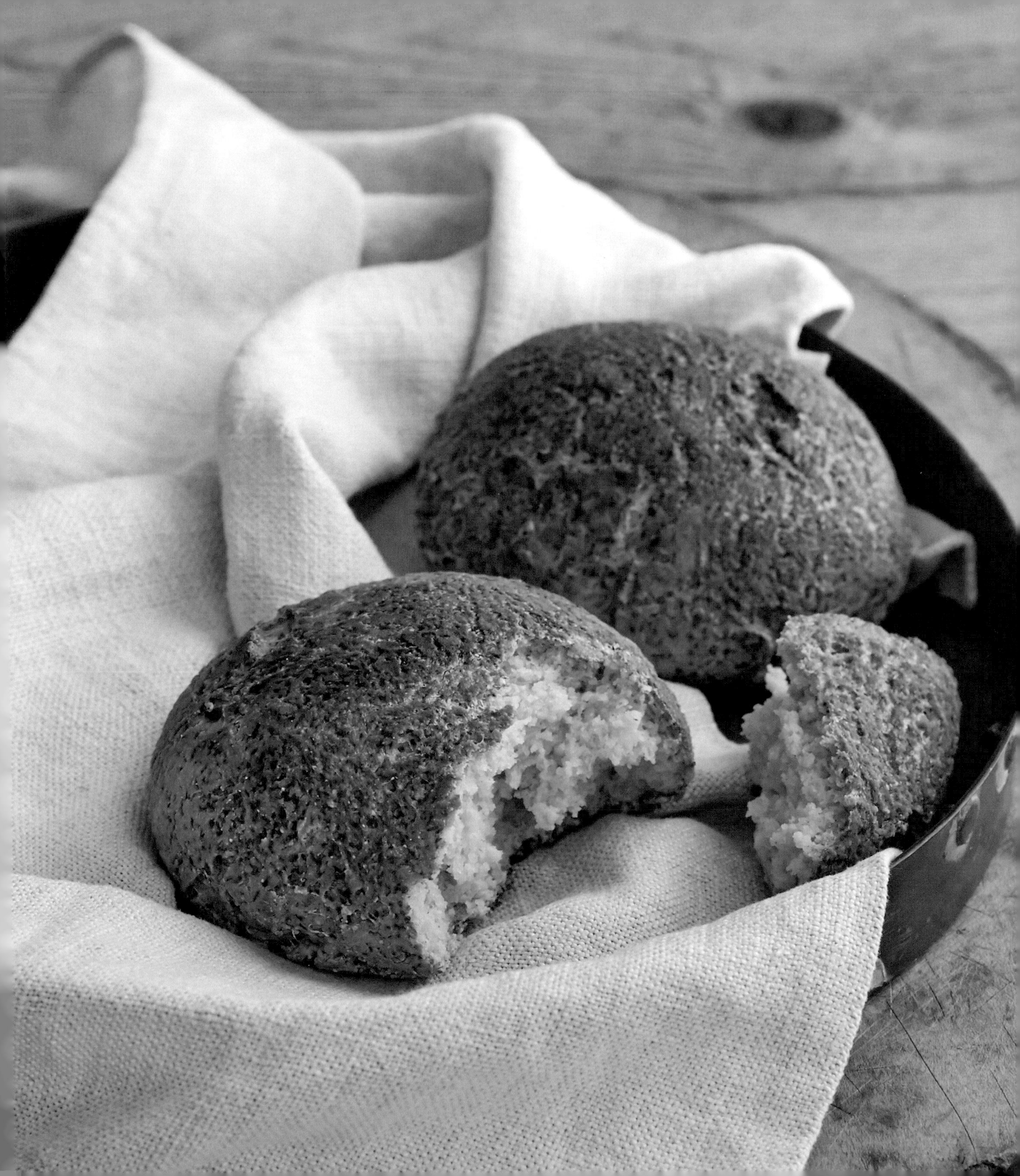

shape into balls or boules. Dust 2 bread proofing baskets (also known as *bannetons* or *brotforms*) with some of the all-purpose flour blend. Gently lower the dough balls into the proofing baskets. Cover with a slightly damp towel and let the dough proof for 4 hours.

Prepare to bake. Preheat the oven to 475°F. When the oven has come to temperature, put a Dutch oven in and allow it to grow hot (just before smoking).

Bake the bread. When the Dutch oven is hot, pull it out of the oven carefully. Plop one of the dough balls into the hot Dutch oven and cover it immediately. Bake for 30 minutes. Take the lid off. Put a pan filled with ice cubes on the rack below the Dutch oven. Bake until the crust is dark golden brown, almost veering toward charred, and the internal temperature is 200°F. Take the bread out of the oven.

Put the Dutch oven back into the oven. When it has returned to full heat, bake the second loaf the same way. Allow the bread to come to room temperature before slicing it. That's hard but worth it.

To Make Baguettes

Follow the same procedure here for day one. On day two, instead of forming the dough into 2 balls, use the bench scraper to cut the dough into 4 pieces. Shape the dough pieces into 4 baguettes. To form a baguette, shape one piece of dough into a rectangle about the size of a piece of paper (8 x 11) on a floured surface. Fold the top part of the dough down onto the rectangle, then the bottom half over that, as though you are folding a letter. Pat a line in the middle of the dough shape you have made, then fold the dough in half on itself again. Seal the edges, moving the dough around a bit to make this happen. Sprinkle the surface with flour. Working with your hands in the middle of the loaf, rock the loaf and slowly roll it into a baguette shape, about 12 inches long. Transfer the dough to a parchment-lined baguette pan and repeat with the remaining dough. Let the dough rest for another 2 hours.

Bake at 475°F until the crust is golden brown and the internal temperature is 200°F, about 30 minutes.

Note: Gluten-free bread does not last as long on the counter as gluten bread. It's great the day of baking, pretty good the next day, and then stale by the third day. We bake two loaves at once, eat one for dinner and breakfast the next day, then freeze the remaining bread in slices. With baguettes, slice them in half in the middle, then slice them lengthwise. Freeze them this way for toasting later for sandwiches.

SANDWICH BREAD

Makes 1 loaf

Above all else, Americans who find out they have to avoid gluten seem to miss sandwich bread. Sandwiches are, after all, the perfect handheld food. For decades, Americans lived on grocery store white bread, so starchy and full of chemicals that it balled up in the hand and could be thrown across the room. Some speculate that it was Americans' need for stiff sandwich bread that could stay on store shelves for weeks that pushed the hybridization of wheat, which today contains more gluten than the wheat of the early part of the twentieth century. (European bread tends to be far denser and more strangely shaped than American bread.) Like it or not, most of us like sandwich bread and miss it.

After years of making gluten-free bread, on the search for an easy-to-make recipe for flavorful sandwich bread that didn't crumble or taste like a brick, Danny and I came up with one we love for our last cookbook. We made it at least once a week for a couple of years, mostly for sandwiches and toast for our daughter. After Gluten-Free Girl Every Day *was published, I started playing again. Maybe I could find another way, a better recipe? We played again for over a year and found that . . . this recipe still makes the best sandwich bread we've tried. Why mess with success?*

Fat for greasing the pan

½ cup warm water (no hotter than 110°F)

1 envelope (2¼ teaspoons) active dry yeast

1 teaspoon honey

235 grams All-Purpose Gluten-Free Flour Blend (page 17)

100 grams Grain-Free Flour Mix (page 19)

2 teaspoons psyllium husks

1½ teaspoons fine sea salt

3 large eggs, at room temperature

½ cup hot water

¼ cup extra-virgin olive oil

1 large egg, beaten

Prepare to bake. Grease a 5 x 9-inch loaf pan.

Proof the yeast. In a small bowl, whisk together the ½ cup of warm water, yeast, and honey. When a bubbly foam forms on the surface of the water, the yeast is alive and ready to use.

Combine the dry ingredients. In another bowl, whisk together the flours, psyllium husks, and salt until they are one color. Set aside.

Mix the wet ingredients. In the bowl of a stand mixer with the paddle attachment, whip up the eggs on medium speed. Add the ½ cup of hot water and the oil. Mix until the water has cooled to room temperature, about 5 minutes.

Make the batter. With the mixer running on medium speed, pour in the dry ingredients a bit at a time, followed by the yeast mixture. Let the mixer continue to run to incorporate some air into the batter. The final dough will resemble thick pancake batter. (If the dough feels thicker than that, add a dribble of water until your batter is the consistency of pancake batter.)

Let the batter rise. Pour the batter into the prepared pan. Allow the batter to rise until is nearly at the top of the pan, about 1 hour.

Bake the bread. Preheat the oven to 450°F. Brush some of the beaten egg onto the top of the bread dough. Slide the loaf pan into the oven and bake the bread until the top is brown, the edges of the bread are pulling away from the pan, and the internal temperature registers 200°F on an instant-read thermometer, 30 to 45 minutes.

Allow the loaf to cool. Let the bread cool in the pan for 20 minutes, then turn the bread out onto a wire rack. Do NOT slice the bread until it has cooled completely.

Feel like playing?

If you like a more butterfly loaf of bread, substitute 3 tablespoons of melted butter for the olive oil. If you'd like more grains in your bread, substitute 50 grams of the all-purpose flour blend with 50 grams of cooked grains, such as millet, or pseudo cereals, such as quinoa or millet.

HAMBURGER BUNS

Makes 6 buns

Once you've made your own hamburger and hot dog buns, you'll never long for the additive-filled, cardboard-textured grocery store buns again. All you need is the recipe we created for sandwich bread and a hamburger bun pan. (If you don't have that pan, we'd recommend it. You're going to want to eat pulled pork sandwiches, page 87, as well.) Soft, pliable hamburger buns without gluten are yours to make.

3 tablespoons (45 grams) unsalted butter, melted, plus extra for greasing

1 batch Sandwich Bread (page 53) batter

¼ cup (27 grams) sesame seeds

½ teaspoon fine sea salt

Prepare to bake. Grease a hamburger bun pan with butter.

Let the dough rise. Pour the batter for the sandwich bread, which will have the consistency of pancake batter, halfway up each well of the hamburger pan. Distribute the batter evenly among the wells. Allow the batter to rise and hydrate until it is just under the lip of the pan, about 45 minutes.

Preheat the oven to 400°F.

Bake the hamburger buns. When the batter has risen, the tops will have stiffened into something akin to traditional bread dough. Gently, very gently, brush the melted butter on top of each bun, then sprinkle with the sesame seeds and salt. (If you can't eat butter, then brush the tops of the buns with olive oil.) Bake until the tops are browned and set and the internal temperature of the bread reaches 180°F on an instant-read thermometer, about 20 minutes.

Allow the hamburger buns to cool entirely on a wire rack before slicing them open.

Hot Dog Buns

With a few small changes, these can be hot dog buns. Allow the dough to rise in a large bowl in a warm place. When the dough has hydrated enough that it is kneadable, divide the dough into 6 portions. Form each into a *bâtard*-style roll (essentially, a long, even cylinder), about 6 inches long. Nestle them next to each other in a large, wide bread pan (such as a hearth bread pan) or small casserole pan. You want a pan the right size in order to put the hot dog bun dough pieces next to each other with no room to spread. Allow them to rise for 1 hour. Brush the tops with melted butter and bake at 400°F until the tops feel set and the sides have a spring, about 15 minutes. Allow the buns to cool in the pan for 15 minutes, then transfer them to a wire rack. They should pull apart easily at room temperature. Also, if you're looking for crunchier hot dog buns, make small hoagie rolls (see page 60).

Feel like playing?

If you don't own a hamburger bun pan, allow the dough to rise in a large bowl in a warm place. When the dough has hydrated enough that it is kneadable, divide the dough into 6 portions. Make each portion into a large ball, then gently form it into buns. Nestle them next to each other in a few skillets and let them rise together. Bake in the same fashion as above.

PIZZA DOUGH

Makes 2 (12-inch) pizza crusts

Our friends Brandon and Molly own a tremendous pizza place/neighborhood restaurant called Delancey in Seattle. You might have heard of it: they've grown pretty famous for the thin-crust pizza pie, the always fresh vegetables, and the delicious cocktails at Essex, the bar next door. Brandon makes incredible vegetable dishes in the same wood-fired oven where he bakes the pizzas, and those are more than enough for me. But I've been working on my ideal gluten-free pizza crust for nine years. Finally, just before the deadline for this book, I started working on a new one, based on the recipe from Roberta's pizza in Brooklyn, thanks to a piece in the New York Times. *If I bring a dough ready to go, and call ahead so Brandon can set aside toppings for me, Brandon can make me and Lucy a gluten-free pizza that never makes us sick. I brought him in this dough, feeling pretty good but assuming he'd tell me it still needs work. Brandon brought me a gorgeous pizza with braised beef tongue, local mushrooms, and a lot of crusty cheese melted toward the edges. When he came back, I gave him a slice. He kept nibbling as we talked about it. And eating more. I expected him to offer suggestions, but eventually he just said, "This one's good. Don't change it." And he took another slice.*

Brandon is steeped in pizza, traveling all over the world to every great slice he could find before he started Delancey, and eating pizza nearly every day for six years since then. Brandon approves of this pizza dough.

We do too.

150 grams All-Purpose Gluten-Free Flour Blend (page 17)

150 grams Grain-Free Flour Mix (page 19)

1½ teaspoons psyllium husks

1 teaspoon sea salt

¾ teaspoon active dry yeast

1 teaspoon olive oil, plus extra for drizzling

1 cup (225 grams) lukewarm water

Make the dough. Combine both flours, the psyllium husks, salt, and yeast in the bowl of a stand mixer with the paddle attachment. Whirl them up.

With the mixer running on low, pour in the oil, then the water, very slowly. When everything has been added and the dough feels soft and pliable (but far wetter than a typical gluten dough), turn the mixer onto medium and let it run for a few more moments. Turn off the mixer and scrape down the sides of the bowl with a rubber spatula.

Let the dough rise. Cover the bowl with plastic wrap and let it sit in a warm place for 1 hour. Then, put the dough in the refrigerator and let it sit overnight.

CONTINUED

Prepare to bake. The next day, pull the dough out of the refrigerator 1 hour before you intend to roll it.

Divide the dough into 2 balls. Put one dough ball between two lightly greased pieces of parchment paper. Roll out the dough until it is about 12 inches across. Take the top piece of parchment paper off the dough and transfer the dough to a baking sheet. Repeat with the remaining dough ball.

Prebake the pizza dough. Put the baking sheets in the oven—one on the lower rack and one in the middle—and turn the oven on to 350°F. After 30 minutes, trade the baking sheets between the racks. Continue baking until the tops and edges of the dough feel set, about 30 minutes more. This will steam the water out of the dough and give you a great dough for baking.

Top the pizzas. At this point, remove the crusts from the oven and top the crusts with a drizzle of oil and any toppings you wish. (Here are some of our favorites: chèvre and sautéed cremini mushrooms with fresh thyme; fresh mozzarella with burrata and prosciutto; a tomato sauce with warm garlic, lardo, and an egg cracked on it at the end; fresh tomatoes with marjoram, mozzarella, and Italian sausage; and for Lucy, always lots of cheese with pineapple.) One thing Brandon taught us that improves the crust: cover the edges of the pizza with grated Parmesan cheese. Crusty melted cheese makes the crust of a gluten-free pizza even better.

Finish baking the pizzas. Bump up the temperature to as high as your oven will go. Ours stops at 550°F. If you have a baking stone in the oven, that raises the heat even more. Put the pizzas in the oven when it's truly hot, then watch them. Wait until the cheese bubbles, then turn on the broiler at the end. Watch the pizzas closely. Don't let them burn. But bake them to just before that point.

Voilà! Pizza.

Feel like playing?

Of course, you could use any flours you wish here, based on what works in your kitchen. But this ratio of flours to yeast to salt to psyllium to oil to water has worked for us every time, no matter what the combination of flours. It's pizza dough.

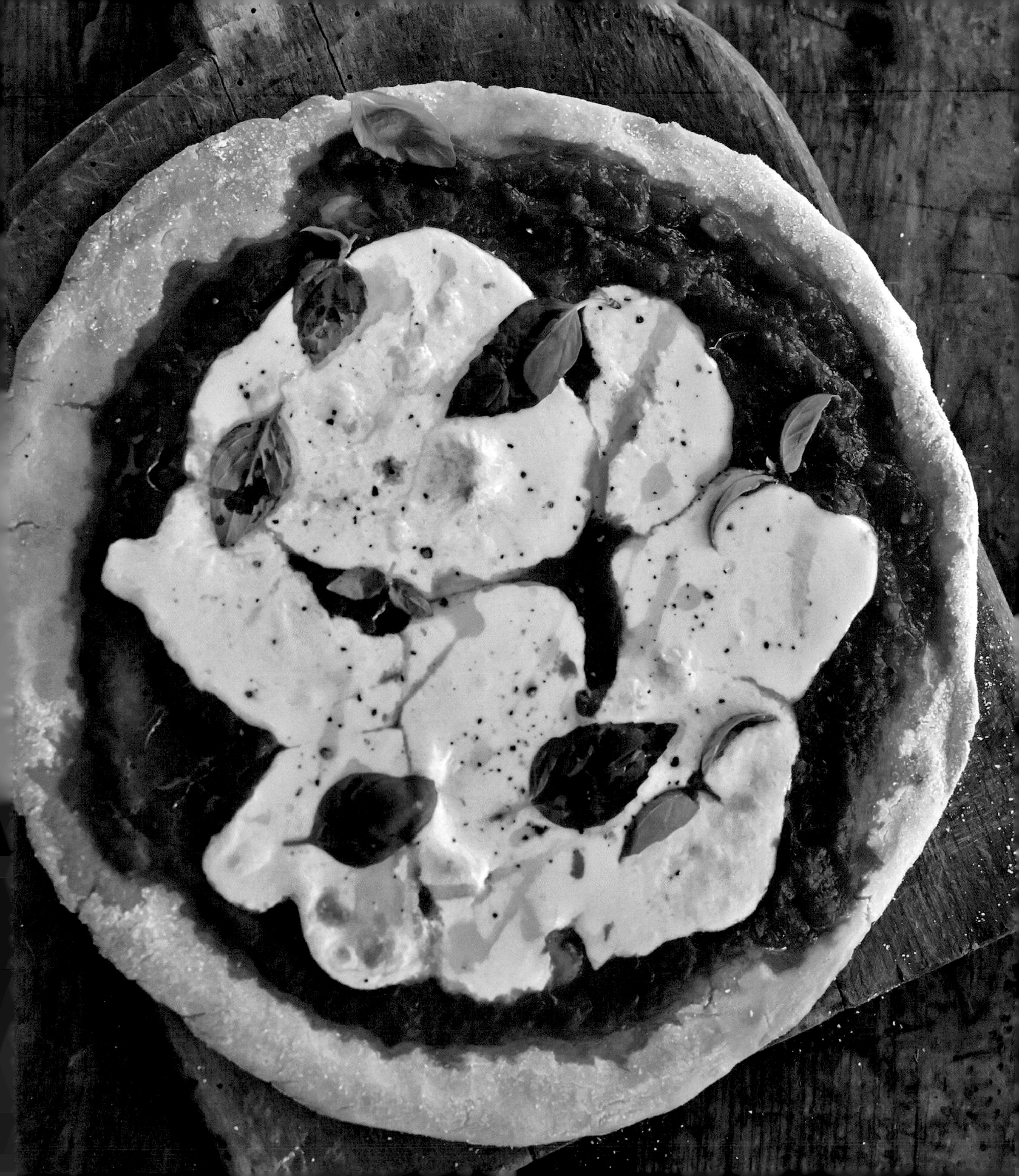

HOAGIE ROLLS

Makes 8 hoagie rolls

Hoagie rolls are a delicious vehicle for moving lobster, Philly cheesesteaks, Italian beef, breaded pork tenderloin, and Cuban sandwich ingredients to your mouth. Sure, you could eat the insides of those sandwiches on a salad or a bed of rice and eat like a queen. But sometimes you want soft bread around beef dripping in its own juices. Here's the roll for most of the sandwiches in this book. Of course, you can also use one of these to make a hoagie, a sandwich that originated in Philadelphia with ham, prosciutto, salami, and provolone cheese with a strong oregano dressing. Why not?

1⅓ cup warm water

2 teaspoons organic cane sugar or honey

2 teaspoons active dry yeast

350 grams All-Purpose Gluten-Free Flour Blend (page 17)

200 grams Grain-Free Flour Mix (page 19)

1 tablespoon psyllium husks

1 tablespoon fine sea salt

3 tablespoons (45 grams) unsalted butter, softened

⅔ cup whey (see Note), at room temperature

1 large egg, beaten

Proof the yeast. In the bowl of a stand mixer with the paddle attachment, whisk together ⅓ cup of the warm water, the sugar, and yeast. Let the mixture sit for 15 minutes, until it is foamy and slightly rises in size.

Add the dry ingredients. Add the all-purpose flour blend, grain-free flour mix, psyllium husks, and salt to the yeast mixture. Mix until the dough is fluffy and slumps off the paddle, about 4 minutes.

Finish the dough. With the stand mixer running on low, add in bits of the butter, one at a time, making sure the butter is fully incorporated before adding more. Scrape down the sides of the bowl with a rubber spatula. Add the whey and the remaining 1 cup of warm water, until the dough is soft and pliable, a bit shaggy. It will not be the consistency of traditional bread dough. Don't add more flour to make it look like the bread dough you know. Cover the bowl with plastic wrap and refrigerate it overnight.

Divide and proof the dough. The next day, bring the dough out of the refrigerator. Let it come to room temperature, about 1 hour. Scoop the dough out of the bowl onto a clean surface. It should be fairly kneadable at this point. Gently, move the dough around until the air is deflated and you have a smooth dough ball. Divide the dough into 6 balls. Flatten and work a ball of dough until is about 8 inches long. Starting from the top long side, roll the dough into a cigar shape. Roll the seams on the counter to seal it. Set aside the roll and finish the rest of the balls of dough. Let them rest on a baking sheet lined with parchment paper until they have plumped out, 60 to 90 minutes.

Prepare to bake. Preheat the oven to 425°F. Brush each hoagie roll with some of the beaten egg. If you wish, gently make a small shallow slash on the top of each roll. Slide the baking sheet into the oven. Bake until the rolls are golden brown and firm to the touch, 18 to 25 minutes. Take the hoagie rolls out of the oven and let them cool on the baking sheet for 10 minutes. Move them to a wire rack and allow them to cool completely.

Note: Whey is the liquid left over after you make cheese. Whenever we make fresh ricotta, we save the leftover whey for making these rolls. The protein and flavor in whey strengthen all gluten-free breads. If you don't want to make ricotta, you can also pour off the liquid from whole-milk plain yogurt and use it here.

Feel like playing?

If you cannot eat butter, try lard here. It will work just as well. Vegetable shortening works okay too. If you want, you can use the entire dough to make a buttery sandwich bread by baking it in a 5 x 9-inch loaf pan.

DINNER ROLLS

Makes 8 dinner rolls

It's one of the enduring images of Thanksgiving, the most beloved American holiday: warm, browned fluffy dinner rolls on the table, ready to sop up that gravy. You might think a fluffy dinner roll is impossible without gluten. It's not, of course. These are grain-free too, so feeding someone who cannot tolerate grains well at your Thanksgiving feast just grew easier.

The key here is the psyllium husks. This natural insoluble fiber absorbs water in a way you won't believe the first time you use it. The dough here will be wet, thickly wet, and it will dribble off the whisk. After you have let the dough rise and the flours hydrate for 90 minutes, the dough will be still tacky but much closer to bread dough. Tuck those dough balls into each other in a pie plate and you will have soft, fluffy dinner rolls.

1 cup warm water (about 110°F)

1 envelope (2¼ teaspoons) active dry yeast

1 teaspoon honey

450 grams Grain-Free Flour Mix (page 19)

2½ teaspoons psyllium husks

1 teaspoon fine sea salt

8 tablespoons (115 grams) unsalted butter, melted and cooled

Fat for greasing the pan

1 large egg, beaten

Proof the yeast. Whisk together the warm water, yeast, and honey in the bowl of a stand mixer with the paddle attachment. When a bubbly foam forms on the surface of the water, the yeast is alive and ready to use.

Combine the dry ingredients. In a bowl, whisk together the flour mix, psyllium husks, and salt. With the stand mixer running on low, slowly add the dry ingredients to the yeast mixture.

Finish the dough. With the stand mixer running on low, pour in the melted butter slowly until everything is evenly combined. The texture of the dough will be a little like paint spackle—it should be wet. The batter should drip off the paddle when you lift it, not quickly, but in slow motion.

Rise the dough. Cover the bowl with plastic wrap and let it sit in a warm place in the kitchen for 90 minutes. The dough will have risen in volume, but mostly the flours will have hydrated. It will feel less like a batter and more like a dough. It will still be a little tacky to the touch.

Prepare to bake. Preheat the oven to 425°F. Grease a 9-inch pie pan.

Bake the rolls. If you have a 2-inch ice cream scoop, use it here to scoop a ball of dough. If you don't have one, wet your hands and grab a big ball of dough. Plop it in the middle of the pie pan. Repeat until you have filled the pie pan. Wet your hands and smooth the tops of the dough balls.

Brush the beaten egg, very gently, over the tops of the dough balls.

Bake until the tops of the rolls are browned and firm to the touch and the internal temperature registers 200°F on an instant-read thermometer, 15 to 20 minutes. Remove the rolls from the oven and let them cool in the pie pan. Serve immediately.

Feel like playing?

If you cannot tolerate eggs, you can brush the tops of the rolls with olive oil instead. To make these dairy-free, substitute melted coconut oil for the butter. If you would prefer to use the All-Purpose Gluten-Free Flour Blend (page 17) instead, add 1 more tablespoon of melted butter to the recipe.

ENGLISH MUFFINS

Makes 6 English muffins

Growing up on English muffins that came packaged in a rectangular box at the grocery store, I was shocked to find how easy they are to make, even without gluten. Taking a little time to make these for your family means Smoked Salmon Eggs Benedict (page 26) could be yours for breakfast soon. (Also, egg and cheese muffin sandwiches for busy mornings.)

315 grams All-Purpose Gluten-Free Flour Blend (page 17)

1½ teaspoons psyllium husks

1½ teaspoons organic cane sugar

1¼ teaspoons active dry yeast

¾ teaspoon fine sea salt

½ to ¾ cup low-fat buttermilk

1 tablespoon (15 grams) unsalted butter, softened

Cornmeal for dusting (make sure it's gluten-free)

Fat for greasing the skillet

Combine the dry ingredients. Whisk together the flour blend, psyllium husks, sugar, yeast, and salt in the bowl of a stand mixer with the paddle attachment.

Combine the wet ingredients. With the mixer running on low, add ½ cup of the buttermilk and the butter to the dough. Let the mixer run for a couple of moments. Stop the mixer and scrape down the sides of the bowl with a rubber spatula. If there is any visible flour remaining, dribble in a bit more milk, until the dough is soft and cohesive. Let the mixer run for 5 more minutes. Once you scrape the dough into a ball, it should be smooth and a bit sticky.

Rise the dough. Cover the bowl with plastic wrap and set it in a warm place. Let the dough rise until the dough is more kneadable and has risen some, at least 90 minutes.

Proof the dough. Move the dough to a clean surface. Cut the ball of dough into 6 pieces. Knead each piece to release any air pockets and roll it into a ball. Repeat with the remaining balls. Scatter cornmeal generously over a baking sheet. Put the 6 balls of dough on the sheet and cover them with a slightly damp kitchen towel. Let them proof for 1 hour.

Prepare to bake. Preheat the oven to 350°F. Gently, dust both sides of each dough ball with cornmeal.

Griddle the English muffins. Set a large cast-iron skillet over medium heat. Lightly grease the pan with a touch of fat. Put 3 balls of dough into the skillet and flatten them a bit with the palm of your hand. Cook until the bottoms of the English muffins are browned, 5 to 8 minutes. Flip them and cook for another 5 to 8 minutes.

Finish the English muffins. Put the skillet in the oven and bake until the sides of the English muffins feel set, about 5 minutes.

Transfer the baked English muffins to a wire rack and use the skillet to make the remaining English muffins.

Cool completely before splitting open and eating.

Feel like playing?

You could try making these with the Grain-Free Flour Mix (page 19). They'll have a more assertive flavor.

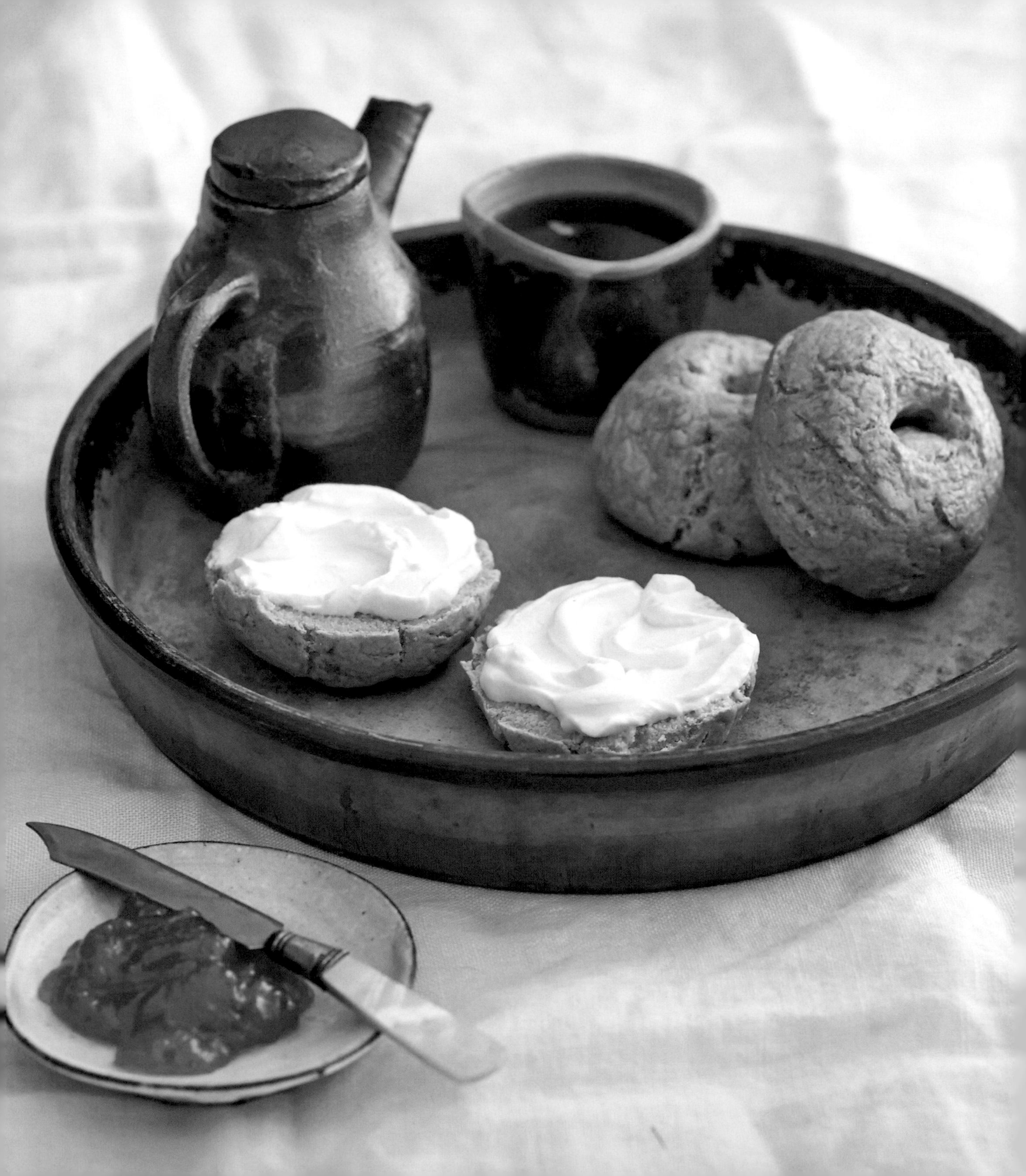

BAGELS

Makes about a dozen bagels

For years, I've been working on gluten-free bagels. Let's make this clear: gluten-free bagels will never be the same as the best bagels in New York City. But these are much better than the commercial gluten-free bagels available in stores. For warm bagels, slathered with cream cheese and smoked salmon, these are the best without gluten I've ever eaten. They are a bit crisp on the outside and soft and chewy on the inside. They're old-school New York bagels, smaller than the enormous bagels of warehouse stores. Making a sponge, then letting the dough sit in the refrigerator overnight, develops a wonderful flavor in the bagels. (Thank you to Bruce Ezzell from The Breadlist in North Carolina for his lucid explanation of how to make bagels.)

FOR THE SPONGE

250 grams All-Purpose Gluten-Free Flour Blend (page 17)

250 grams Grain-Free Flour Mix (page 19)

¾ teaspoon active dry yeast

2¼ cups lukewarm water

FOR THE BAGELS

250 grams All-Purpose Gluten-Free Flour Blend (page 17)

240 grams Grain-Free Flour Mix (page 19)

50 grams tapioca flour

1 tablespoon psyllium husks

2 teaspoons fine sea salt

1 tablespoon molasses or dark honey

1 tablespoon baking soda

1 large egg, beaten

Make the sponge. Whisk together the flours and yeast in a large bowl. Slowly drizzle in the lukewarm water. Stir them together until everything is thoroughly combined. Cover the bowl with plastic wrap and set in a warm place. Allow it to sit for at least 2 hours and up to 4 hours.

Make the dough. Put the sponge into the bowl of a stand mixer with the paddle attachment. Add the additional flours, psyllium husks, salt, and molasses and mix them together on low speed until the dough is light and sticking to the sides of the bowl. Scrape down the sides of the bowl with a rubber spatula and push the dough into a ball in the bowl. Let it sit and rest for 90 minutes.

Form the bagels. Put the dough onto a clean counter and push it around to knead out any air bubbles. Cut the dough into 4-ounce pieces. (There should be 12 or 13 balls of dough.)

There are two options for forming the bagels. 1) Flatten each ball of dough, slightly, with the palm of the hand. Make a hole in the center with your thumb. (This is the easiest way.) 2) Roll each ball of dough into an 8-inch rope. Wrap the ends of the dough around each other, leaving a small hole in the middle, and overlap the edges. Press the ends together, rocking the dough back and forth a bit to seal the edges. (This may seem more difficult at first, but we think it makes for better-looking bagels.)

CONTINUED

Put the bagels on two parchment-lined baking sheets and cover them loosely with a very lightly damp towel. Slide the baking sheets into the refrigerator and let them rest overnight.

Prepare to bake. The next day, pull the dough out of the refrigerator. Let it sit on the counter for 1 hour to come to room temperature. Preheat the oven to 475°F. Set a large pot of water over high heat to come to a simmer. Add the baking soda and stir.

Boil the bagels. Gently, lower 3 or 4 bagels into the simmering water. The bagels should float to the top of the water fairly immediately. Let the bagels simmer for 1 to 2 minutes. (The longer you let them simmer, the chewier the bagels will be.) Flip them over and allow them to simmer for 1 more minute. Using a Chinese spider or slotted spoon, transfer the bagels to the parchment-lined baking sheet. Repeat with the remaining bagels.

Bake the bagels. Brush the egg over the tops of the bagels. Put the baking sheets into the oven and bake for 9 minutes. Switch the baking sheets between racks and bake until the bagels are golden brown and the tops are starting to set, another 8 to 11 minutes.

Allow the bagels to cool. Serve immediately.

Feel like playing?

Feel free to top the egg wash with sesame seeds, poppy seeds, or salt. I'm a bit of a bagel purist, so I'd never put raisins or cinnamon or anything else in my bagels. You might be different. If you are, add any ingredients to the dough when you add the additional flour and psyllium husks.

BUTTERMILK BISCUITS WITH CHEDDAR AND JALAPEÑO

Makes 6 to 8 biscuits

I don't know about you, but sometimes we just want biscuits for breakfast. Light and flaky biscuits seem a thing of the past when you first realize you need to be gluten-free. But find the right combination of flours, a touch of psyllium, and the usual accompaniments of buttermilk and quick cold hands when working with the dough? You have biscuits. Add some sharp Cheddar and fresh jalapeños and you have a Texan/Southwestern/Mexican-inspired biscuit. Call it what you want. I call this a good breakfast.

Fat for greasing the skillet

280 grams All-Purpose Gluten-Free Flour Blend (page 17)

2 teaspoons baking powder

1 teaspoon fine sea salt

8 tablespoons (115 grams) cold unsalted butter, cut into ½-inch cubes

5 ounces (1¼ cups) freshly grated sharp Cheddar cheese

¾ cup cold low-fat buttermilk

2 tablespoons finely chopped jalapeños

4 tablespoons (55 grams) unsalted butter, melted (optional)

Prepare to bake. Preheat the oven to 425°F. Grease a 9-inch cast-iron skillet.

Combine the dry ingredients. In a large bowl, whisk together the flour, baking powder, and salt. Put the bowl in the freezer. Put the cold cubed butter in the freezer for 15 minutes too, along with the bowl of the food processor (if using).

Make the biscuit dough. When the oven is fully heated, take the flour mix and butter out of the freezer. Put them both into the cold bowl of the food processor. (You can also do this by hand.) Pulse the food processor until the butter is broken down into pieces the size of lima beans, 5 to 10 times.

Add the cheese, buttermilk, and jalapeños to the bowl of the food processor. Pulse until they are all combined and the dough is starting to cohere. Do not take it as far as a solid ball, however.

Make the biscuits. Sprinkle a little all-purpose flour blend onto a clean, dry surface. Turn out the dough onto the board and sprinkle with just a touch more flour. Working as quickly as you can, gather the dough loosely into a circle. Fold the dough in half, bringing the back part of the dough toward you. Pat the dough into an even round. Turn the dough 90 degrees, then fold the dough in half again and pat. This should make the dough fairly even. If not, you can fold the dough a third time. Pat out the dough to a 1½-inch thickness.

CONTINUED

Dip a 2½-inch biscuit cutter into a bit of flour and push it straight down into the dough, starting from the outside edges. Do not twist the biscuit cutter. Cut out the remaining biscuits. Working quickly, pat any remaining scraps into another 1½-inch-thick piece of dough and cut the last biscuit.

Bake the biscuits. Move the biscuits to the prepared cast-iron skillet, nudging them up against one another. If you nestle the biscuits alongside each other, edges touching, you will have taller biscuits after baking.

Slide the skillet into the oven and bake the biscuits for 6 minutes. Rotate the skillet 180 degrees and continue baking until the biscuits are firm and light golden brown, another 6 to 8 minutes. Remove the skillet from the oven and brush the tops of the biscuits with the melted butter, if you wish. Let the biscuits cool for 10 minutes.

Remove from the skillet and serve immediately.

Feel like playing?

You could make these with smoked salmon instead of cheese and jalapeños (try 6 ounces of flaked smoked salmon), if you want Pacific Northwest biscuits. Any kind of cheese is delightful here, depending on your taste. If you want plain biscuits (and those are great too), take out the cheese and jalapeños and add enough thick full-fat yogurt to make the biscuit dough cohere.

BROWN BREAD

Makes 1 loaf

We had so many requests from New England folks to make gluten-free brown bread that we knew it had to go in this book. Dense and dark with molasses, this is a quick bread without yeast. It's a very particular taste and texture, which we were able to re-create with our all-purpose flour mix, teff flour, and cornmeal. I love the fact that it bakes up best in a coffee can, set over boiling water in the oven so that it steams. There's no other recipe quite like this. Still, not having grown up on this bread, I didn't quite understand why so many people wanted it back. When we were in Boston on our potluck road trip tour, I sat down in a beautiful gluten-free bakery named Glutenus Minimus (you have to love that name), surrounded by over a hundred happy people. When I asked the people at my table about brown bread, their faces grew alive with excitement. "My father made the same dinner for us every Saturday night," one woman told me. "It was pork and beans and slices of brown bread fried in butter. The thought of never having brown bread again means I can never have that dinner my father made me." After that, I understood. Boston, this is for you.

2 tablespoons (29 grams) unsalted butter, softened

80 grams teff flour

70 grams All-Purpose Gluten-Free Flour Blend (page 17)

70 grams finely ground cornmeal (make sure it's gluten-free)

½ teaspoon baking powder

½ teaspoon baking soda

½ teaspoon ground allspice

¼ teaspoon ground cloves

1 cup low-fat buttermilk

½ cup unsulfured molasses

½ cup raisins

Prepare to bake. Preheat the oven to 325°F. Set a large pot of water over high heat and bring to a boil. Turn down the heat to low and let the water simmer. Liberally grease the inside of a 1-pound coffee can with the butter.

Combine the dry ingredients. In a large bowl, whisk together the teff flour, all-purpose flour blend, cornmeal, baking powder, baking soda, allspice, and cloves.

Combine the wet ingredients. In another bowl, whisk together the buttermilk and molasses.

Finish the batter. Make a well in the center of the dry ingredients. Pour in the molasses and buttermilk and whisk the batter together. Add the raisins. The batter will be thick, just a touch too thick to pour easily.

Bake the bread. Scrape the dough into the prepared coffee can. The batter should be no more than two-thirds of the way up to the rim of the coffee can. Cover the coffee can with aluminum foil. Put the coffee can in a large baking pan and slide that into the oven. Carefully, pour enough of the simmering hot water into the baking pan so it comes up one-third the sides of the coffee can. Bake the brown bread until a toothpick inserted into the middle comes out clean, about 2 hours and 20 minutes.

Remove the baking pan from the oven and let it sit for 10 minutes. Carefully, with oven mitts, transfer the coffee can to a wire rack and let it cool for 1 hour before sliding the brown bread out of the coffee can.

Slice into the brown bread. It's good as it is, but it seems to be most loved fried up in more butter.

Feel like playing?

For those of you looking for a substitution for the teff, it's going to be hard. Teff flour gives this bread its dark color and distinct taste. You could use another whole-grain flour like sorghum or brown rice in its place, but it won't replicate the feeling of brown bread. Then again, you could just make yourself a new tradition. Why not?

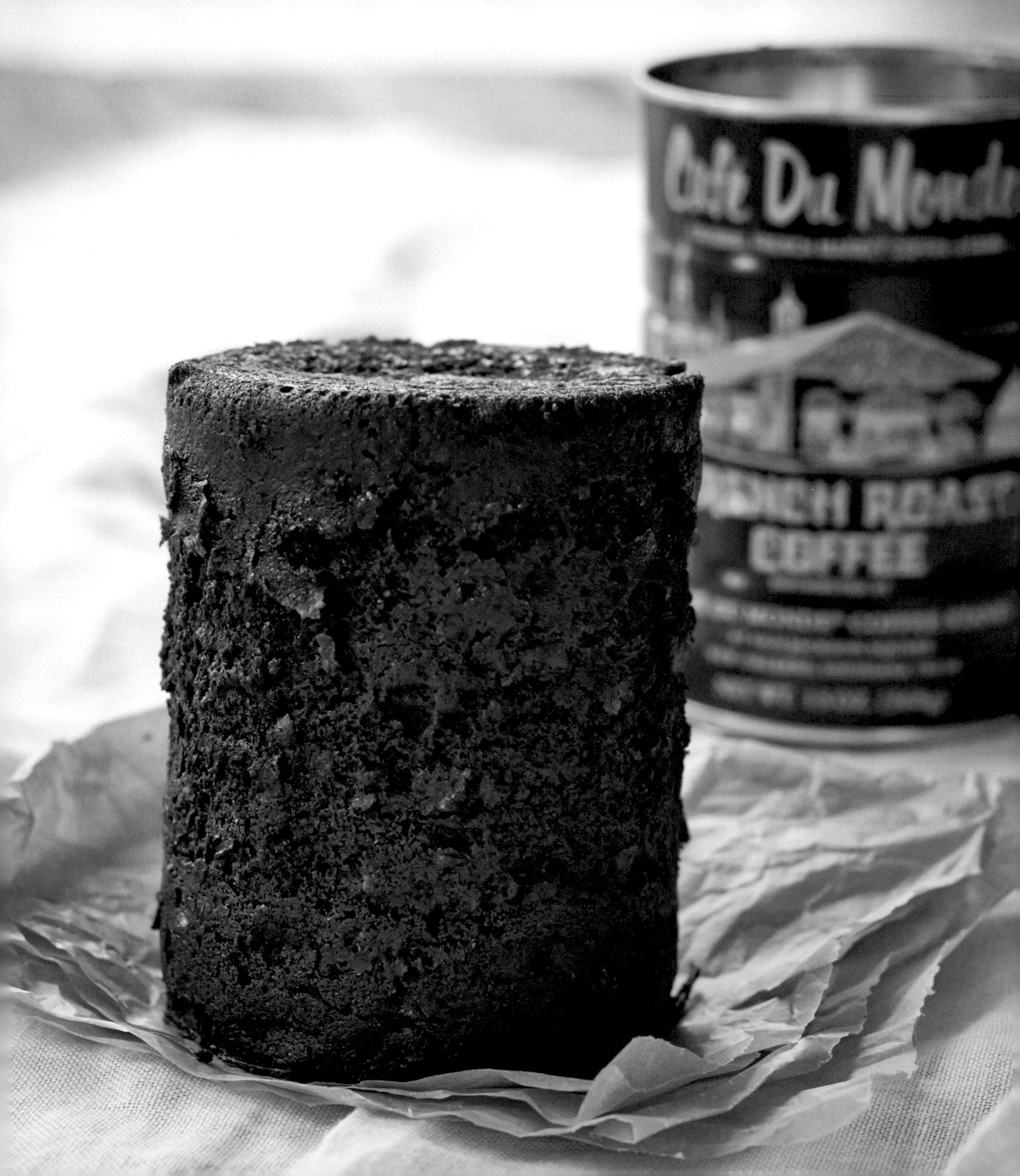
COFFEE

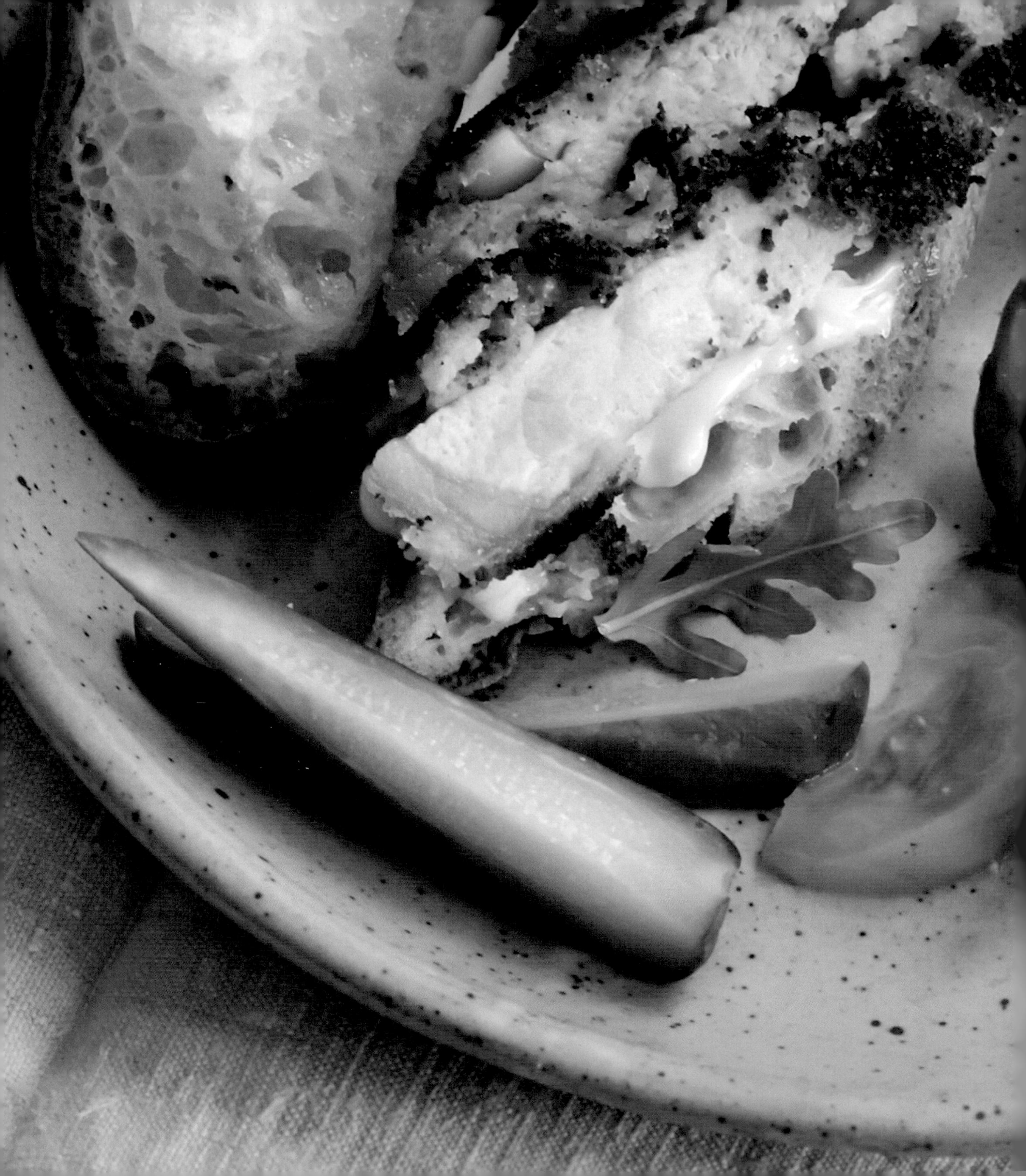

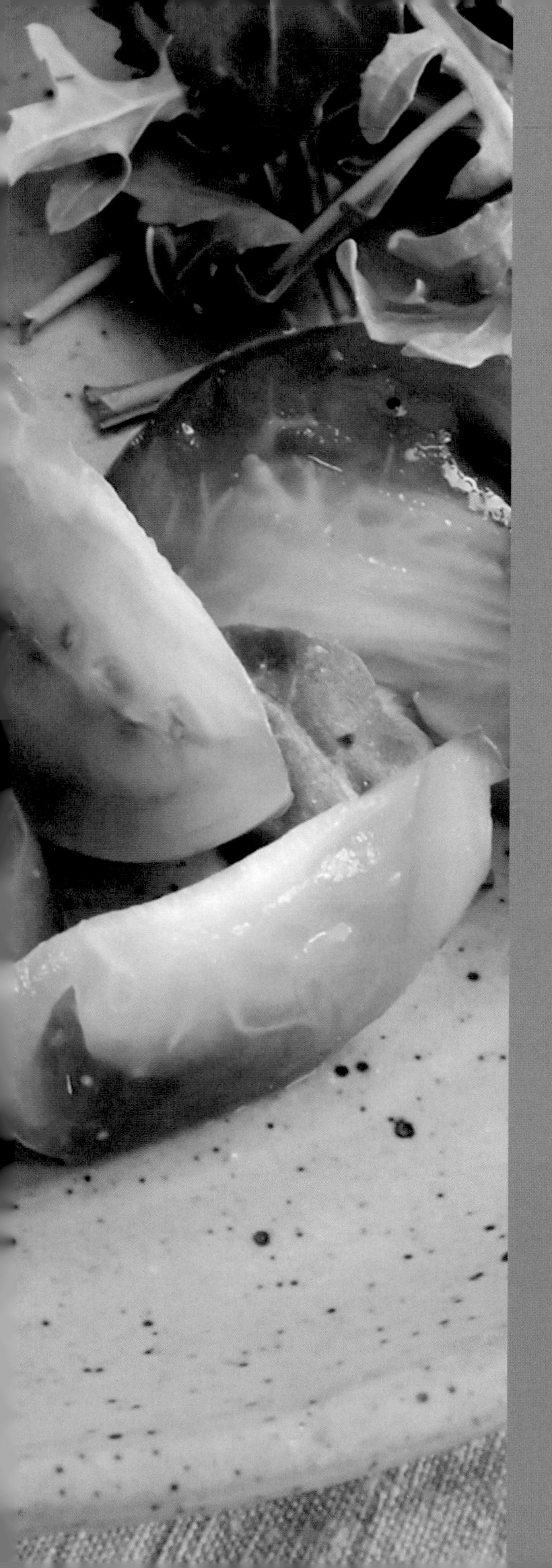

SANDWICHES

THE GREAT AMERICAN BURGER

We all have our own platonic ideal of the burger— small and smooshed beneath a crinkly white bun; large and oozing juice under an enormous sesame seed bun; made of buffalo meat or beef chuck or turkey or filled with bacon or mushrooms or caramelized onions—and there is quite a bit of heated conversation around what makes a great burger. We're simply offering our favorite kind of burger and the ways to reach it.

Choose the meat. We believe the best burgers are not lean. If you're going to eat a burger, go all in. It's harder these days to find beef in the meat section of the grocery store that isn't labeled "extra-lean." That meat does not make a great burger. It makes a mealy burger. Ideally, the meat is 80 percent meat and 20 percent fat. The best bet is to ask the butcher in that meat department (or at a good local butcher shop) to coarsely grind chuck for you, which ensures you're going to get good fat in there. If you can afford grass-fed beef, there are solid reasons to believe that beef may be better for you. But if you can't afford it, this isn't necessary. Some chefs we know use different mixes of beef cuts in their burgers: a friend in Maine uses chuck, brisket, and bacon together. That's a darned fine burger. But it's not necessary. We love the taste of buffalo meat, and that truly is an American burger. But buffalo tends to run leaner, so you'll want to cut in more fat with frozen bacon (see page 79).

Form the patties. Remember this: a hamburger is not meat loaf. The more you handle the meat, the tougher the burger will be. Treat the meat gently. Take it out of the refrigerator, season it with salt and pepper, then divide the meat and form loose patties. These should be hamburger patties that look as though they might fall apart.

Choose the right surface. We find that the absolute best cooking surface for a burger is a cast-iron skillet, especially one you've cooked with for a while. (You've probably noticed that we cook much of our food in a cast-iron skillet.) It conducts heat well, making for even cooking at high heat. Some chefs swear that cast-iron is better than the grill, so if they are having a barbecue, they put the cast-iron on the grill. (We still put ours directly on the grill.) And don't be afraid of the heat.

Add fat. For decades, Americans lived in fear of fat. But fat is not the enemy, as the medical profession and traditional media are recognizing now. Besides, if you're having a burger, there's no point in going halfway and trying to make a low-fat burger. Enjoy this. We like greasing the skillet with beef suet before laying down the patties.

Now, with all this, you're going to have a great burger. Let's look at a couple of options.

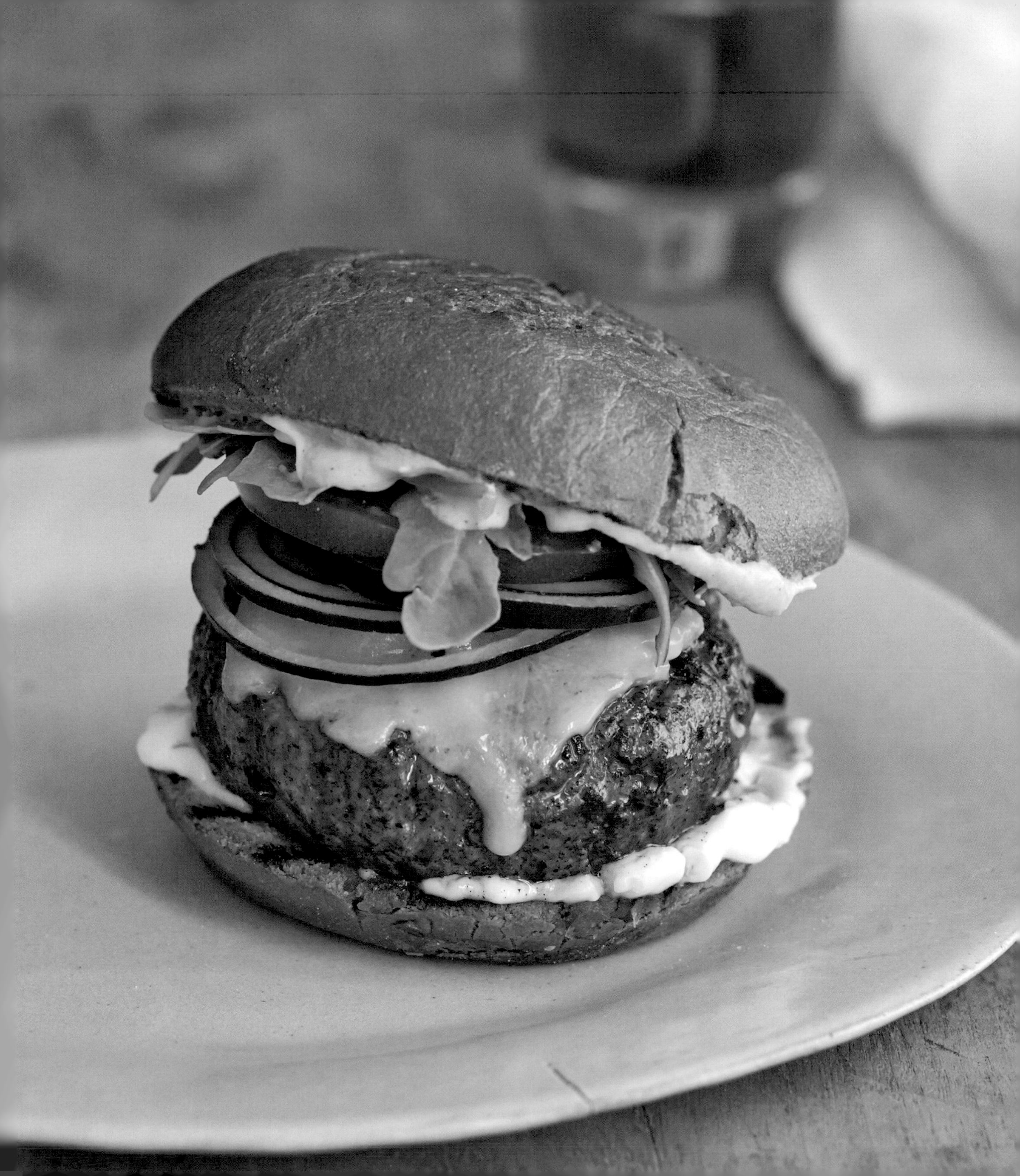

BASIC BEEF BURGERS

Feeds 4

1¾ pounds recently ground beef chuck (80% meat and 20% fat)

Kosher salt and freshly ground black pepper

2 tablespoons beef suet

Season the meat. Take the meat out of the refrigerator. Season the meat with salt and pepper. Gently, divide it into 4 parts. Loosely, barely touching the meat, form each part into a round patty. Set the patties on a plate.

Cook the burgers. Set a large cast-iron skillet over medium-high heat. Add the suet to the pan. When the suet is hot, gently place the patties in the pan. (You might need two skillets, if yours are small.) Cook for 3 minutes. Flip the burgers and cook until medium-rare, another 3 or 4 minutes. (If you are adding cheese, add it as soon as you flip the burgers.) If you want the burgers more well done, cook them for another 3 to 5 minutes. Take the burgers off the heat and eat them.

BUFFALO-BACON BURGERS

Feeds 4

6 ounces bacon

22 ounces ground buffalo meat

Kosher salt and freshly ground black pepper

2 tablespoons beef suet

Prepare the bacon. Chop the bacon into 1-inch pieces. Put them in the freezer. After 30 minutes, take the bacon out of the freezer and put it in the bowl of a food processor. Pulse until the frozen bacon looks like ground meat.

Make the burgers. Combine the ground bacon and buffalo meat gently. Season with salt and pepper. Gently, divide the dough into 4 parts. Loosely, barely touching the meat, form each part into a round patty. Set the patties on a plate.

Cook the burgers. Set a large cast-iron skillet over medium-high heat. Add the suet to the pan. When the suet is hot, gently place the patties in the pan. (You might need two skillets, if yours are small.) Cook for 3 minutes. Flip the burgers and cook until medium-rare, another 3 or 4 minutes. (If you are adding cheese, add it as soon as you flip the burgers.) If you want the burgers more well done, cook them for another 3 to 5 minutes. Take the burgers off the heat and eat them.

Note: For an entertaining and exhaustive look at burgers across America, pick up a copy of John T. Edge's *Hamburgers and Fries*.

Feel like playing?

Once you have the basic template, add any spices or flavorings that work for you or the region of the country in which you live. In New Mexico, we ate a tremendous green chile burger, with Hatch green chiles and white Cheddar cheese, at a legendary place called Bobcat Bite. In southern California, I've been served juicy burgers with a mound of guacamole. Toppings? Sliced red onions, pickles, any kind of cheese you want, bacon, aioli, arugula instead of lettuce—there are endless variations. Also, there are burgers fast-food style, with special sauce. We're going to let you figure those out on your own. These are our favorite burgers.

ITALIAN BEEF SANDWICHES

Feeds 8

I ate the most memorable sandwich of my life hunched over the back of a rental car in a parking lot in South Chicago. When my friend Sharon and I drove across the country, from New York City to Oregon, we plotted the routes we would take based on legendary foods we couldn't miss. For lunch one day, we stopped at Al's #1 Italian Beef in Little Italy, the home of (what some said was) the best Italian beef sandwich in America. Think of a French dip, but with thicker meat, sweet peppers, and dipped in the beef juices. Sharon and I stood over the trunk of our white rental car, eating and making happy noises. The drippings from those sandwiches stayed on the car until Wyoming, when we hit an epic thunderstorm. The memory still stays.

3 pounds boneless beef roast (sirloin, top round, or chuck)

6 cups beef stock (if you're using boxed stock, make sure it's gluten-free)

1 tablespoon freshly ground black pepper

2 teaspoons chopped fresh basil or 1 tablespoon dried

2 teaspoons chopped fresh oregano or 1 tablespoon dried

1 teaspoon onion powder

½ teaspoon red pepper flakes

6 cloves garlic, peeled and cut into small slivers

4 tablespoons extra-virgin olive oil

½ medium yellow onion, peeled and finely chopped

3 large red bell peppers, sliced into slivers

8 gluten-free Hoagie Rolls (page 60)

Prepare to cook. Preheat the oven to 400°F. Cut small slits in the roast, about every 2 inches. Set a large pot over high heat. Pour in the beef stock. Bring it to a boil, then turn down the heat and keep it at a low simmer.

Make the rub. In a bowl, whisk together the pepper, basil, oregano, onion powder, and red pepper flakes.

Rub the roast. Rub three-quarters of the spice mixture all over the roast. Push the slivers of garlic into the slits you made in the roast.

Sear the beef. Set a large cast-iron skillet over medium-high heat. Pour in 2 tablespoons of the olive oil. Put the roast into the skillet and cook until the bottom is browned, about 3 minutes. (Watch it carefully. The garlic could burn quickly.) Flip the roast and continue searing each side until it is browned. Turn off the heat and take the roast out of the pan.

Roast the beef. Pour the hot stock into the bottom of a 9 x 13-inch roasting pan. Scrape all the remnants of the beef from the skillet into the stock. Put a raised rack into the pan. Put the roast on the rack, above the juice. Roast the beef until the temperature has reached 130°F for medium-rare, about 1½ hours. Take the beef out of the oven and put it on a plate to rest for 15 minutes, then put it in the refrigerator. Let it grow entirely cold. Set aside the stock for later.

Cook the peppers. While the meat is cooking, set a large skillet over medium-high heat. Add the remaining 2 tablespoons of olive oil. Add the onions, peppers, and remaining spice mixture and cook, stirring occasionally, until they are browned and softened, about 15 minutes. Take them off the heat and let them cool.

Reduce the stock. Set a large pot over high heat. Pour in the beef stock. Bring it to a boil, then turn the heat down to low. Allow the stock to cook until it reduces by one-third.

Slice the beef. Using the sharpest knife you have, slice the beef into the thinnest pieces you can make. Go slowly. Overly thick slices of meat will overpower the sandwich. Now, you're ready to make sandwiches.

Make the sandwiches. Slice the hoagie rolls to open them partially. Dip as many slices of meat as you want on your sandwich into the hot stock with tongs and let it stay there for 1 minute. Pile it on the roll. Add some of the onions and peppers. Spoon juice over it all, or you can go the entire way and dip the sandwich into the juices.

Eat immediately with a lot of napkins handy.

Feel like playing?

This is the long, slow way, the Italian way. You can easily use already roasted beef, green peppers, and store-bought stock and gluten-free rolls to make these quickly. Heat up the stock with basil, oregano, pepper, and red pepper flakes to get some of the flavor in there and make it easy on yourself.

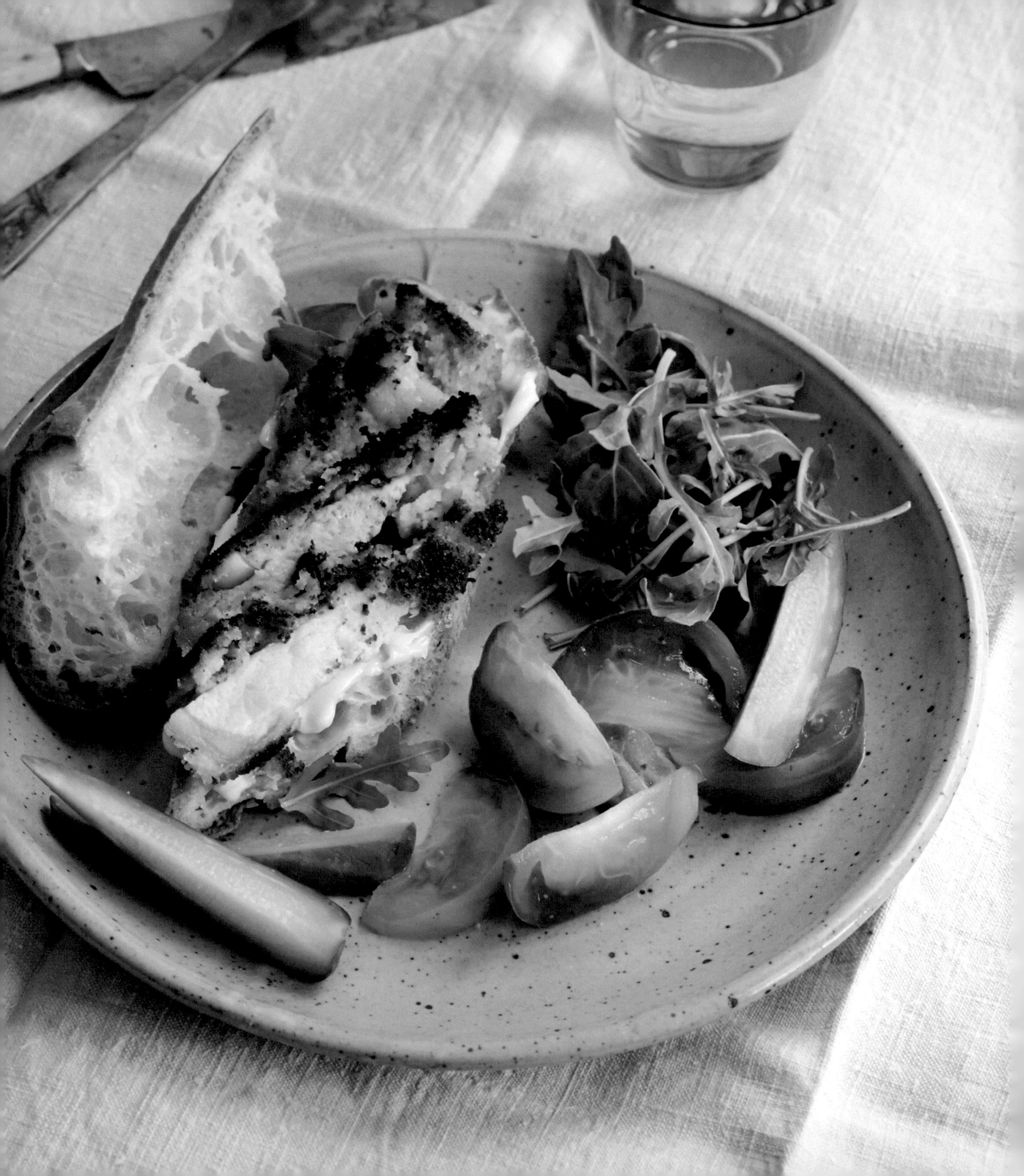

BREADED PORK LOIN SANDWICHES

Feeds 4

We're big fans of the Hoosier state around here. We have some dear friends, Debra and Rod Smith, who live in Indiana, and they assured us this recipe simply had to be in this American cookbook. "It's classic Indiana! You have to make a breaded pork loin sandwich." Many of our most fervent fans agreed. After making this—a flattened piece of tender pork, dunked in flour, eggs, and breadcrumbs, and then fried until crispy—we certainly agreed.

2 pounds boneless pork loin

2 cups low-fat buttermilk

2 cloves garlic, peeled and crushed

2 teaspoons onion powder

Kosher salt and freshly ground black pepper

280 grams All-Purpose Gluten-Free Flour Blend (page 17)

2 cups finely ground gluten-free breadcrumbs

Fat or oil of your choice for frying (we like rice bran oil, peanut oil, or lard)

4 Hamburger Buns (page 55) or Hoagie Rolls (page 60)

Feel like playing?

You can easily make this with the Grain-Free Flour Mix (page 19), if you wish. If you have to be dairy-free, add the juice of 1 lemon to your favorite dairy-free milk to make "buttermilk" for the marinade.

Pound the pork. Cut the pork into 4 pieces. Cut each piece horizontally across, stopping before you cut through entirely, then open the piece. It should look like a butterfly. Put each piece between 2 pieces of plastic wrap and pound the pork with a meat mallet until it is only 1⁄4 inch thick.

Marinate the pork. In a large bowl, whisk the buttermilk, garlic, and onion powder together. Nestle the pounded-out pork pieces in the buttermilk mixture. Let it marinate in the refrigerator overnight.

Dredge the pork. The next day, remove the pork from the buttermilk and wipe off each piece. Season each piece with salt and pepper. Put the flour in a wide bowl, set the buttermilk mixture next to it, and set the breadcrumbs in a third bowl next to that. Dredge a pork piece on both sides in the flour, then into the buttermilk mixture again, and then dredge it on both sides in the breadcrumbs. Lay the pork piece on a plate while you finish the rest of the pork.

Fry the pork. Set a large wok or Dutch oven over medium-high heat. Pour in 1 inch of the oil or fat you chose for frying. When it has come to 360°F on an instant-read thermometer, gently place 2 of the pieces of pork in the hot fat. Fry on one side for 3 minutes, then flip the piece. Cook until the pork loin is golden brown and crisp, about another 3 minutes. Remove from the oil and drain on a paper towel–lined plate. Repeat with the remaining pork.

Make the sandwiches. Open the hamburger buns or hoagie rolls and put the fried loin inside. Top and slather with your choice of ingredients and condiments: we like homemade mayonnaise, dill pickles, tomatoes, and arugula. That choice is up to you.

GRILLED PIMIENTO CHEESE SANDWICHES

Feeds 4

When I first heard Southern friends talking about pimiento cheese in holy terms, I was confused. Did they mean that processed cheese spread with flecks of red peppers in the glass jar that my mother bought for parties in the 1970s? No, they did not. Our Southern friends and readers who requested this sandwich in droves longed for real pimiento cheese, an intoxicating spread of mayonnaise, cheddar cheese, and pimientos. Here's the only problem: no one agrees on the right way to make it. Some folks like orange cheese and others like white. Some like grated onion and some want nothing to do with that. (I'm in that camp.) In the South, there's a big fight over the bottled mayonnaise: Hellmann's! No, Duke's! Being new to this, we felt free to play here. We use homemade mayonnaise made of olive oil, extra sharp and sharp Cheddar cheeses, pimientos, and a tiny touch of our secret ingredient: fish sauce. Before you start yelling bloody hell at us, know that it adds an incredible savory taste without any fish taste. Promise. Take this stuff and make grilled cheese out of it? Oh man. I finally understand the fuss.

FOR THE PIMIENTO CHEESE

1 cup mayonnaise (homemade mayo tastes the best but the stuff in a jar works too)

4 ounces pimiento, drained of liquid

½ teaspoon fish sauce (make sure it's gluten-free)

Tiny pinch cayenne pepper

8 ounces (2 cups) freshly grated extra-sharp Cheddar cheese

8 ounces (2 cups) freshly grated sharp Cheddar cheese

FOR THE SANDWICHES

8 slices gluten-free Sandwich Bread (page 53)

2 tablespoons unsalted butter, softened

Make the pimiento cheese. Place the mayonnaise, pimiento, fish sauce, and cayenne pepper in a large bowl. Stir them together well. Stir in the extra-sharp Cheddar cheese and sharp Cheddar cheese. Refrigerate overnight.

Make the sandwiches. Set a large cast-iron skillet over medium heat. Slather one side of all the slices of bread with the softened butter. Put 4 slices into the hot pan, buttered side down. Dollop a generous scoop of the pimiento, cheese onto the bread slices in the skillet and top with the remaining 4 slices. Cook until the bottom slice is browned, about 4 minutes. Flip the sandwiches and cook until the bottom is browned and the pimiento cheese is melty. Cut the sandwiches in half and serve.

Feel like playing?

I will say that this is a great filling for deviled eggs. It's good on crackers, on toast in the morning when you don't want something sweet, and as a decadent base for the cheese sauce for macaroni and cheese.

CRAB MELTS

Feeds 4

When I lived in New York City, my favorite late-night meal with friends at a diner was pretty simple: a tuna melt with a chocolate shake. Eating that after 1 a.m. felt like decadence. Now I realize that the real decadence is eating a crab melt on bread that doesn't make me sick, with good Cheddar cheese instead of that nasty processed cheese product the diners used. This one's better.

8 ounces fresh lump crabmeat, shells entirely removed

2 stalks celery, finely chopped

½ small red onion, peeled and finely chopped

¼ cup mayonnaise (homemade mayo tastes the best but the stuff in a jar works too)

2 tablespoons chopped fresh tarragon

1 tablespoon chopped fresh chives

1 tablespoon freshly squeezed lemon juice

Kosher salt and freshly ground black pepper

4 slices gluten-free Sandwich Bread (page 53) or Hoagie Rolls (page 60)

4 slices Cheddar cheese

Prepare to melt. Preheat the broiler.

Make the crab salad. In a bowl, mix together the crab, celery, red onion, mayonnaise, tarragon, chives, and lemon juice. Season with salt and pepper.

Toast the bread. (Remember to use a dedicated gluten-free toaster if you are feeding a celiac.)

Make the crab melts. Pile each slice of toast with crab salad, then top with the cheese. Gently push down the cheese a bit. Put the open-face sandwiches under the broiler and watch the cheese melt over the crab.

Pull those sandwiches out and eat.

Feel like playing?

You can substitute high-quality tuna or chicken for the crab. Most restaurants use American cheese for a crab melt. Danny and I can't stomach the stuff, but it does melt easily. Go ahead, if you must. Also, if you can't eat dairy, skip the cheese and eat this as a cold sandwich.

CHEESESTEAKS

Feeds 4

Legend has it that the Philly cheesesteak was invented by a hot dog vendor in the 1930s who was making himself some lunch. He put some beef from his butcher on the grill to use in one of his hot dog buns. The smell was so great that a cab driver pulled up and asked the owner to make him one. Word spread, and soon the hot dog vendor opened up a lunch place and the rest is history. I don't know how much of that is true, but I do know that folks from Philadelphia are very passionate about their cheesesteaks. I've been told by some folks that there will never be a proper Philly cheesesteak made outside that city. If that's true, then just make this darned fine sandwich and call it whatever you want.

2 pounds top round steak

4 tablespoons extra-virgin olive oil

2 large red bell peppers, thinly sliced

1 large yellow onion, peeled and thinly sliced

Kosher salt and freshly ground black pepper

4 gluten-free Baguettes (page 52), sliced open

8 slices provolone cheese

Prepare the steak. Roll the steak into a tight log. Truss it with kitchen string to keep it tight. Put it in the freezer until the meat is firm to the touch but not quite frozen, about 45 minutes. Slice the meat as thinly as possible, moving quickly, shaving it if you can. Put the slices of meat in the refrigerator.

Prepare to cook. Preheat the broiler.

Cook the peppers and onions. Set a large cast-iron skillet over medium-high heat. Pour in 2 tablespoons of the olive oil. Add the peppers and onions to the hot oil. Cook, stirring frequently, until the onions are soft and translucent and the peppers are browning, about 7 minutes. Transfer the vegetables to a plate.

Cook the meat. Season the meat with salt and pepper. Add the remaining 2 tablespoons of olive oil to the skillet. When the oil is hot, fill the skillet with slices of meat. Cook for 30 seconds, then flip the slices and cook for another 30 seconds. Put the cooked meat onto a plate and cook the rest of the meat this way.

Assemble the sandwiches. Put the bottoms of the baguettes on a parchment-lined baking sheet. Pile the meat on the baguettes. Top with the cooked peppers and onions. Lay 2 slices of cheese on top of each baguette. Put the sandwiches under the broiler until the cheese is melted and oozy. Top with the remaining baguette slices and eat immediately.

Feel like playing?

Some folks love sautéed mushrooms on their cheesesteaks. Some like ketchup. Others insist on marinara sauce. You can't go wrong any way here.

PULLED PORK SANDWICHES

Feeds 4

One of the best meals I've ever eaten was at Franklin Barbecue, in Austin, Texas. Formerly housed in a food truck, Franklin makes better barbecue than I had ever eaten before. We stood in line for several hours, in 100°F heat, cooled only by the occasional glass of sweet tea. The wait was worth it. The look of those ribs, sausages, brisket, and pulled pork, cooked low and slow, made everyone around the table stand on our chairs to take photographs of the meal. (We were all food writers. We're weird.) Watching the astonished faces of the people around us—all saying one thing: get off your damn chairs and eat, you fools—made us sit down and start eating. And oh, the eating. That was some damned fine barbecue.

Tell truth, barbecue that good without a pit and a pit master seemed beyond us. When we started doing research for this book, we found a British writer who had become obsessed with pulled pork and asked every barbecue expert she could find how to make it at home. Her basic rub you see here and the technique for roasting at high heat, then low and slow, then another 10 minutes of high heat, was so good that we started making our pulled pork this way. (Funny that we learned how to make pulled pork from a Brit.) And then Danny made a barbecue sauce we love. Add patience to all of that and you might not have the pulled pork from Franklin Barbecue, but you'll have some incredible homemade pulled pork.

FOR THE MEAT

3½ pounds Boston butt pork shoulder

2 tablespoons kosher salt

2 tablespoons packed dark brown sugar

1 tablespoon smoked paprika

FOR THE BARBECUE SAUCE

1 cup ketchup

1 cup rice wine vinegar

1 cup gluten-free oyster sauce

¼ cup sliced scallions

3 cloves garlic, peeled and smashed

1 small nub fresh ginger, peeled and chopped

½ cup chopped fresh cilantro

FOR THE SANDWICH

4 gluten-free Hamburger Buns (page 55)

CONTINUED

Prepare the meat. Pull the pork out of the refrigerator and let it come to room temperature. Preheat the oven to 425°F.

Make the rub. In a bowl, combine the salt, brown sugar, and smoked paprika. Rub half the mixture all over the meat.

Roast the meat. Put the pork into a large baking pan and put it in the oven. Roast until browned, about 40 minutes. Turn down the heat to 250°F and pull the meat out of the oven. Make a loose tent of aluminum foil over the pork shoulder. Put the meat back in the oven and roast until the meat is soft enough to pull apart with a spoon and has reached an internal temperature of 190°F, about 7 hours. Pour off the juices and set them aside.

Turn the heat back up to 425°F. Take the foil tent off the pork shoulder and roast uncovered for 10 minutes. Take the pork out of the oven and cover it with the foil again to rest for at least 30 minutes.

Let the pork rest. Pull apart the pork with two forks. This should be easy. Spread the meat out over a baking sheet. Sprinkle the rest of the seasoning rub over it, and any leftover juices from roasting, and stir them both into the meat. Set the baking sheet in the refrigerator and let it rest for 24 hours to soak up those flavors.

Make the barbecue sauce. Set a large pot over medium-high heat. Put the ketchup, rice wine vinegar, oyster sauce, scallions, garlic, and ginger into the pot. Bring the liquids to a boil, then turn down the heat to low and let the sauce simmer for 30 minutes, stirring occasionally. Add the cilantro and continue simmering for another 10 minutes, stirring occasionally. Strain the sauce. Let it also sit overnight, for best flavors.

Heat up the sauce and pork. Set a large pot over medium heat. Pour in the barbecue sauce. Bring the sauce to a simmer, then stir the meat into the sauce. When the meat is entirely heated, pile it onto the bottom half of the hamburger buns. Spoon any remaining sauce over the pork. Top with the other half of the hamburger buns and eat.

Feel like playing?

You can easily use a bottled barbecue sauce instead of making your own. But this one is so easy that it would be a shame to do that. Plus, this is great sauce for any barbecue you want to make: brisket, sausages, chicken, or even meaty white fish. Have fun with it.

LOBSTER ROLLS

Feeds 4

When Danny and I drove through New England in a minivan with our daughter, we both gawked at nearly everything in Maine. Craggy coastline, gorgeous green fields, good people, and a real back-to-the-land ethic that stirred us both. On top of that, in every gas station? Whoopie pies (page 282) and lobster rolls. At first, I thought Danny was a little crazy to get a lobster roll from a gas station. Isn't that the path to food poisoning? But in Maine, fresh lobster, good lobster, is everywhere. Many Mainers told us that lobster is no big deal. It's working man food, easily available and cheap. Of course, for the rest of us, lobster is a real treat. And that gas station lobster roll was great, Danny told me. So we came home and made our own version with a gluten-free hoagie roll. We both felt the same: we wanted the taste of the lobster to shine through the salad. Some people put chopped celery in their lobster roll, and you're free to add it here. But this lobster roll? It's as pure as the water off the coast of Maine.

1 pound cooked lobster meat

¾ cup mayonnaise (homemade mayo tastes the best but the stuff in a jar works too)

Freshly squeezed juice of ½ lemon

1 tablespoon chopped fresh tarragon

1 tablespoon chopped fresh Italian parsley

Kosher salt and freshly ground black pepper

4 gluten-free Hoagie Rolls (page 60)

Make the lobster salad. You want big chunks of meat, so you should barely touch the meat from the claws. Tail meat can come as one big piece, so cut that up a bit. In a bowl, combine the lobster meat with the mayonnaise, lemon juice, tarragon, and parsley. Season the salad with salt and pepper.

Make the sandwiches. Stuff the lobster salad into the hoagie rolls. And go ahead and really stuff. This is not a streamlined sandwich. It's messy and glorious and full of lobster. Eat immediately.

Feel like playing?

Lobster rolls seem to inspire quite a bit of heated feelings about how they should be made, including the buns in which the salad should sit. New Englanders (but particularly the ones who don't live there anymore, it seems) insist that only split-top New England hot dog buns are correct. We bought a special hot dog pan to make those buns, gluten-free, and the buns were good. But the pan made such small buns that we felt a little cheated. So we put these on hoagie rolls instead. You're welcome to use the hot dog buns on page 56, or you can eat your lobster on any bun you want!

KENTUCKY HOT BROWNS

Feeds 4

At the Brown Hotel in Louisville, Kentucky, the dining room makes nearly 1,200 of these sandwiches in the three days surrounding the Kentucky Derby. 1,200! Invented at the Brown Hotel in the 1920s as another savory dish for the late-night room service menu, this much-loved sandwich has endured well into the twenty-first century. Unlike the other sandwiches in this chapter, the Kentucky Hot Brown is too messy to eat with hands. You'll need a knife and fork with this one. This is also a great way to use all that leftover turkey after Thanksgiving.

One 2-pound turkey breast

2 tablespoons extra-virgin olive oil

Kosher salt and freshly ground black pepper

4 thick slices gluten-free Sandwich Bread (page 53) (make the slices about 1½ inches thick)

3 tablespoons unsalted butter

27 grams All-Purpose Gluten-Free Flour Blend (page 17)

2 cups whole milk (you can use dairy-free milk, if it's unsweetened)

4 ounces (1 cup) freshly grated Gruyère cheese

4 ounces (1 cup) freshly grated Pecorino Romano cheese

Pinch freshly grated nutmeg

2 large ripe tomatoes, thickly sliced

4 slices cooked bacon

½ cup chopped fresh Italian parsley

1 teaspoon Hungarian paprika

Prepare to cook. Preheat the oven to 325°F.

Roast the turkey. Drizzle the turkey with the olive oil, then season it with salt and pepper. Put the turkey breast into a large cast-iron skillet. Roast the turkey breast until it reaches an internal temperature of 155°F, about 1½ hours. Let the turkey rest until it is cool enough to handle.

Toast the bread. Since the slices of bread need to be thick to stand up to the sandwich, toast them in the oven at 400°F until they are brown on the top, about 3 minutes. Flip them over and toast the other side. Take them out of the oven and cut them diagonally, to make triangles.

Make the Mornay sauce. Set a Dutch oven over medium heat. Add the butter. When the butter has melted, add the flour and whisk them together continuously for 2 to 3 minutes. When a warm cooked-flour scent is released, add the milk to the pot, ½ cup at a time, stirring constantly. Whisk out any lumps and keep stirring, about 5 minutes. When the sauce starts to thicken, add the Gruyère and ½ cup of the Pecorino Romano. Stir until the cheeses are entirely melted. Season the sauce with the nutmeg and salt and pepper.

Assemble the sandwiches. Put all the triangles of the toasted bread on a parchment-lined baking sheet. Slice the cooked turkey into thick slices (about 1 inch thick). Lay turkey slices on top of each triangle, then tomato slices, then pour a ladleful of the Mornay sauce over each slice. Put the baking sheet under the broiler until the sauce melts over the turkey.

Pull the sandwiches out of the oven. Top with the cooked bacon slices, a few pinches of the fresh parsley, the remaining ½ cup of Pecorino Romano, and the paprika. Serve immediately.

Feel like playing?

You can easily omit the bacon on the top, if you want. This dish is rich enough! And you could use any cheese you want to make this sauce, although Parmesan might be too acidic for the final dish. The Mornay sauce here makes a great cheese sauce for pasta or macaroni and cheese.

CUBAN PORK SANDWICH

Feeds 8

This is a much-loved sandwich in Florida and beyond. Slow-roasted pork with Cuban spices, pickled jalapeños, pan-roasted onions, and garlicky aioli, all spilling out of a long, crisp roll. This is joy. There are a thousand variations in flavors and technique but this one works for us.

FOR THE PORK

1 tablespoon ground cumin

1 teaspoon ground allspice

6 cloves garlic, peeled and minced

Freshly grated zest and freshly squeezed juice of 3 oranges

Freshly grated zest and freshly squeezed juice of 2 limes

3 pounds pork shoulder

FOR THE PICKLED JALAPEÑOS

1 cup apple cider vinegar

1 tablespoon organic cane sugar

Good pinch kosher salt

8 ounces jalapeños, seeds removed and thinly sliced

FOR THE GARLIC AIOLI

1 large egg, at room temperature

3 cloves garlic, peeled and minced

Freshly squeezed juice of 1 lemon

½ teaspoon kosher salt

Pinch freshly ground black pepper

½ cup extra-virgin olive oil

FOR THE REST OF THE SANDWICH

4 tablespoons olive oil

2 large yellow onions, peeled and thinly sliced

4 gluten-free Baguettes (page 52), sliced in half horizontally and then lengthwise

8 romaine lettuce leaves

Toast the spices. Set a small skillet over medium-high heat. Add the cumin and allspice. Heat, stirring frequently, until they release their scents, about 2 minutes.

Make the marinade. Combine the toasted spices, garlic, and orange and lime zest and juice in a large bowl.

Marinate the pork. Put the pork shoulder into a large plastic bag or bowl. Pour the marinade over the pork. Refrigerate overnight.

Pickle the jalapeños. Set a small pot over high heat. Pour in the vinegar, sugar, and salt. Whisk until the liquids just come to a boil and the sugar is fully dissolved. Pour the hot liquid over the jalapeños in a large bowl. Refrigerate overnight.

Make the aioli. Add the egg, garlic, lemon juice, salt, and pepper to a strong blender. Blend until everything is well combined. With the blender running, drizzle in the olive oil, very slowly (more slowly than you would imagine), until the olive oil is gone and there is mayonnaise in the blender. Refrigerate overnight.

Prepare to cook. The next day, preheat the oven to 425°F. Take the pork shoulder out of the refrigerator. Pat the roast dry with a paper towel.

Sear the pork shoulder. Set a large skillet over medium-high heat. Pour in 2 tablespoons of the olive oil. When the oil is hot, put the pork shoulder in the skillet. Sear until the bottom of the roast is browned, 3 to 4 minutes. Turn the shoulder and sear until all sides are browned. Turn off the heat and move the pork shoulder to another cast-iron skillet.

Roast the pork shoulder. Put the pork shoulder in the oven and roast until the pork has reached an internal temperature of 150°F, about 1½ hours. Take the pork out of the oven and let it rest. Tear at the pork roast with two forks, shredding up the meat.

Pan roast the onions. Meanwhile, as the pork roasts, set the skillet with the browned bits in it back over medium-high heat. Pour in the remaining 2 tablespoons of olive oil. When the oil is hot, scrape up all the browned bits from the bottom of the skillet and add the onion slices. Cook, stirring frequently, until the onions are browned and softened, about 15 minutes. Set them aside.

Make the sandwiches. Grab 2 baguette pieces. Slather each of them with the garlic aioli, then on one baguette side pile the pork, the pickled jalapeños, and the pan-roasted onions. Top with a romaine lettuce leaf and put the other side of the baguette on top. Repeat with the remaining baguette pieces.

Eat immediately. Don't worry if it all slides and slathers on you. That's half the fun.

Feel like playing?

If you don't want to bake four baguettes, or you want to skip the bread entirely, make this as a salad over white rice or lots of crisp green lettuce. Once you have the hang of making aioli yourself, instead of buying it in a jar, you're likely to be hooked. And guess what! If you take out the garlic, you have a great homemade mayonnaise.

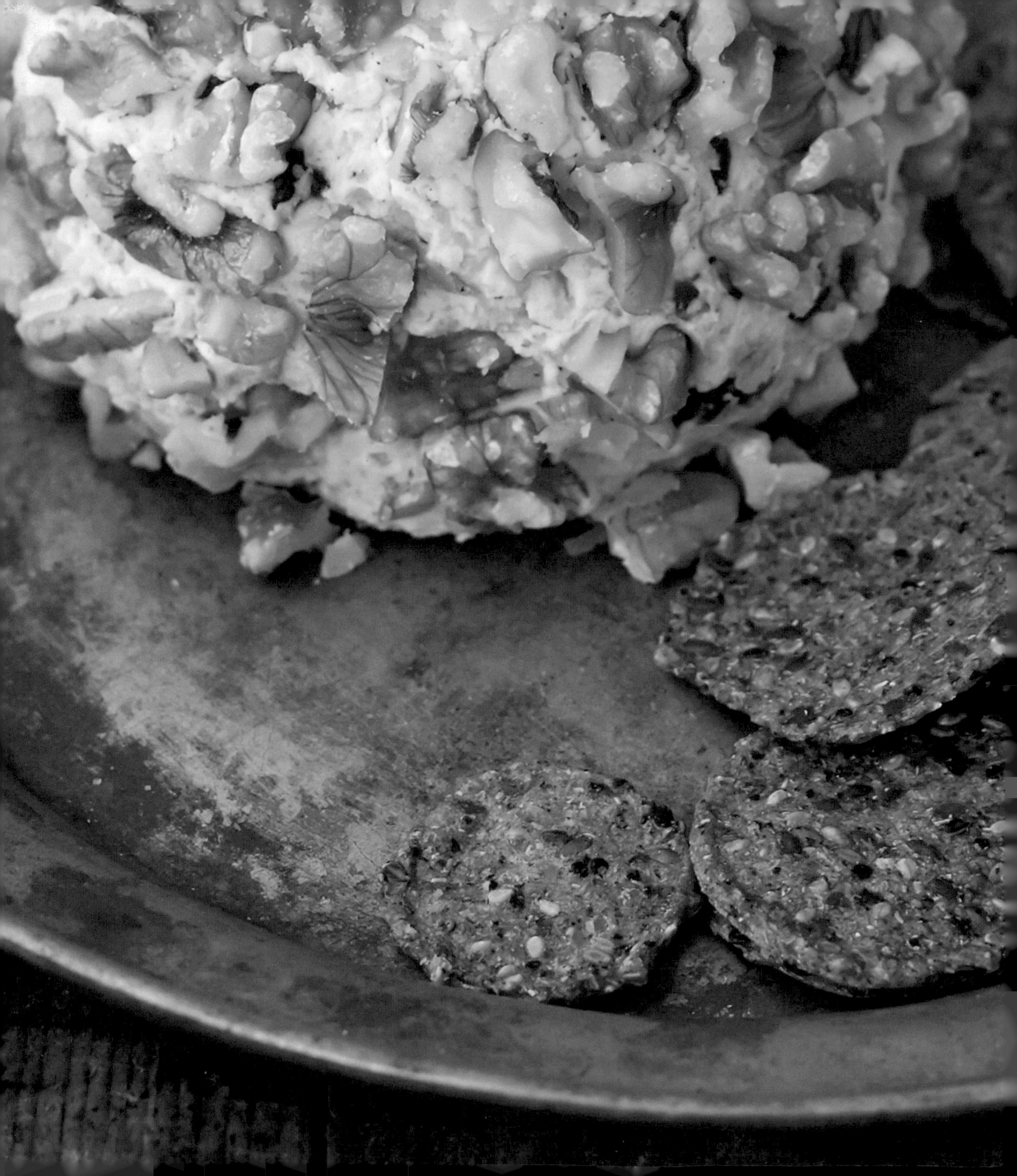

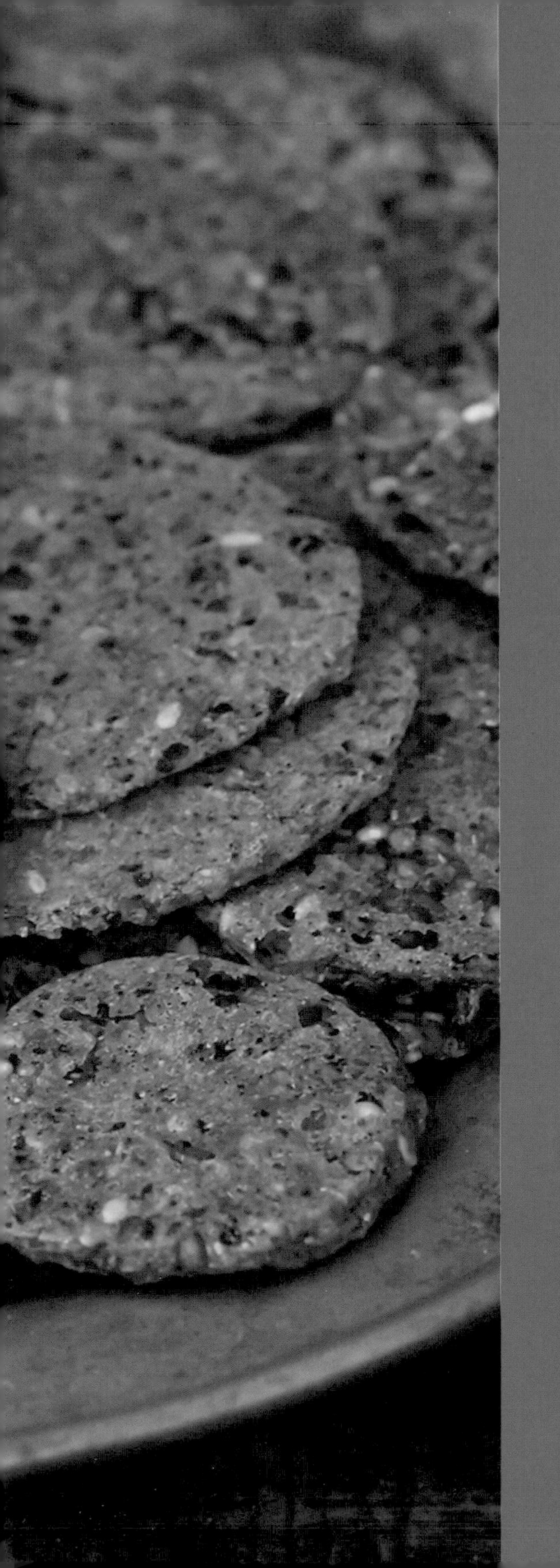

APPETIZERS AND SNACKS

BAKED ARTICHOKE DIP

Feeds 6

I have been to parties where everyone in the home seems to be gathered around the hot artichoke dip. There's something enticing about this combination of good cheeses, artichoke hearts, and warmth. We jazzed up ours by adding some heat with red pepper flakes, and more warmth with nutmeg and bay leaf, and making it safe for everyone who has to avoid gluten by building it with a gluten-free roux.

6 cups whole milk

1 bay leaf

⅛ teaspoon freshly grated nutmeg

6 tablespoons unsalted butter, softened

35 grams All-Purpose Gluten-Free Flour Blend (page 17)

3 ounces (¾ cup) freshly grated Asiago cheese

3 ounces (¾ cup) freshly grated Gruyère cheese

1 medium yellow onion, peeled and chopped

2 cloves garlic, peeled and chopped

3 pounds frozen artichoke hearts, thawed, sliced, and dried

2 tablespoons finely chopped fresh Italian parsley

2 teaspoons finely chopped fresh thyme

½ teaspoon red pepper flakes

Freshly grated zest of 1 lemon

Kosher salt and freshly ground black pepper

2 ounces (½ cup) freshly grated Parmesan cheese

Simmer the milk. Set a small pot over medium heat. Pour in the milk, bay leaf, and nutmeg. Bring the milk to a low boil, stirring to make sure it doesn't burn, then turn down the heat to low. Simmer for 10 minutes, then turn off the heat and let the milk sit on the back of the stove for 30 minutes. Strain the milk through a fine-mesh sieve into a bowl, then transfer the milk back to the pot. Turn on the heat to low again and return the milk to a very gentle simmer. Stir it occasionally while you make the roux.

Make the roux. Set a deep skillet over medium-high heat. Add 4 tablespoons of the butter to the skillet and melt it. Add the flour to the butter and stir them together until the flour has started to brown and cook. Slowly, add ½ cup of the simmering milk to the butter and flour, whisking quickly to incorporate the milk fully. Repeat until all the milk has been added. If the milk is not thick, continue cooking until it has reduced, stirring constantly to avoid burning. Add the Asiago and Gruyère to the skillet. When they are fully melted into the sauce, turn off the heat and let the cheese sauce sit while you prepare the artichokes.

Cook the artichokes. Set a large skillet over medium-high heat. Add the remaining 2 tablespoons of butter to the skillet. Add the onions and garlic and cook, stirring occasionally, until the onions are soft and translucent, about 7 minutes. Add the artichoke heart pieces and cook, stirring occasionally, until they are hot, about 5 minutes. Add the parsley, thyme, and red pepper flakes and cook until the scent is released, about 1 minute. Add the lemon zest, turn off the heat, and season with salt and pepper.

CONTINUED

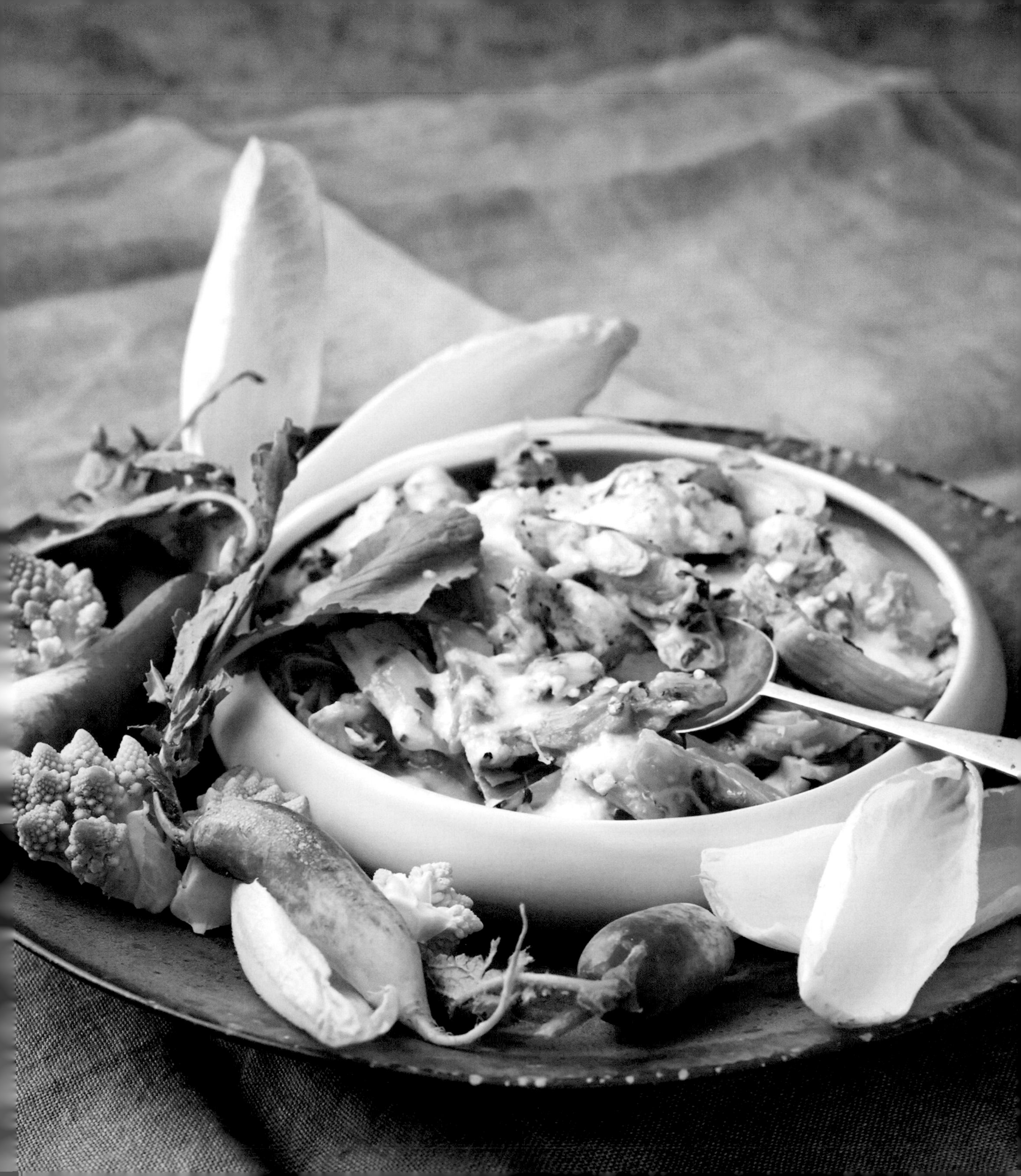

Prepare to bake. Preheat the oven to 400°F.

Bake the artichoke dip. Pour the artichoke mixture into a 9 x 13-inch baking dish. Pour the cheese sauce over it and stir to combine it all thoroughly. Sprinkle the Parmesan on top. Bake until the cheese is almost melted and bubbling golden brown, about 15 minutes.

Serve immediately with crackers, slices of crusty bread, or vegetables.

Feel like playing?

This is a dairy-heavy dish. There's no way around it, since that's the allure for repeated dipping: all that cheese. You could try a nondairy milk and nondairy cheese here. We haven't tried it, but I'm certain your dairy-free guests would like it.

ROSEMARY-THYME CRACKERS

Feeds 6

Over the past 10 or 15 years, interesting crackers started showing up at picnics and dinners around the country. No longer relegated to processed cracker circles out of a box, Americans have come to love rough-hewn shards of crackers, full of flavor and toppings like sesame seeds and olive oil. This cracker recipe, adapted from Gale Gand's Lunch!, *comes from Paul Kahan, executive chef at Blackbird and Avec in Chicago. They are a little fussy, since the recipe requires making a sponge, then a dough, both of which sit and rise for a couple of hours. But trust me—most of the work is in the waiting. Full of flavor, crisp at the edges with just a tiny bit of chew in the middle, these crackers are far more delicious than the flavor of boxed crackers could ever be.*

560 grams All-Purpose Gluten-Free Flour Blend (page 17)

1½ teaspoons active dry yeast

1 teaspoon honey

1¼ cups warm water

1 tablespoon kosher salt

1 tablespoon psyllium husks

2 teaspoons chopped fresh rosemary

1 teaspoon chopped fresh thyme

5 tablespoons extra-virgin olive oil

½ teaspoon freshly ground black pepper (optional)

Make the sponge. In a large bowl, whisk together 200 grams of the flour and the yeast. Add the honey and slowly pour the warm water into the bowl. Using a rubber spatula, gently mix it all together. Cover the bowl with plastic wrap and set it in a warm place. Let the sponge sit for 2 hours.

Make the dough. Put the remaining 360 grams of flour, the salt, psyllium husks, rosemary, and thyme into the bowl of a stand mixer with the paddle attachment. With the mixer running on low, drizzle in 4 tablespoons of the olive oil. Add the sponge and mix the dough until it is well combined. It should slump off the paddle a bit when the mixer stops running. Cover the bowl with plastic wrap and set it in a warm place to rise for at least 1 hour and no more than 2 hours.

Let the dough rise again. Gently, move the dough to a clean surface. It should be fairly kneadable at this point. Knead the dough a bit to work out any air bubbles. Form a smooth dough ball, put it in a bowl, and let the dough proof for another 2 hours.

Prepare to bake. Preheat the oven to 400°F.

Ready the dough. Cut the dough in half. Roll out one dough ball between two pieces of lightly greased parchment paper, rolling it out as thinly as possible into a long sheet of dough. (Make the sheet of dough as long as your baking sheet.) Peel off the top parchment,

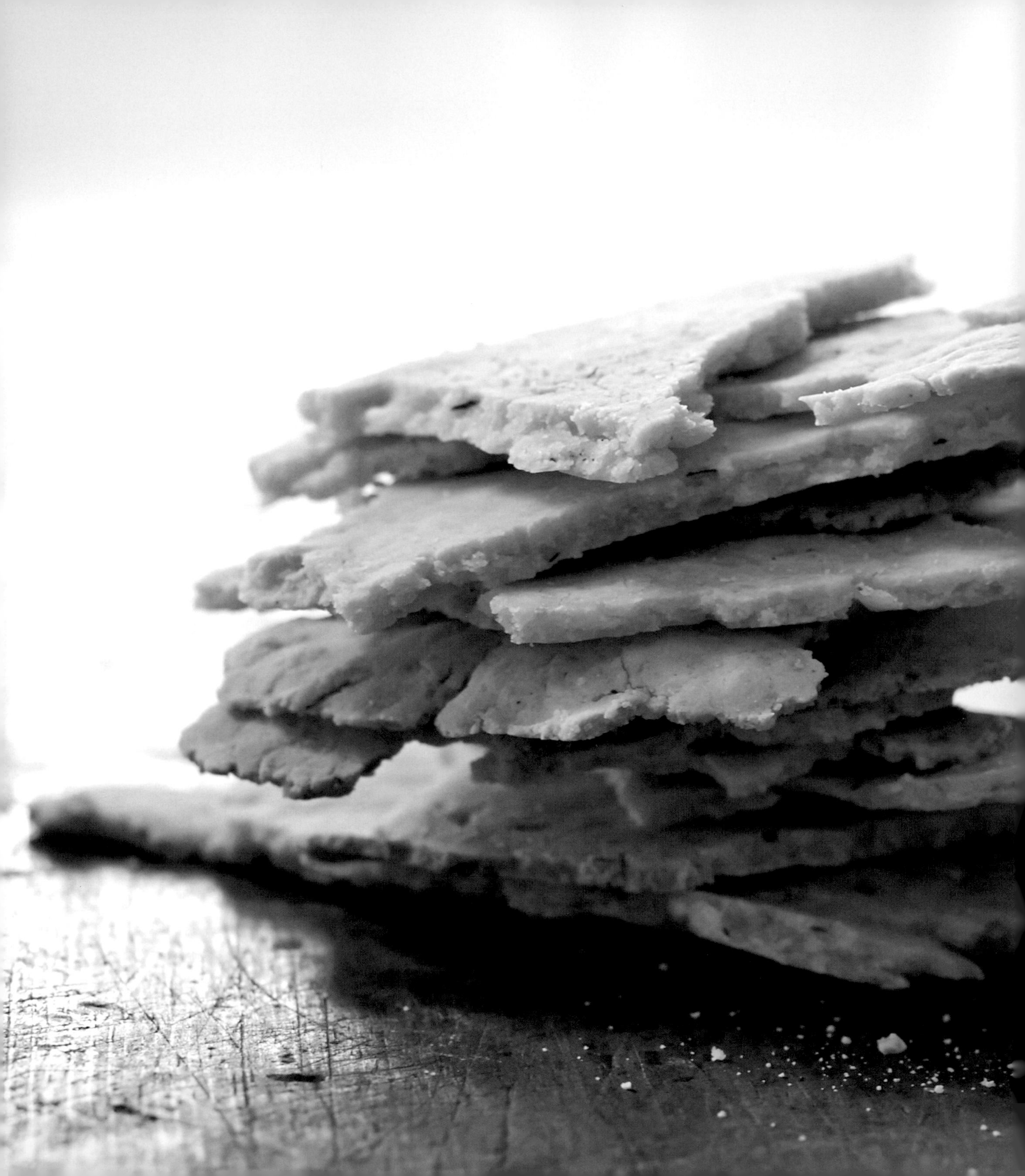

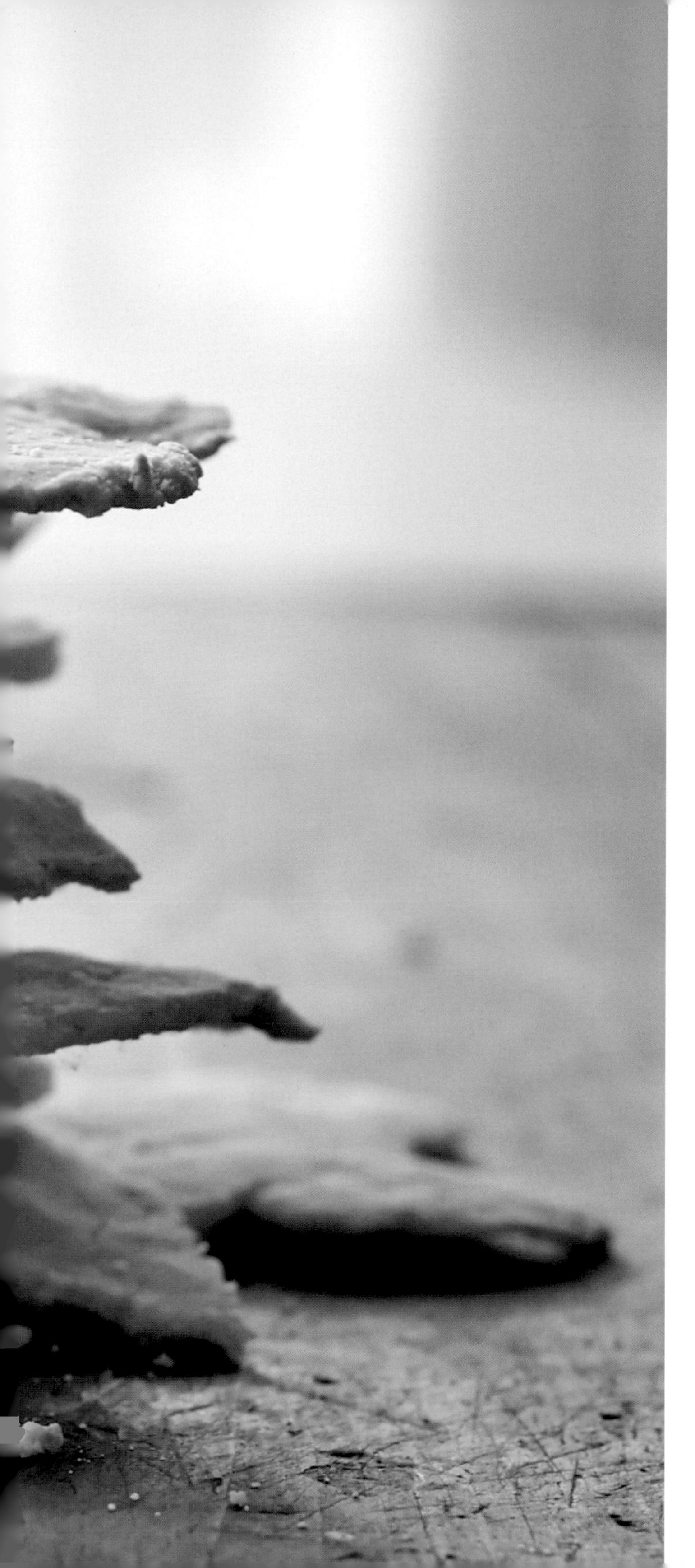

and move the bottom piece of parchment paper with the sheet of dough to the baking sheet. Repeat with the remaining dough ball, carefully moving the sheet of dough onto the baking sheet. Poke both sheets of dough with a fork over the entire sheet. Sprinkle the remaining 1 tablespoon of olive oil over the dough, and sprinkle with a bit of salt and the pepper, if you wish. Bake until the crackers are golden brown, 20 to 25 minutes. Allow the crackers to cool on the pan, then break them into rough shards about 3 inches long.

Feel like playing?

Would you like a grain-free cracker? This recipe works really well with the Grain-Free Flour Mix (page 19). Use the same weight of either of those flours in this recipe. Feel free to change the herbs freely here. Tarragon would work well. So would oregano. Try topping them with fennel seeds or sesame seeds too. Play.

PIGS IN A BLANKET

Feeds 6

Did you grow up on pigs in a blanket the way Danny and I did? This was party food. Our moms bought crescent rolls in a can, wrapped that packaged dough around cocktail weenies, and baked them. As kids, we thought these were fantastic, and we know we weren't the only ones. How do we make them gluten-free? Homemade pizza dough works great. Instead of cutting the dough into little triangles to make them into crescent roll shapes, we save time by simply wrapping a piece of the dough around each wiener and baking. If you make an extra ball of pie dough when you are making pie, you'll have a quick appetizer when friends are coming over. And our daughter loves pigs in a blanket now too.

1 disk chilled Pizza Dough (page 57)

1 package cocktail wieners (make sure they are gluten-free)

1 large egg, beaten

Prepare to bake. Preheat the oven to 400°F. Line a baking sheet with parchment paper.

Prepare the dough. Divide the dough into 16 pieces. Roll out each one to about a 1-inch length. Wrap each piece of dough around 1 wiener, sealing the ends. Brush each pig in a blanket with some of the beaten egg. Put each one on the baking sheet, spacing them out evenly. Put the baking sheet in the freezer for 15 minutes.

Bake the pigs in a blanket. Bake the pigs in a blanket until the dough is golden brown, about 10 minutes. Serve immediately.

Feel like playing?

If you want to be more meticulous and make these look like crescent rolls, roll out the dough and cut it into 4 rectangles. Cut into triangles 2 inches wide by 6 inches long.

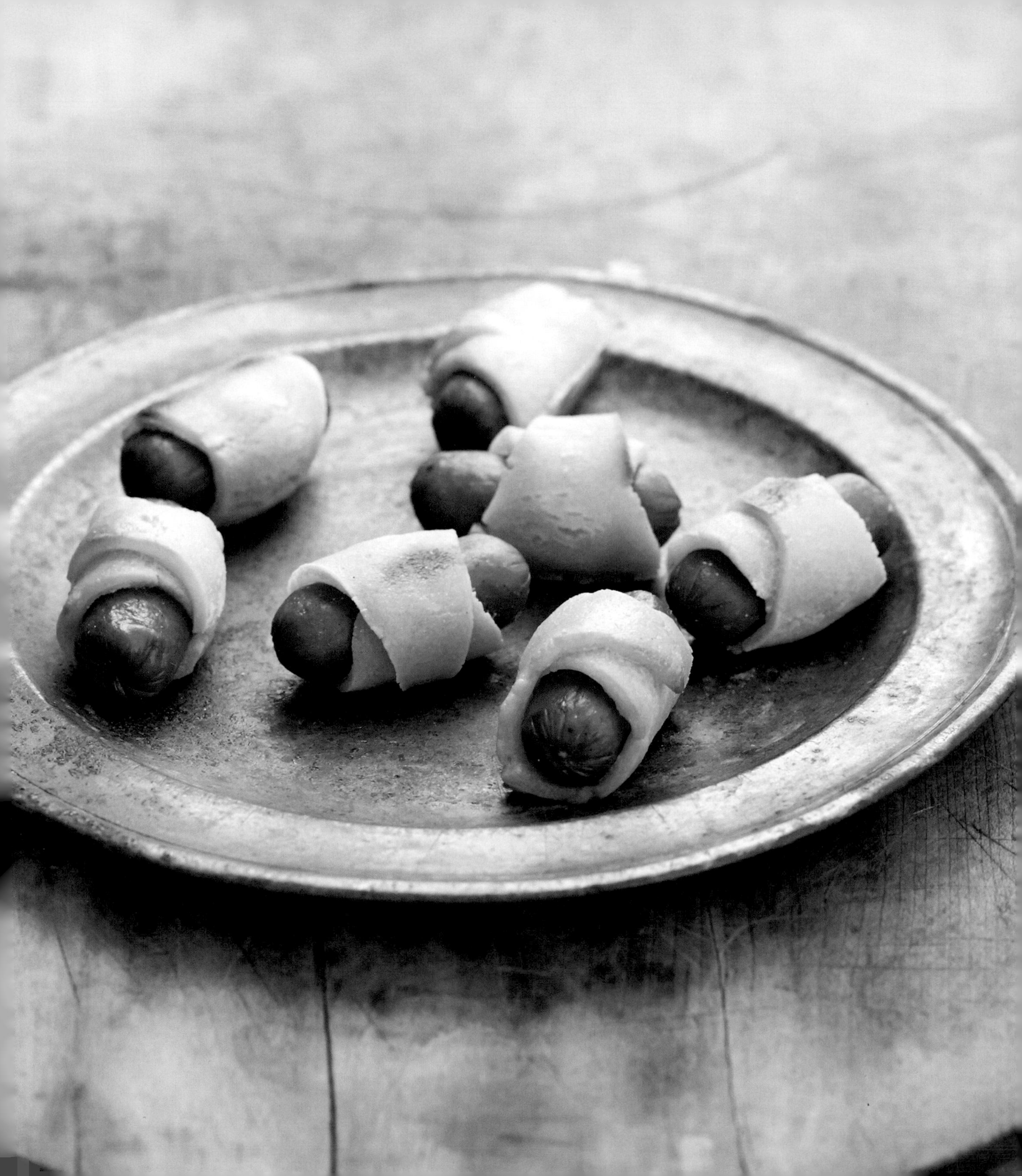

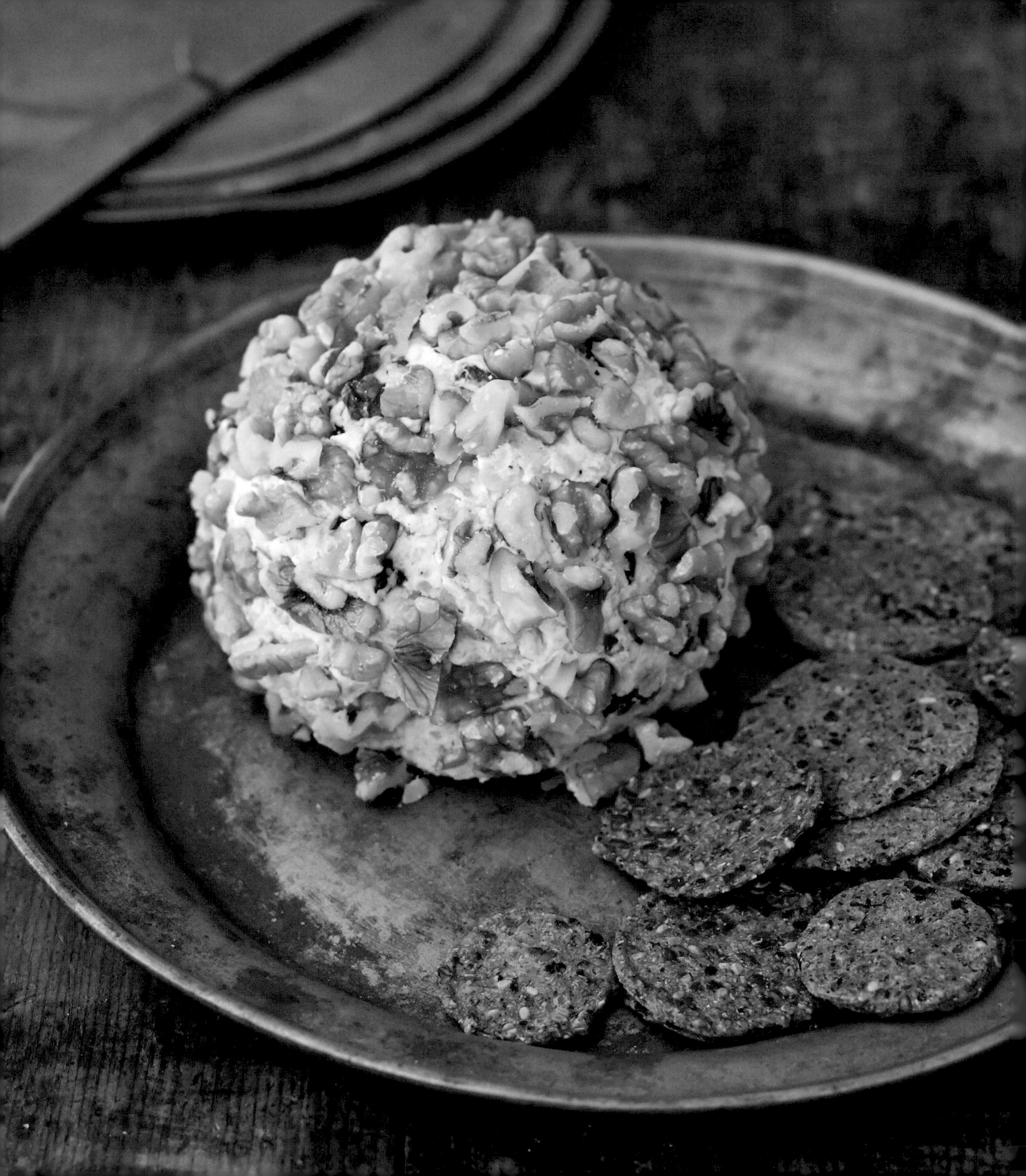

CRANBERRY-CHUTNEY CHEESE BALL

Feeds 6

My parents used to buy a cheese ball studded with nuts on the outside for nearly every party they held. I had no idea then that it was something we could make ourselves. I might not have to tell you this, but this homemade version is far better than the one from the store. (Thanks to Michelle Buffardi, for her book Great Balls of Cheese, *which was the inspiration for this recipe.)*

8 ounces cream cheese

8 ounces (2 cups) freshly grated sharp Cheddar cheese

½ cup dried cranberries

2 tablespoons Major Grey chutney (make sure it's gluten-free)

2 teaspoons Dijon mustard

1 teaspoon freshly grated lemon zest

½ teaspoon kosher salt

Freshly ground black pepper

¾ cup (75 grams) chopped walnuts

Mix and form the cheese ball. In the bowl of a stand mixer with the paddle attachment, combine the cream cheese, Cheddar cheese, cranberries, chutney, mustard, and lemon zest. When they are thoroughly combined, taste the mixture. Season with the salt and pepper. Form the mixture into a ball, cover it in plastic wrap, and let it sit overnight in the refrigerator.

Finish the cheese ball. Before serving, take the cheese ball out of the refrigerator and unwrap it. Lay the chopped walnuts on a plate. Set the cheese ball in the center of the walnuts and carefully roll the cheese ball around until it is entirely coated with walnuts. Serve immediately.

Feel like playing?

Use this basic template to create any flavor of cheese ball you want. Substitute goat cheese for the Cheddar, dried cherries for the cranberries, more mustard for the chutney, and any nut you want for the coating.

TUNA POKE

Feeds 4

This deeply flavorful dish originates in Hawaii, where the tuna is so fresh that there's really no use in cooking it. If you're concerned about eating raw tuna, may we remind you of something? Sushi. You'll just wish you had more as soon as you are done eating this serving.

1 red onion, peeled and finely chopped

⅓ cup gluten-free tamari

3 scallions, finely chopped

2 large cloves garlic, peeled and minced

1 tablespoon chopped pickled ginger

1 teaspoon sesame oil

1 pound tuna, cut into ½-inch chunks

1 tablespoon black and white sesame seeds

Combine the ingredients. In a bowl, whisk together the red onion, tamari, scallions, garlic, ginger, and sesame oil. Pour this over the chopped tuna and mix to combine. Let the tuna sit for 30 minutes to marinate.

Serve. Sprinkle the sesame seeds over the top of the tuna and serve.

Feel like playing?

You could play with fish sauce, yuzu, fresh ginger, or white onions here. Consider this a template, and you can play to find your dish within it.

CORNISH PASTIES

Feeds 6

It's a given that much of American culture was adopted from the British. We use the same language (well, sort of), we share a similar legal system, and our country's founders were inspired by some of the great thinkers of Great Britain. However, far too few people in this country have come to love one of the best foods of the United Kingdom: the Cornish pasty. In the upper peninsula of Michigan, however, people know better. This lovely, crusty meat hand pie came to Michigan with folks who emigrated in the mid-nineteenth century. These have a tender dough and a filling of tiny dices of beef, vegetables, and herbs. These pocket pies are a wonderful afternoon snack for hungry children and adults, and not just the Anglophiles.

FOR THE PASTY DOUGH

525 grams All-Purpose Gluten-Free Flour Blend (page 17)

2½ teaspoons psyllium husks

1 teaspoon fine sea salt

5 tablespoons (70 grams) cold lard, cut into chunks (or beef suet)

8 tablespoons (115 grams) cold unsalted butter, cut into small pieces

FOR THE FILLING

2 pounds sirloin tip steak (or top blade, flatiron, or rib-eye if you're feeling rich), finely chopped

2 pounds sweet potatoes, peeled, quartered, and thinly sliced

1 small rutabaga, peeled and finely chopped

1 medium yellow onion, peeled and finely chopped

18 grams All-Purpose Gluten-Free Flour Blend (page 17)

1 teaspoon chopped fresh thyme

1 large egg, beaten

Make the dough. In a large bowl, whisk together the flour, psyllium husks, and salt. Drop the chunks of lard and butter onto the flour. Work the fat into the flour with your fingers, coating each piece and slowly making it smaller until the fat is the size of lima beans. Pour in a couple of tablespoons of cold water, slowly, working the dough, then pouring in 1 or 2 tablespoons more. You want the dough to be just moistened. The dough might look a little dry, but when you pinch some of it between your fingers, it should stick together. Do not overwet the dough. (If you make this in the food processor, quickly pulsing the flour and fat together, then adding water, you're more likely to get the dough's texture right.)

Dump the dough onto a clean surface. Gather all the dough together and form into a large rectangle. Cover with plastic wrap and refrigerate.

Make the filling. In a bowl, combine the beef, sweet potatoes, rutabaga, onion, flour, and thyme.

Fill the pasties. Take the dough out of the refrigerator and cut it into 6 pieces. Roll out each piece between two pieces of lightly greased parchment paper into an 8-inch circle. Put 1 cup of filling onto the side of the dough. Tap around all the edges of the dough with slightly wet fingertips. Lift the side of the pasty without the filling up, over the filling, and onto the other side. Crimp all the edges of the pasty to seal it like a turnover. (If it looks like the letter D, that's the traditional shape for a Cornish pasty. If you want to make it easier on yourself, lift the two sides of the pasty to seal on top.) Put the pasty on a parchment-lined baking sheet. Repeat with the remaining balls of dough and filling. Put the baking sheet in the freezer for 30 minutes.

Prepare to bake. Preheat the oven to 400°F.

Bake the pasties. Remove the pasties from the freezer. Brush each one with a bit of the egg. With a sharp little knife, make two slits in the top of each pasty. Bake for 30 minutes, then turn down the heat to 350°F and continue baking until the crust is golden brown and firm and the filling is piping-hot, about 30 more minutes. Cool the pasties on the baking sheet for 10 minutes, then transfer to a wire rack.

You can eat the pasties warm, right away, and you will want to do this. But they also freeze well and can be reheated for a hearty after-school snack.

Feel like playing?

The traditional filling for a Cornish pasty is beef, rutabaga (called a Swede in the UK), potatoes, and herbs. But you? Oh, you can do what you want here. Carrots, fennel, turnips—they'd all be great. You could easily make these vegetarian by bulking up on the vegetables. And you could add cheese. Once you have the technique down, you can make these your own.

QUESADILLAS WITH GLUTEN-FREE FLOUR TORTILLAS

Makes 12 tortillas and 6 quesadillas

Quesadillas are this nation's best quick snack food, in our opinion. Take two tortillas, fill with cheese of any kind and another filling, warm it on a skillet until the cheese is oozy, and a hungry kid is satisfied within 5 minutes. Of course, you can use corn tortillas for quesadillas, and we often do. But sometimes, the most satisfying quesadilla is a warm, homemade flour tortilla. Flour tortillas are most favored in northern Mexico, which may be why they are so loved in the United States. This is a simple recipe, worth the time to make. After you have made a few batches, you'll have the hang of homemade tortillas and you might never buy them from a store again.

280 grams All-Purpose Gluten-Free Flour Blend (page 17)

1½ teaspoons kosher salt

½ teaspoon baking powder

3 tablespoons lard (seek out lard from your butcher or farmers' markets)

About ½ cup warm water

Fillings, as desired

Combine the dry ingredients. In a large bowl, whisk together the flour, salt, and baking powder.

Make the tortilla dough. Drop small spoonfuls of the lard into the flour mixture. Rub the lard into the flour, which should yield a crumbly, sandy flour. Slowly, drizzle in the warm water, stirring the water into the dough with a rubber spatula as you go. The dough should come together roughly but not into a wet ball. If the dough feels too dry, add a bit more water. If it feels too wet, add more flour.

Dump the dough onto a clean surface. Gather the dough into your hands and work it until it comes together in a ball. Knead the dough back and forth five or six times, until the dough feels smooth. Cut it into 12 pieces. Put each piece on a baking sheet and cover them with a damp towel. Let the dough rest for 30 minutes.

Roll and cook the tortillas. Set a cast-iron skillet over medium-high heat. While the skillet is heating up, roll out one of the pieces of dough to about 6 inches in diameter. Use a bench scraper or rubber spatula to gently lift the tortilla in your hand and transfer it to the skillet. If there isn't a little sizzle, take the tortilla off the skillet and turn up the heat. When the bottom of the tortilla has brown charred spots, flip the tortilla. When the other side is cooked, transfer the warm tortilla to a basket lined with a kitchen towel.

CONTINUED

Close the towel over the tortilla and cook the rest of the tortillas in the same fashion.

Make the quesadillas. When all the tortillas are cooked, turn the heat down to medium-low. Put one tortilla on the skillet, spread about 2 tablespoons of filling on it, and top with another tortilla. Cook until the bottom is warmed and a little more charred, then flip the quesadilla and cook for another minute or so. Serve immediately.

Feel like playing?

Of course, you can make a quesadilla out of any filling you like. We like sharp white Cheddar cheese and tomatillo salsa. Or chèvre and pickled vegetables. Or Monterey Jack and avocado. Really, you can make this up any way you want!

ARTICHOKE CRAB CAKES

Makes 8 crab cakes

Danny grew up in Colorado and I grew up in southern California. We're from the left half of the country. And in this half of the country, and particularly in the Pacific Northwest, there is only one crab worth mentioning: Dungeness crab. Fresh crabmeat is a treat around here, something we splurge on for birthdays and particular celebrations. Danny's three favorite foods are crab, artichokes, and avocado, so on his birthday, I make him these crab cakes. They taste mostly of crab, uncluttered by other flavors but for artichokes and tarragon, which help the flavor of the crab sing.

6 ounces fresh Dungeness lump crabmeat

¾ cup gluten-free breadcrumbs

¼ cup mayonnaise (homemade mayo tastes the best but the stuff in a jar works too)

½ cup frozen artichoke hearts, thawed and finely chopped

1 large shallot, peeled and finely chopped

2 tablespoons chopped fresh tarragon

1 teaspoon freshly squeezed lemon juice

Dash Tabasco sauce

Kosher salt and freshly ground black pepper

1 large egg, beaten

Fat or oil of your choice for sautéing (we use olive oil)

1 large avocado, pitted, peeled, and chopped into small pieces

Prepare to bake. Preheat the oven to 425°F.

Make the crab cakes. Pick through the crabmeat carefully, removing any stray shells or cartilage. In a bowl, combine ¼ cup of the breadcrumbs and the mayonnaise. Add the crab to the bowl. Add the artichoke hearts, shallot, tarragon, lemon juice, and Tabasco and stir until well combined. Taste, then season with salt and pepper. The mixture will feel a little too loose to hold together in a ball, so add the egg and stir well to combine. Season again if you wish.

Cook the crab cakes. Make 2-ounce balls of the crab mixture, then pat each one into a thick round cake. Coat each crab cake with the remaining ½ cup of breadcrumbs on both sides.

Set a large cast-iron skillet over medium-high heat. Add 2 tablespoons of the fat of your choice. Put 4 of the crab cakes into the hot fat. When the bottoms of the cakes have browned, about 3 minutes, flip the crab cakes and put the skillet in the oven. Cook until the crab cakes are firm and browned, 5 to 7 minutes.

Repeat with the remaining crab cakes and serve immediately, topped with the chopped avocado.

Feel like playing?

The crab cakes made in Maryland seem to be made most often with Old Bay seasoning, mustard, and Worcestershire. Add those flavors here instead.

BROILED KUMAMOTO OYSTERS WITH GARLIC-BUTTER BREADCRUMBS

Feeds 4 to 6

Here in the Pacific Northwest, it's an embarrassment of riches when it comes to oysters. We've had the luck of visiting the oyster beds on the Olympic Peninsula of Washington, where Taylor Shellfish Farm grows Shigoku oysters (firm and large), Olympia oysters (tiny and smoky), Pacific oysters (super briny), and Kumamoto oysters, which have a clean, sweet taste. Originally from Japan, these oysters have come to be the favorites for many of us in the Pacific Northwest. (When our daughter first tasted these at two years old, she ate a dozen.) It's hard to improve upon a cold, fresh oyster that has been just shucked. But sometimes, we like to broil them with garlic-butter breadcrumbs and serve them to our friends immediately.

8 tablespoons unsalted butter

2 heaping tablespoons minced garlic

2 cups gluten-free breadcrumbs

12 Kumamoto oysters, shucked and on the half-shell

Prepare to make. Preheat the broiler.

Make the breadcrumbs. Set a large skillet over medium heat. Add the butter. When the butter has melted, add the garlic. Cook, stirring frequently, until the garlic scent is released, 1 minute. Add the breadcrumbs, toss to coat, and remove from the heat.

Broil the oysters. Top each oyster with about 1 tablespoon of the breadcrumb mixture. Arrange the oysters in an oven-safe pan. Put them under the broiler until the breadcrumbs brown, about 2 minutes. Serve immediately.

Feel like playing?

Feel free to add fresh herbs like thyme or rosemary to the breadcrumbs.

KNISHES

Makes 16 knishes

When I first moved to New York City, I was amazed by everything. (That's not atypical for the first year in New York City.) The smell of the streets, the faces of thousands of people coming toward me on the sidewalks, and the food. Oh, the food. Mostly, the food. When I first stepped foot into Zabar's, a gourmet grocery store on the Upper West Side of Manhattan, I wanted one of everything. But what amazed me most was the corner in the back of the store dedicated entirely to knishes. What the heck was a knish? This soft, savory pastry, filled with a variety of fillings such as mashed potatoes and caramelized onions, seemed to be first served in street carts on the Lower East Side in the late nineteenth century. This Jewish delicatessen staple is wonderful comfort food. The original—and still the best—knish is made with schmaltz, the chicken fat skimmed off the top of homemade chicken stock. Your butcher might be able to sell you schmaltz. It's worth seeking out as the fat for this delicacy. You could try butter or oil in place of the schmaltz, but that won't be an authentic knish. Then again, neither is a gluten-free knish. It's good, though.

300 grams All-Purpose Gluten-Free Flour Blend (page 17)

1½ teaspoons psyllium husks

1 teaspoon baking powder

1 teaspoon kosher salt

1 large egg, at room temperature

½ cup schmaltz (chicken fat)

1 teaspoon apple cider vinegar

½ cup warm water

3 tablespoons extra-virgin olive oil

2 tablespoons (29 grams) unsalted butter

3 large yellow onions, peeled and sliced in even-size slices

1 teaspoon sugar

½ teaspoon kosher salt

3 pounds russet potatoes (about 3 large potatoes), peeled and chopped

2 teaspoons chopped fresh thyme

Combine the dry ingredients. In a large bowl, whisk the flour, psyllium husks, baking powder, and salt together.

Make the dough. Make a well in the center of the dry ingredients. Add the egg, chicken fat, vinegar, and warm water. Using a rubber spatula, mix everything into a dough. The dough will be a bit shaggy and maybe feel a bit greasy to the touch. That's okay. Make sure the dough is entirely combined. Let it sit out for 1 hour. Refrigerate the dough overnight.

Caramelize the onions. The next day, set a Dutch oven over medium-high heat. When the air above the pot feels hot to your touch, pour in the oil. Add the butter. When the butter has melted and the oil shimmers in the pot, add the onions. Toss them to coat in the oil and butter, and cook, stirring occasionally. Turn the heat down to medium. After 10 minutes, pinch the sugar and salt over the top of the onions and stir well to coat. Continue to cook the onions, stirring every 10 minutes or so, until they soften and then begin to reduce in volume. After 30 minutes of total cooking time, the onions will shrink into themselves, browning. Stir the onions again, scraping the bottom of the pot with a metal spoon, to catch all that brown caramelized goodness. Don't let the onions burn. Continue to cook the onions, stirring and scraping the bottom of the pot every 2 to 3 minutes to make sure the onions don't burn. After 45 minutes of total cooking time, the onions will be lovely. After 60 minutes, the onions will be dark brown, wafting a slight sweetness. Cook them as long as you wish, knowing the onions will grow darker and sweeter the longer you cook them. Turn off the heat and set aside to cool.

Cook the potatoes. Set a Dutch oven on the stovetop. Fill it three-quarters full with cold water and add enough salt to make it taste like the ocean. Add the potatoes to the cold water. Bring the water to a boil over high heat, then reduce the heat to medium. Simmer until a knife slides right through one of the potatoes without any force, 10 to 15 minutes. Drain the potatoes into a colander in the sink. Let the potatoes steam there for about 5 minutes to allow them to dry.

Rice the potatoes. If you own a potato ricer or food mill, push the potatoes through it. Or, you could push the potatoes through a fine-mesh sieve with the back of a ramekin or wooden spoon.

Mash the filling. Put the potatoes back in the Dutch oven. Fold 1½ cups of the caramelized onions and the thyme into the potatoes. (Save the rest of the onions for the tops of the knishes.)

Make the knishes. Take the knish dough out of the refrigerator. Let it sit out for 20 minutes to come to room temperature. Between two pieces of lightly greased parchment paper, roll the dough out to a large thin rectangle, about 15 x 30 inches.

Spoon the potato filling onto the top of the rectangle of dough, forming a log along the long side. Fold in the sides of the dough. Using the bottom piece of parchment paper as a push, roll the dough into a log over the potato filling, and continue rolling until you have reached the end of the dough. Seal the ends. Cut the log into 16 pieces.

Put one piece into your hand. As you can, press inward, gathering the dough toward the top of the knish to seal it. Put the knish dough side down on a parchment-lined baking sheet. Make an indentation on the top of the knish and shape the dough to make a more even circle. Repeat with the remaining knishes.

Put the baking sheet into the freezer for 30 minutes.

Prepare to bake. Preheat the oven to 450°F.

Bake the knishes. Bake the knishes for 15 minutes, then turn the baking sheet 180 degrees in the oven and bake until the tops are golden brown, about 10 more minutes.

Top each knish with more caramelized onions and serve.

Feel like playing?

Knishes freeze well. Reheat them by baking in a 450°F oven until they are warm in the center, about 5 minutes. You can fill the knishes with any traditional filling, such as kasha (roasted buckwheat), mushrooms, or meat. Try sweet potatoes in place of the potatoes, if you wish.

SOFT PRETZELS

Makes a dozen pretzels

Soft pretzels did not originate in the United States. In fact, it's said that the first soft pretzel was made in 610 A.D. by an Italian monk determined to inspire his students to study. (That would probably work for me.) However, pretzels became an American classic in the late 1800s in Pennsylvania, where Julius Sturgis opened the first commercial pretzel bakery. Today, 80 percent of all hard pretzels eaten in America are baked in Pennsylvania, with each person from Philadelphia eating 12 pounds of pretzels a year, on average. Those of you in Philadelphia who cannot eat gluten, this recipe is for you.

1½ cups warm water

1 tablespoon honey

1 envelope (2¼ teaspoons) active dry yeast

430 grams All-Purpose Gluten-Free Flour Blend (page 17)

200 grams Grain-Free Flour Mix (page 19)

1 tablespoon (12 grams) psyllium husks

4 tablespoons (60 grams) unsalted butter, melted

2 teaspoons kosher salt

1 cup (300 grams) baking soda

1 large egg yolk

Coarse, flaky salt for sprinkling

Proof the yeast. In the bowl of a stand mixer with the paddle attachment, whisk together the warm water, 1 teaspoon of the honey, and the yeast. Let them rise until the top is frothy and the yeast has doubled in volume, about 15 minutes.

Make the dough. Add the flour blend, grain-free flour, and psyllium husks to the yeast mixture and mix until combined. Add the melted butter and salt. Let the mixer run until the dough is aerated and slumps off the paddle, about 5 minutes. Scrape down the sides of the bowl with a rubber spatula.

Let the dough rise. Cover the bowl with plastic wrap and allow it to rest in a warm place in the kitchen for 2 hours.

Shape the pretzels. Scoop the dough out of the bowl. Divide the dough into balls of 85 grams each (between the size of a golf ball and a baseball). Dust the countertop with flour blend. Roll each dough into a tight ball, fully pushing out all air pockets, then roll the ball of dough between your hands to make a thick cigar-shaped piece. Starting from the middle, slowly roll the dough back and forth, moving your hands gently toward the ends of the dough as you do. The dough should lengthen into a fairly even rope. Stop when the rope is about 15 inches long. Press along the length of the rope to make sure it is solid and not about to tear.

Pick up the rope of dough and form it into a large U, with the two ends at the top. Wind the two ends around each other, twice, then fold them onto the bottom of the rope. This should look like a pretzel. (It might take a few tries until this feels familiar.)

Freeze the dough. Put the completed pretzel onto a plate. Repeat until the plate is full. Put the full plate in the freezer for 30 minutes. Continue filling plates and putting them in the freezer until you have rolled the entire batch of dough into pretzels.

Make the baking soda water. Set a large pot filled with about 10 cups of water and the baking soda over high heat. Stir the water and baking soda together until the water comes to a full boil. Reduce the heat to medium-low and keep the water at a steady simmer.

Prepare to bake. Preheat the oven to 450°F. Line a baking sheet with parchment paper.

Dunk the pretzels. Take one plate of frozen pretzels out of the freezer. One at a time, lower a pretzel into the baking soda water, on a slotted spoon, for about 30 seconds. Don't let the pretzel stay in the water for longer than 1 minute or the dough will start to fall apart. Lift the dunked dough, still in its original shape, onto the lined baking sheet. Continue until the baking sheet is full.

Bake the pretzels. In a small bowl, whisk together the egg and the remaining 2 teaspoons of honey. Brush the egg-honey wash over each pretzel. Top with coarse salt. Continue until all the pretzels on the baking sheet are washed. Bake until the pretzels are firm to the touch and dark brown, 15 to 18 minutes. Remove the pretzels from the oven and cool them on the baking sheet for 10 minutes. Move them to a wire rack and let cool until they are only slightly warm.

Keep going with the remaining pretzels until you have baked them all.

Feel like playing?

If you cannot eat eggs, you can wash the pretzels with only honey. Just watch them closely when you bake them, as the honey might make them brown too quickly. If you want to make pretzel rolls—delicious for sandwiches—shape the dough into 4-ounce balls and shape into oval rolls. Bake the same way you bake the pretzels.

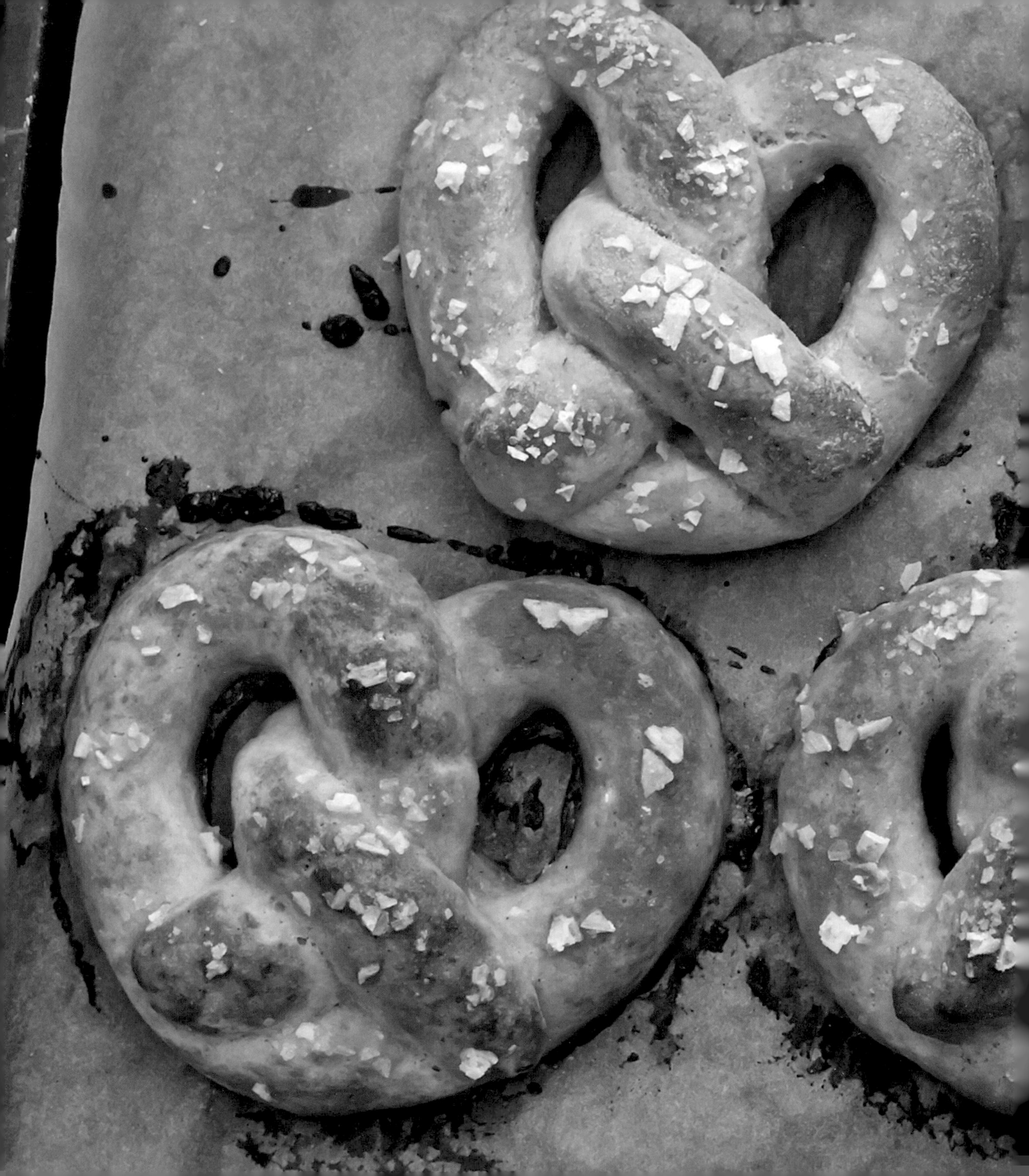

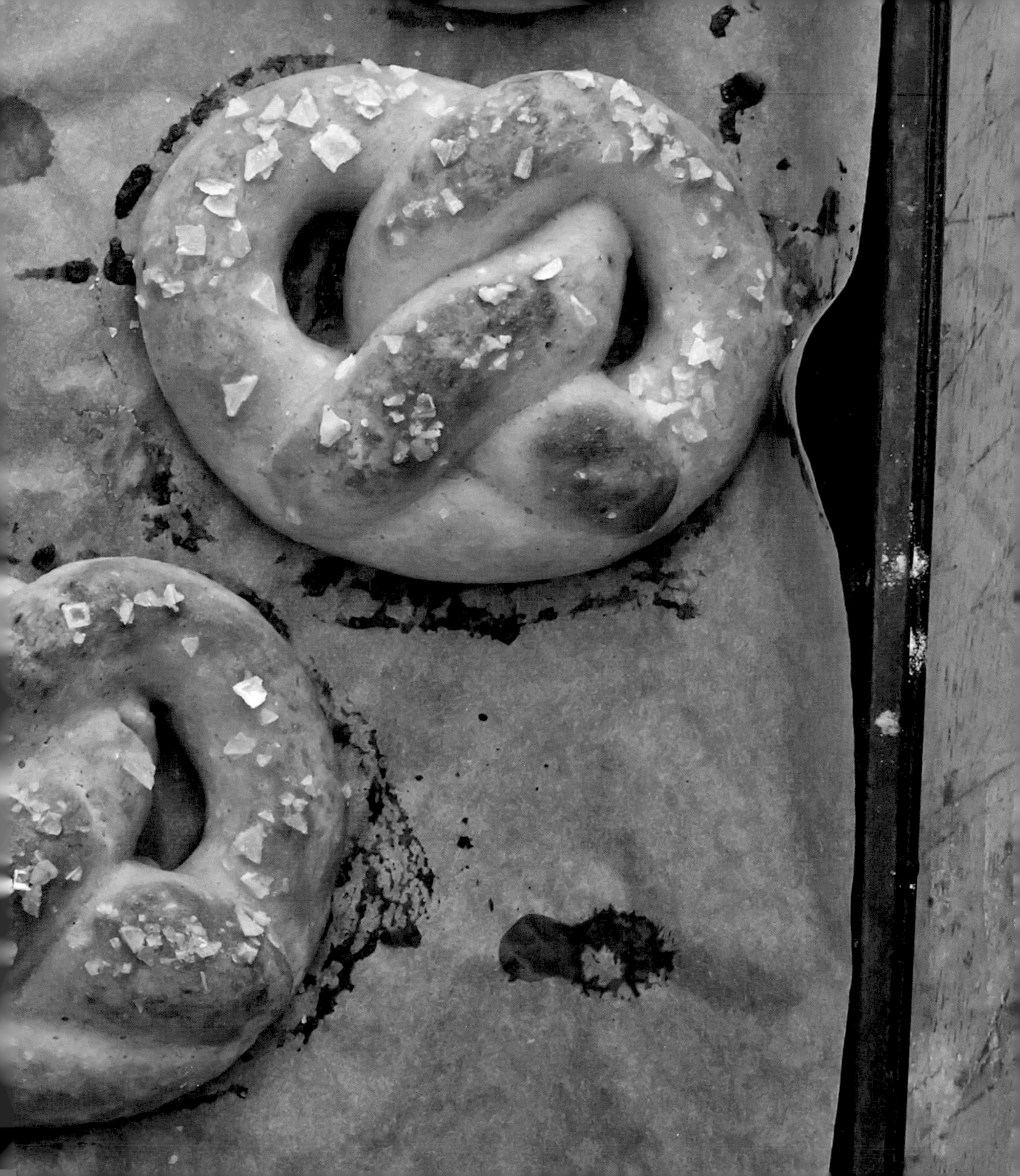

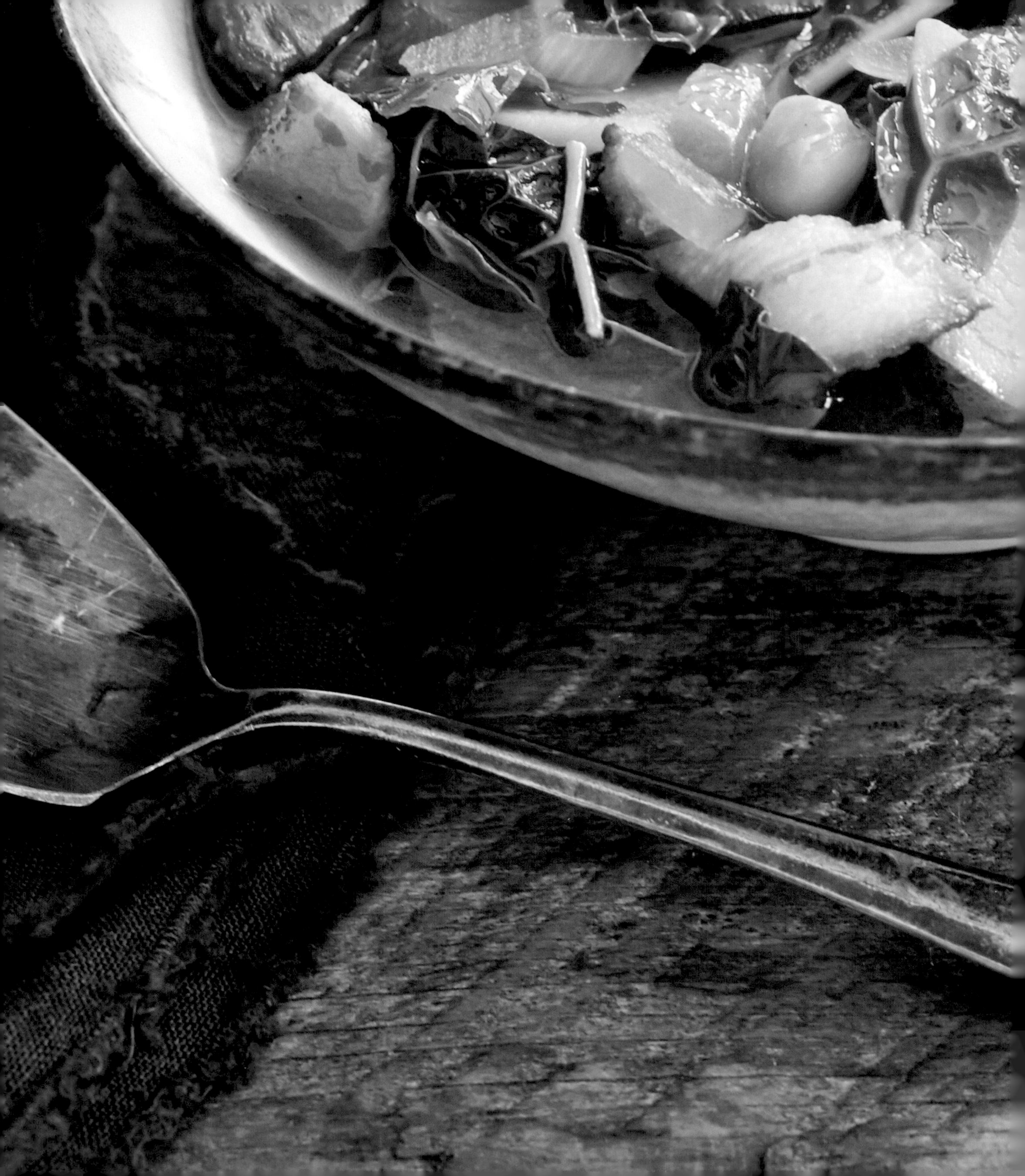

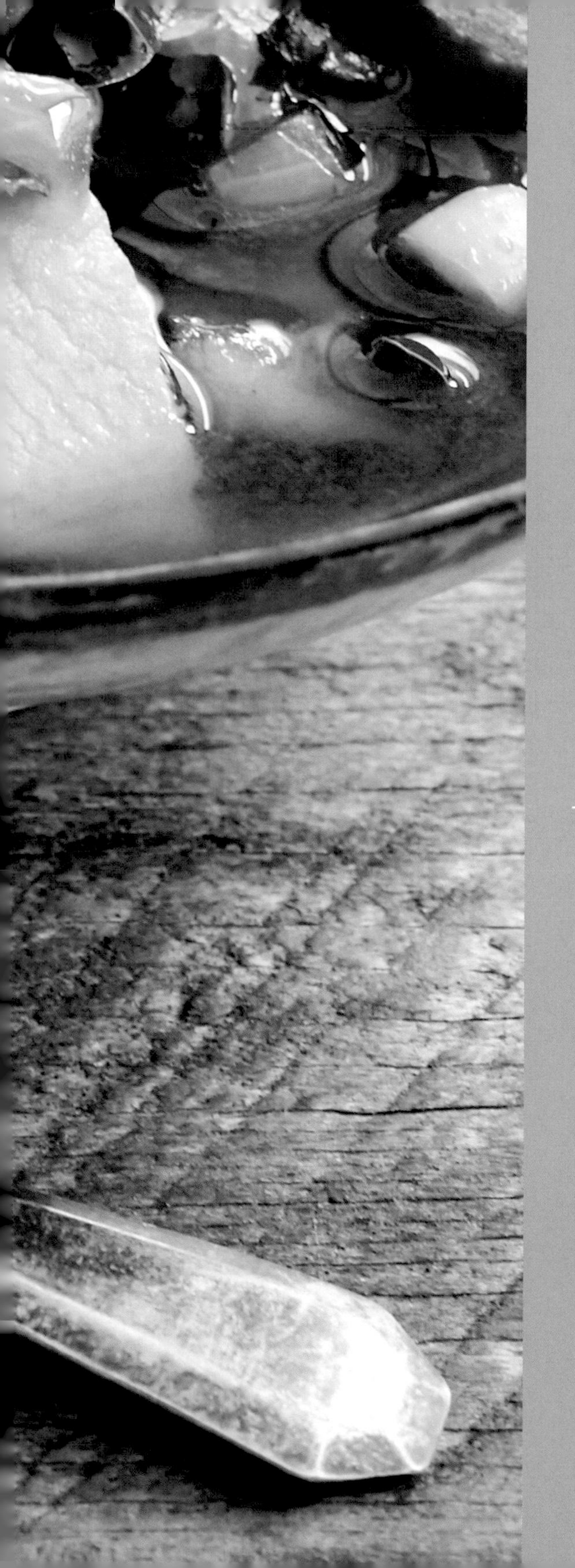

SOUPS AND STEWS

NEW ENGLAND CLAM CHOWDER

Feeds 6

This clam chowder is full of clam flavor, thick and creamy, and it also happens to be dairy-free. How do you make a creamy New England clam chowder without cream? A knife-tender russet potato, clam juice, and a good blender yield a luscious soup. And, if you have access to them, fresh clams added at the end. No one will ever suspect this is a gluten-free, dairy-free soup. They'll just ask for more.

1 tablespoon extra-virgin olive oil

4 thick slices bacon, diced

1 medium onion, peeled and finely chopped

3 stalks celery, chopped

2 cloves garlic, peeled and minced

2 tablespoons finely chopped fresh thyme

1 large russet potato, peeled and chopped

18 grams All-Purpose Gluten-Free Flour Blend (page 17)

Two 10-ounce cans clams, drained

4 cups clam juice

4 ounces fresh clams in their shells (optional)

Freshly squeezed juice of 1 lemon

¼ teaspoon cayenne pepper

Kosher salt and freshly ground black pepper

Cook the bacon. Set a Dutch oven over medium-high heat. Pour in the oil. When the oil is hot, add the bacon. Cook, stirring frequently, until the meat is crisp, about 5 minutes. Remove it from the oil.

Cook the aromatics. Turn down the heat to medium. Add the onions, celery, and garlic to the hot oil. Cook, stirring occasionally, until the onions are soft and translucent, about 7 minutes. Stir in the thyme and cook until the scent is released, about 1 minute.

Cook the potato and flour. Add the potato pieces and the flour. Cook, stirring frequently, until the flour starts to brown, about 3 minutes.

Simmer the soup. Add the canned clams and clam juice. Bring the soup to a low boil, then turn down the heat to low. Simmer the soup for 20 minutes, stirring occasionally.

Puree the soup. Pour one-quarter of the soup into a strong blender. Cover well. Remember the soup will be hot, so take care. Puree the soup. Pour the pureed soup back into the Dutch oven.

Steam the clams. Set a large pot with 1 inch of water on the stove. Lower a steamer basket into the pot. Carefully put the clams in their shells into the steamer basket. Cover the pot and turn the heat on high. Steam the clams in the boiling water until the shells have opened, 5 to 10 minutes. Toss any clams whose shells did not open.

Finish the soup. Add the lemon juice and cayenne pepper and simmer the soup for a moment. Season with salt and pepper. Turn off the heat. Stir in the steamed clams and serve.

Feel like playing?

If you have access to fresh shellfish stock or clam stock, use that in place of the bottled clam juice, by all means.

HEIRLOOM TOMATO SOUP WITH GOAT CHEESE CROUTONS

Feeds 6

It's pretty clear that the juiciest, biggest tomatoes grow in the Midwest. (Or is it New Jersey? Or Florida?) Here in the Pacific Northwest, tomato season is ridiculously brief and entirely reliant on the sometime sun we receive in the summer. Our tomatoes may not be as firm-fleshed as the ones grown so easily in Iowa, but we love the heirloom tomatoes that arrive in August: large, a little squished and funny looking, and much longed for all year long. In that brief slice of time, we make this tomato soup with local goat cheese and feast until October.

5 tablespoons extra-virgin olive oil

1 medium yellow onion, peeled and chopped

2 stalks celery, chopped

1 large carrot, peeled and chopped

3 cloves garlic, peeled and sliced

2 tablespoons chopped fresh basil

2 teaspoons smoked paprika

2½ pounds heirloom tomatoes, chopped

4 cups chicken stock (if you're using boxed stock, make sure it's gluten-free)

Kosher salt and freshly ground black pepper

CROUTONS

½ loaf day-old Sandwich Bread (page 53)

2 ounces chèvre

Prepare to bake. Preheat the oven to 425°F.

Cook the aromatics. Set a Dutch oven over medium heat. Pour in 2 tablespoons of the olive oil. When the oil is hot, add the onions, celery, carrot, and garlic. Cook, stirring occasionally, until the onions are soft and translucent, about 7 minutes. Stir in the basil and smoked paprika and cook until the scents are released, about 1 minute.

Cook the tomatoes. Add the chopped tomatoes to the soup. Cook, stirring occasionally, until the tomatoes have started to soften, about 3 minutes. Pour in the stock and turn up the heat to medium-high. Bring the stock to a boil, then reduce the heat to low. Simmer the soup for 20 minutes, stirring occasionally.

Puree the soup. Pour one-third of the soup into a blender, adding 1 tablespoon of the olive oil. Cover well. Remember the soup will be hot, so take care. Puree the soup. Pour it into a bowl. Continue with another third of the soup, adding another tablespoon of olive oil. Repeat with the remaining soup and olive oil. Pour the pureed soup back into the Dutch oven.

Finish the soup. Bring the soup back to a boil over medium-high heat, then reduce the heat to low. Season with salt and pepper. Simmer the soup while you make the croutons, stirring occasionally.

CONTINUED

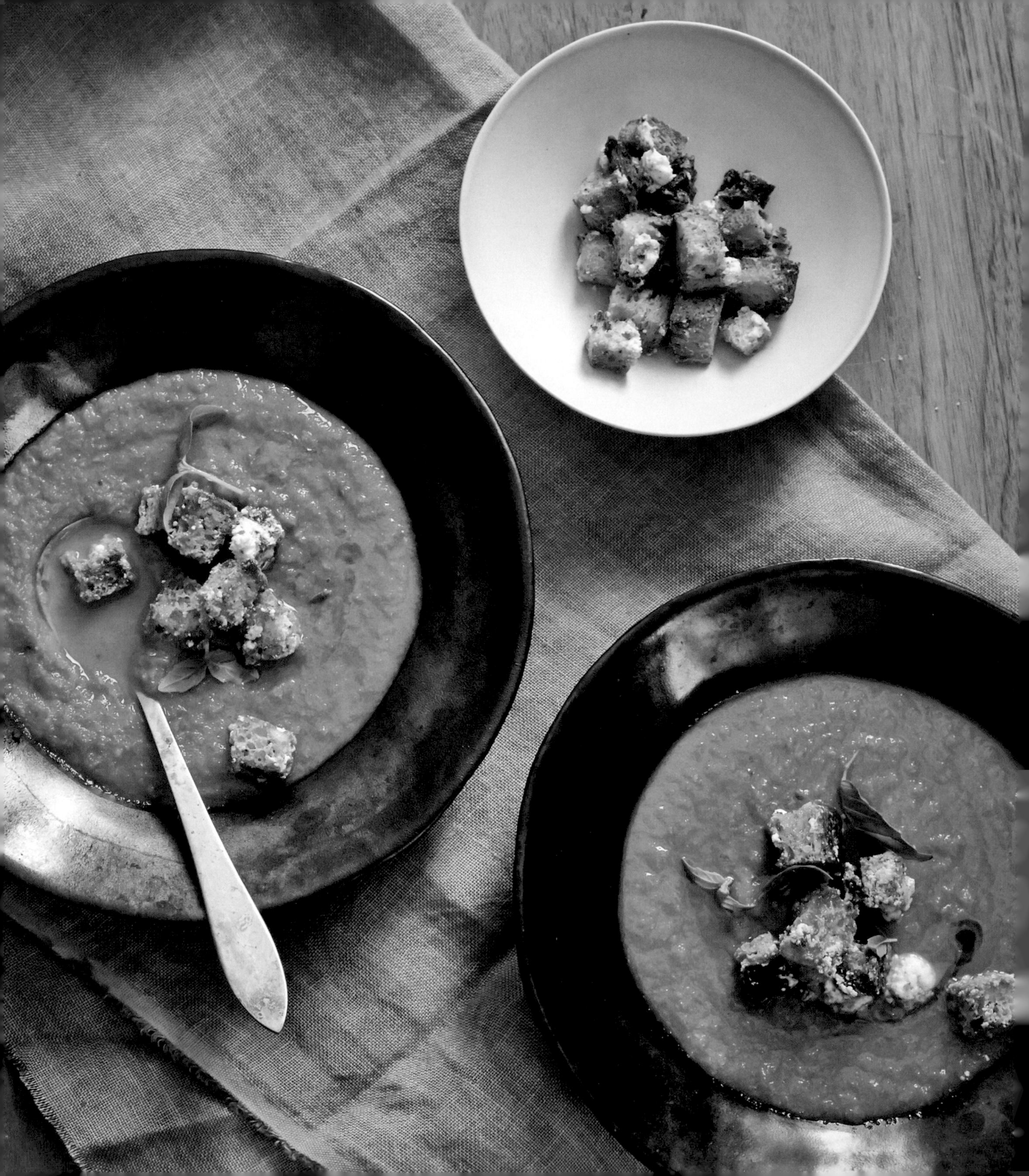

Make the croutons. Cut the loaf of sandwich bread into 1-inch slices. Cut each slice into 1-inch cubes. Put the cubes of bread onto a parchment-lined baking sheet. Toast the cubes of bread until they are browned and starting to harden, about 10 minutes.

Take the croutons out of the oven. Turn on the broiler. Slather each crouton with a bit of the chèvre. Put the croutons in the oven and watch carefully. Take them out of the oven when they are melty and bubbly.

Serve the soup. Ladle a generous portion of soup into each bowl, then dot the top with the goat cheese croutons. Serve immediately.

Feel like playing?

Since heirloom tomatoes that taste of summer are only available here for a couple of months a year, when we feel like tomato soup the rest of the year, we use canned San Marzano tomatoes from Italy. If you can't eat dairy, the croutons are still good without the cheese.

CREAM OF MUSHROOM SOUP

Feeds 6

Mushrooms, sherry, fresh thyme, chicken stock, and coconut milk—it all sounds utterly wonderful to me. But here's the gift of this recipe. Once you have made it, you can make any of the familiar casseroles from the Midwest that some of us love so much. Tater Tot Hot Pot (page 181), here we come!

3 tablespoons unsalted butter

2 tablespoons high-quality olive oil

1½ pounds cremini mushrooms, chopped

1 large onion, peeled and chopped

2 stalks celery, chopped

1 carrot, peeled and quartered

5 cloves garlic, peeled and smashed

2 tablespoons finely chopped fresh thyme

27 grams All-Purpose Gluten-Free Flour Blend (page 17)

½ cup dry sherry

3 cups chicken stock (if you're using boxed stock, make sure it's gluten-free)

One 14-ounce can coconut milk

Kosher salt and freshly ground black pepper

Cook the aromatics. Set a Dutch oven over medium-high heat. Add 1 tablespoon of the butter and the olive oil to the pot. When the fat is hot, add the mushrooms and cook, stirring frequently, until they have browned and shrunk in size a bit, about 3 minutes. Add the onions, celery, carrot, and garlic. Cook, stirring occasionally, until the onions are soft and translucent, about 7 minutes. Add the thyme and cook, stirring, until the scent is released, about 1 minute.

Cook the flour. Add the flour and toss with all the vegetables. Cook, stirring, until the flour has cooked, 2 to 3 minutes.

Simmer the soup. Splash the sherry into the pot. Cook, stirring occasionally, until the sherry has reduced in volume by half, about 5 minutes. Pour in the stock. Bring it to a boil, then cook the soup over medium-high heat for 10 minutes.

Puree the soup. Pour one-third of the soup into a blender. Cover well. Remember the soup will be hot, so take care. Puree the soup. Pour it into a bowl. Continue with another third of the soup. Repeat with the remaining soup. Pour the pureed soup through a fine-mesh sieve back into the Dutch oven.

Finish the soup. Bring the soup to a boil, stirring occasionally. Add the coconut milk and whisk until the milk is heated through. Whisk in the remaining 2 tablespoons of butter and stir until it is fully incorporated. Season with salt and pepper.

Feel like playing?

If you use lard or nondairy butter sticks, this will be an entirely dairy-free soup. You could certainly use vegetable stock or water in place of the chicken stock to make this a vegetarian soup. The consistency of the final soup is fairly thick, to make it work in casseroles. If you would like a thinner soup for eating—because this is a delicious soup—try thinning it out with club soda or chicken stock.

PORTUGUESE KALE SOUP

Feeds 6 to 8

This hearty soup is sometimes called Portuguese penicillin in the New England Portuguese community. I can see why. With this much goodness in it—Spanish chorizo, bacon, beans, and fresh kale—you have to feel good after a bowl of this soup. It's meaty and delicious. In the middle of the winter, this soup satisfies.

1 tablespoon extra-virgin olive oil

1 pound fresh Mexican chorizo, sliced

4 thick slices bacon, diced

2 medium onions, peeled and diced

2 cloves garlic, peeled and minced

1 tablespoon chopped fresh oregano

2 large sweet potatoes, peeled and chopped

2 cups chicken stock (if you're using boxed stock, make sure it's gluten-free)

One 15-ounce can cannellini beans, drained and rinsed

1 pound Lacinato kale, leaves stripped from the stems and cut into chiffonade

Kosher salt and freshly ground black pepper

Cook the chorizo and bacon. Set a Dutch oven over medium-high heat. Pour in the oil. When the oil is hot, add the chorizo and bacon. Cook, stirring frequently, until the meat is crisp, about 5 minutes. Remove it from the oil.

Cook the aromatics. Turn down the heat to medium. Add the onions and garlic to the hot oil. Cook, stirring occasionally, until the onions are soft and translucent, about 7 minutes. Stir in the oregano and cook until the scent is released, about 1 minute.

Cook the sweet potato. Throw the sweet potatoes into the Dutch oven and cover them with the stock. Simmer until the potato is just tender to a knife, about 15 minutes.

Blend part of the soup. Pour one-third of the soup into a blender. Cover well. Remember the soup will be hot, so take care. Puree the soup. Pour it into a bowl. Continue with another third of the soup. Pour the pureed soup back into the Dutch oven.

Finish the soup. Add the cooked chorizo and bacon to the soup, along with the cannellini beans. Heat the soup over medium heat. Add the kale. Cook, stirring occasionally, until the kale is wilted, about 3 minutes. Season with salt and pepper.

Feel like playing?

The sweet potato adds a tiny bit of sweetness to the soup, adding complexity to the taste. But if you wish, you could use russet potatoes instead.

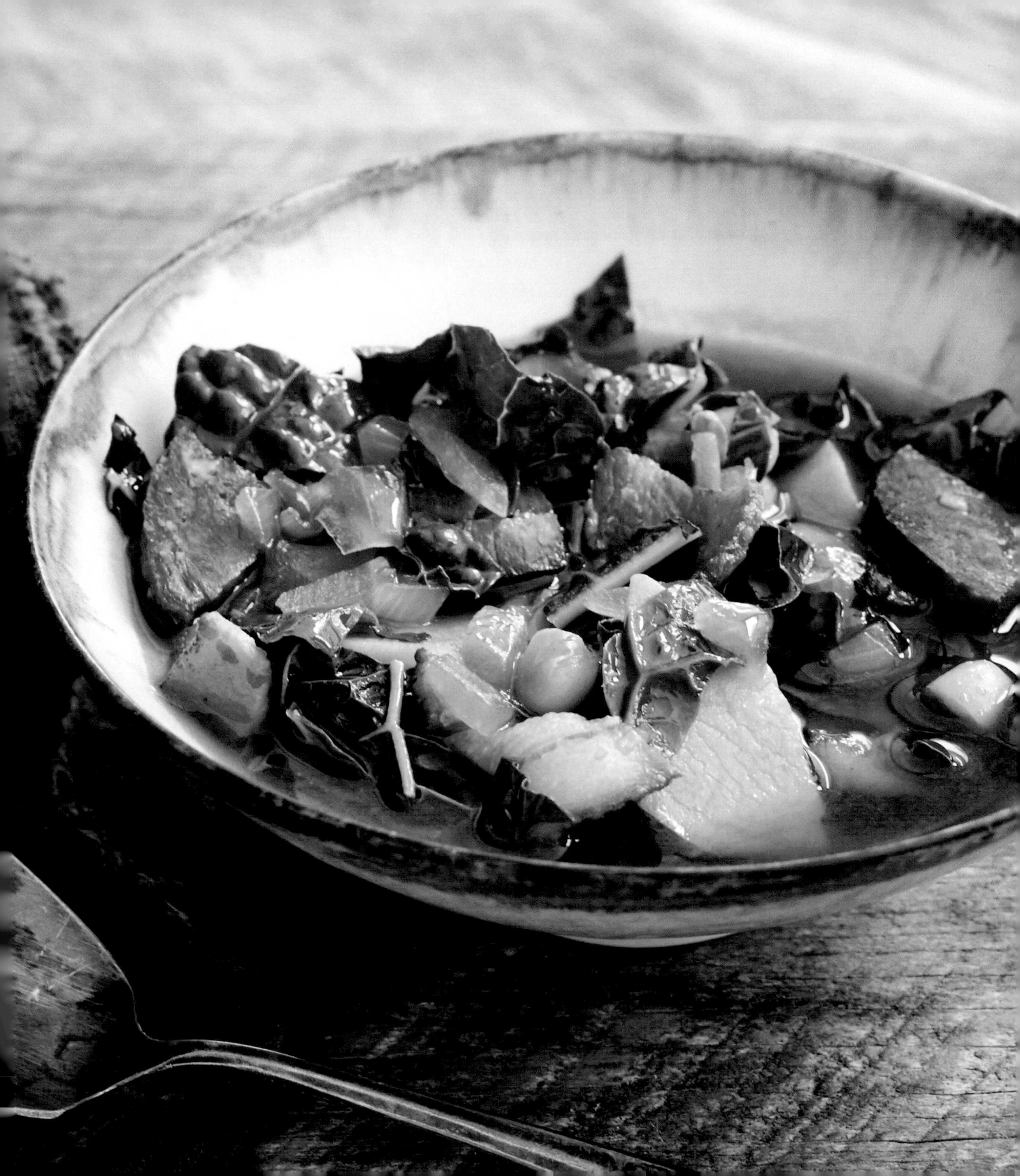

AMISH CHICKEN AND NOODLE

Feeds 6

Years ago now, I drove across the country from New York to Oregon with my best friend, Sharon. It was a trip fueled entirely by food and the desire to experience every regional specialty we could find. One day in Pennsylvania, we made a 60-mile detour off the main highway to visit an Amish diner written about in a guidebook. We drove past slow-moving horse-drawn carriages to park in front of a humble café. Need I say that the pies were spectacular? (This was before I realized I had celiac and needed to be gluten-free.) My favorite part of the long meal we shared was chicken and noodle. I thought I was ordering chicken noodle soup. However, what arrived at the white table was a bowl of rich chicken soup with thick homemade noodle squares. Also known as Amish chicken pot pie, this is the ultimate comfort food. This recipe is adapted from one by David Rosengarten, whose cookbook It's All American Food *has been a great inspiration for this book.*

CHICKEN STOCK

One 3½-pound chicken

6 large carrots, peeled and chopped

1 large onion, peeled and cut into quarters

2 large stalks celery, chopped

5 sprigs fresh thyme

5 sprigs fresh parsley

1 bay leaf

1 teaspoon black peppercorns

½ teaspoon kosher salt

NOODLES

350 grams All-Purpose Gluten-Free Flour Blend (page 17)

1½ teaspoons psyllium husks

Make the chicken stock. Put the chicken, 2 of the carrots, the onions, celery, thyme, parsley, bay leaf, and peppercorns in a large Dutch oven. Cover with enough water to have 1 inch of water above the top of the chicken. Set the pot over medium heat. Bring the water to a boil. Simmer until the chicken is tender to the touch and you can use tongs to slide the leg off the chicken, about 1½ hours.

Strain the stock. Take the chicken out of the pot. Pour the stock through a fine-mesh sieve into a large bowl. Allow the stock to cool to room temperature, skim the fat off the top of the stock, then put the stock in the refrigerator. Allow the chicken to cool on the counter to room temperature. Take the skin off the chicken and discard it. Cut the chicken into bite-size pieces. Throw away the bones. Refrigerate the chicken meat.

Make the dough. Set a small pot over high heat. Pour in 1 cup of the stock. Bring it to a boil, then pour the stock into a large bowl. Stir in the salt. Add 280 grams of the flour and the psyllium husks and stir it together with the stock. This will make a shaggy dough. Add more of the flour, a bit at a time, stirring it all up with your hands to make sure the flour is evenly added until the dough is sticky but coherent. Dump the dough onto a cutting board and bring it all together with your hands. Wrap the dough in plastic wrap and refrigerate it for 1 hour.

Cut the noodles. When the dough has chilled, cut it into four pieces. Roll out one piece of the dough between two pieces of lightly greased parchment paper to a 1⁄4-inch thickness. Cut the dough into 1-inch squares. Lay the squares on another piece of parchment paper. Continue with all the dough the same way. Allow the dough squares to air-dry for 30 minutes.

Make the stew. Set a Dutch oven over medium heat. Pour in the remaining broth. Add the remaining 4 carrots and simmer them in the broth for 5 minutes. With the stock simmering, add a layer of noodle squares to the top of the pot. When the squares have slowly sunk to the bottom of the pot, add another layer, continuing like this until you have added all the squares of noodles. Simmer until the noodle squares are tender, about 5 minutes. Add the chicken pieces and simmer until they are heated through. Serve immediately.

Feel like playing?

Making the chicken stock from scratch, with a whole chicken, yields the richest stock and chicken meat to eat. However, if you are in a rush, you can use 8 to 10 cups of boxed chicken stock instead here. For a classic chicken noodle soup, cut the dough into long noodles instead, or simply use packaged gluten-free noodles here for a quick soup.

CREAM OF ARTICHOKE SOUP

Feeds 6

Just off Highway 1, on the coast of California, between San Francisco and Santa Cruz, is Duarte's Tavern. Open since 1894, Duarte's is emblematic of the cuisine of fresh, local ingredients of northern California. One of the greatest crops of this region is artichokes. Duarte's cream of artichoke soup has been served there since the beginning of the restaurant's history. If we were within driving distance of Duarte's, we'd go every month for some of that soup. (Danny loves artichokes so much that he has an artichoke tattoo on his arm.) With frozen artichokes and hazelnut milk, this soup of ours is a little bit of northern California meets Pacific Northwest.

2 tablespoons unsalted butter

1 small onion, peeled and finely chopped

2 cloves garlic, peeled and minced

1 tablespoon finely chopped fresh thyme

2 pounds frozen artichoke hearts, chopped

1 large russet potato, peeled and chopped

3 cups chicken stock (if you're using boxed stock, make sure it's gluten-free)

1 cup hazelnut milk (rice milk would be great too)

Kosher salt and freshly ground black pepper

6 wedges of lemon

Cook the aromatics. Set a Dutch oven over medium heat. Add the butter. When the butter is melted, add the onions and garlic. Cook, stirring frequently—remember that butter can burn quickly—until the onions are soft and translucent, about 7 minutes. Add the thyme and cook, stirring, until the scent is released, about 1 minute.

Cook the artichokes. Add the chopped artichoke hearts to the pot. Cook, stirring frequently, until the artichokes are hot and coated in the onions and thyme, about 3 minutes.

Cook the potato. Add the diced potato and stir. Cover with the stock. Bring the stock to a boil, then reduce the heat to medium-low. Cook until the potato is tender to a knife, about 15 minutes.

Puree the soup. Pour one-third of the soup into a blender. Cover well. Remember the soup will be hot, so take care. Puree the soup. Pour it into a bowl. Continue with another one-third of the soup. Repeat with the remaining soup. Pour the pureed soup back into the Dutch oven.

Simmer the soup. Simmer the soup over medium heat until the liquid has reduced by one-third its volume, about 45 minutes. When the soup has thickened, stir in the hazelnut milk. When the soup is entirely hot, season with salt and pepper.

Serve, with each person receiving a wedge of lemon to squeeze into the soup before eating.

Feel like playing?

If you cannot find hazelnut milk, you could make your own the night before you make the soup. Cover 1 cup of hazelnuts with fresh water and let them soak overnight. Drain the water from the hazelnuts and put them in a strong blender. Add a squeeze of lemon juice, a pinch salt, and enough fresh water to cover the nuts. Blend until you have a thick milk. Pour the liquid through a fine-mesh sieve and you have hazelnut milk. Of course, if you don't want to do any of this, you could easily use cow's milk or any milk that works for you here.

GREEN CHILE PORK STEW

Feeds 6

When Danny and I visited New Mexico for the first time, we fell in love. We fell in love with the high clear light, the vibrant arts community, and the food. Oh, the food. We were particularly crazy about New Mexico Hatch green chiles, which are milder in heat than jalapeños and almost creamy when roasted. We brought home a bag of frozen green chiles and started playing right away. We made this stew with pork we marinated overnight in some of the spices we tasted in New Mexico, then cooked it up with green chiles, tomatoes, and sweet potatoes. Oh my.

FOR THE SPICE RUB

1 tablespoon toasted ground cumin (see Tip)

2 teaspoons chili powder

½ teaspoon ground cinnamon

¼ teaspoon ground cloves

2½ pounds pork butt, cut into 1-inch cubes

FOR THE STEW

Kosher salt and freshly ground black pepper

3 tablespoons lard

1 medium onion, peeled and chopped

3 cloves garlic, peeled and sliced

2 teaspoons chili powder

2 teaspoons ground cumin

1 teaspoon ground cinnamon

18 grams All-Purpose Gluten-Free Flour Blend (page 17)

One 14-ounce can diced tomatoes

8 ounces green chiles

4 cups chicken stock (if you're using boxed stock, make sure it's gluten-free)

2 large sweet potatoes, peeled and chopped

Rub the pork. In a small bowl, combine the cumin, chili powder, cinnamon, and cloves. Rub the spice mixture all over the pork butt cubes. Let the pork sit in the refrigerator overnight to marinate.

Sear the pork. The next day, take the pork out of the refrigerator and season it with salt and pepper. Set a Dutch oven over medium-high heat. Add the lard. When the lard is melted, lay enough pork cubes into the hot fat to lightly cover the bottom of the pot. (Don't crowd it; you'll have to sear the pork in batches.) Cook until the bottoms of the pork cubes are browned, about 3 minutes. Flip over the cubes and sear the other side. Repeat this until all four sides are seared. Take the pork out of the Dutch oven.

Cook the aromatics. Put the onions and garlic into the hot fat. Cook, stirring frequently, until the onions are soft and translucent, about 7 minutes. Add the chili powder, cumin, and cinnamon and cook, stirring, until the scent is released, about 1 minute.

Cook the tomatoes and chiles. Add the flour to the vegetables. Cook, stirring frequently, until the flour is cooked, about 3 minutes (be careful to not burn the flour). Add the tomatoes and chiles and cook, stirring, until they have started to soften and break down, about 3 minutes.

Simmer the stew. Add the stock to the Dutch oven. Bring the stock to a boil, then turn the heat down to low. Simmer the stew, stirring occasionally, until the meat is tender enough that you can break it apart with a fork, about 2½ hours.

Finish the stew. When the stew is almost finished simmering, add the sweet potatoes to a large pot of salted water. Set the pot over high heat. Bring the water to a boil and cook until the sweet potatoes are tender to a knife, 10 to 15 minutes. Drain immediately. When the stew is ready, add the cooked sweet potatoes and serve.

Tip: To roast spices, set a small skillet over medium-high heat. Add the spice (in this case, cumin). Cook, tossing the spice in the pan once in a while, until it begins to smell toasty, about 3 minutes.

Feel like playing?

You could use any meat you want here: venison, bison, beef, chicken, or veal. They would all work. You could remove the meat altogether and have great vegetarian stew.

HOT AND SOUR SOUP

Feeds 6

On a cold night in New York City, I loved the decadence of ordering Chinese takeout to be delivered to my apartment. Most times, all I wanted was a big white take-out carton full of hot and sour soup. This Szechuan specialty is like a kick-ass chicken soup, filled with soy sauce, tofu, dark Chinkiang vinegar, and fresh ginger. The heat and sourness cleared out my nose and made me happy. Now, we make our own version of this soup at home. Almost all Chinkiang vinegars contain gluten, so we substitute apple cider vinegar and red wine vinegar for that sour element. And we use tamari instead of soy sauce. And good dried mushrooms from the Pacific Northwest make this soup ours now.

1 tablespoon gluten-free tamari

1 tablespoon plus 2 teaspoons arrowroot flour (you could also use cornstarch)

1 teaspoon dry sherry

6 ounces pork loin, cut into 2-inch-long strips

2 ounces dried mushrooms (such as shiitake or porcini)

3½ cups chicken stock (if you're using boxed stock, make sure it's gluten-free)

½ teaspoon kosher salt

6 ounces extra-firm tofu, cut into matchsticks

1 large egg, beaten

3 tablespoons toasted sesame oil, plus more for drizzling

2 tablespoons red wine vinegar

2 tablespoons apple cider vinegar

1½ teaspoons ground white pepper

¼ cup thinly sliced scallions

¼ cup chopped fresh cilantro

2 teaspoons peeled and grated fresh ginger

Marinate the pork. In a small bowl, combine the tamari, 1 tablespoon of the arrowroot, and the sherry. Pour the mixture over the pork slices in a bowl and toss. Marinate for 30 minutes.

Soak the mushrooms. Soak the mushrooms in hot water for 15 minutes. Drain and dry the mushrooms. Slice them into small pieces.

Simmer the stock. Set a Dutch oven over medium heat. Pour in the stock and salt. Stir until the salt is dissolved. When the chicken stock is hot, combine the remaining 2 teaspoons of arrowroot with 2 teaspoons water. Mix them into a slurry, then slowly pour the slurry into the stock and stir it in. Simmer the stock for a few more moments.

Finish the soup. Add the pork, tofu, and mushrooms to the chicken stock and stir them together. Simmer for a few moments. Bring the

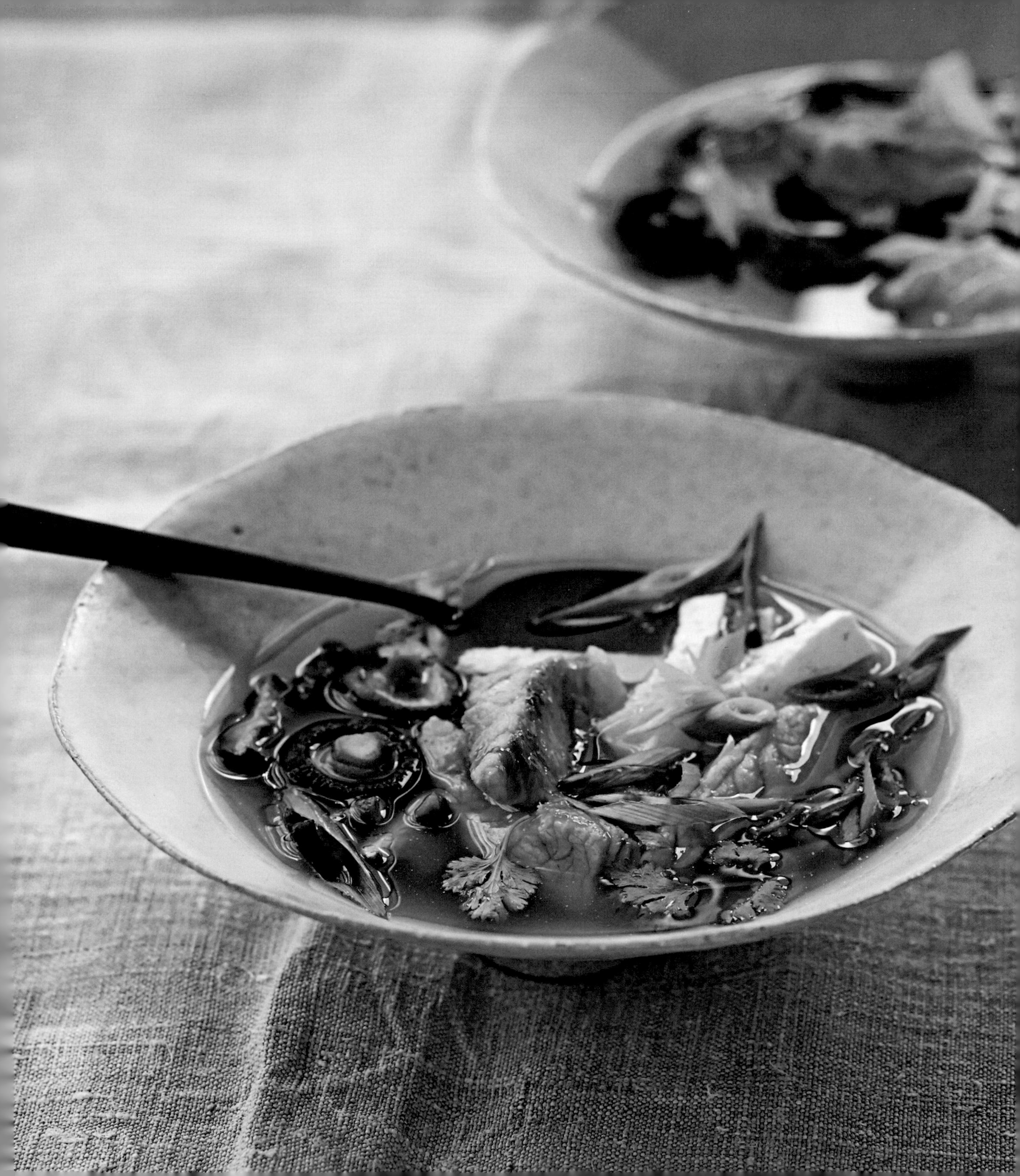

soup to a boil, then reduce to a low simmer. Slowly, pour in the beaten egg. Let the egg sit for 15 to 20 seconds, then stir the stock to incorporate the egg into the soup.

Serve the soup. As soon as you are ready to serve the soup, stir in the sesame oil, both vinegars, and white pepper. Ladle the soup into bowls. Drizzle sesame oil into each bowl, then top the soup with the scallions, cilantro, and ginger. Serve immediately. You might want to have more white pepper, vinegars, and sesame oil on the table for folks to adjust the hot and sour part to their own tastes.

Feel like playing?

Traditionally, hot and sour soup uses dried wood ear mushrooms and lily buds in place of the dried mushrooms here. If you have access to a good Asian market, by all means use those. You could easily make this a vegetarian soup by leaving out the pork and adding more tofu and replacing the chicken stock with vegetable stock.

CHICKEN AND SAUSAGE GUMBO

Feeds 6 to 8

This thick, rich stew from New Orleans is a national treasure, full of flavor and traditions. We can't claim credit for this recipe. Our dear friend Pableaux Johnson kindly gave us his gumbo recipe for this book. Pableaux is an incredible photographer, spending many of his days recording the pageantry of his beloved New Orleans. He's also one hell of a writer. And every Monday night, he opens his home to friends from far and near, who gather for red beans and rice. The man makes a mean pot of gumbo, and he makes something like fifty batches a year. So this? This recipe is a gift.

2 tablespoons lard

1 pound andouille sausage, cut into chunks (you can also use kielbasa or smoked sausage)

1 cup olive oil

140 grams All-Purpose Gluten-Free Flour Blend (page 17)

1½ cups chopped onions

¾ cup chopped celery

¾ cup chopped green bell peppers

3 tablespoons Cajun seasoning

6 cups water

3 bay leaves

One 3½-pound chicken, cut up into 8 pieces (or 6 bone-in chicken breasts)

½ cup chopped scallions

6 tablespoons chopped fresh Italian parsley

Cooked white rice for serving

Cook the sausage. Set a Dutch oven over medium-high heat. Add the lard. When the lard has melted, add the sausage chunks and cook, stirring occasionally, until browned, about 5 minutes. Put the sausage on a paper towel–lined plate and throw out the lard.

Make the roux. Turn the heat to low. Using the same Dutch oven, pour in the olive oil. Heat until the oil is hot, 1 to 2 minutes. Add the flour, one-quarter of it at a time, whisking constantly until each batch is blended in. Cook, stirring frequently and taking care to avoid splatters, until the roux gradually changes color, from pasty beige to peanut butter color to chocolate brown. (Pableaux says this should be the time it takes to drink 2 beers, or about 25 minutes.)

Cook the aromatics. Turn up the heat to medium-high. Add the onions to the roux and cook, stirring frequently, for 2 to 3 minutes. Add the celery and bell peppers. Reduce the heat to low and cook, stirring occasionally, until the vegetables start to soften, about 5 minutes. Stir in the cooked sausage and 1 tablespoon of the Cajun seasoning. Cook, stirring frequently, until the scent is released, about 2 minutes.

Cook the chicken. Pour in the water and add the bay leaves. Stir. Rub the remaining 2 tablespoons of Cajun seasoning all over the chicken. Add the chicken to the Dutch oven and bring the water to a boil. Reduce the heat to low and allow the gumbo to cook at a low simmer, skimming off the fat and stirring occasionally, until the chicken is cooked through and very tender, about 1½ hours. Stir in the scallions and parsley. Fish out the bay leaves. Serve the gumbo over the white rice.

REUBEN SANDWICH SOUP

Feeds 6

One of my absolute favorite sandwiches in the world feels impossible to replicate without gluten. Corned beef, sauerkraut, strong mustard, and Swiss chess? They're all gluten-free, naturally. But a great sour rye bread? That's hard to do without rye flour. I miss the Reuben sandwich. So one day, Danny and I took all the flavors and spices of our favorite sandwiches and made a hearty soup with it instead. This one might just knock off your socks.

2 tablespoons extra-virgin olive oil

2 pounds corned beef, cut into 4 pieces (plus the reserved liquid and spices from the package)

1 medium yellow onion, peeled and chopped

3 cloves garlic, peeled and sliced

2 tablespoons finely chopped fresh rosemary

1 tablespoon finely chopped fresh thyme

1 tablespoon yellow mustard seeds

1 tablespoon caraway seeds

¾ cup red wine, such as Merlot

1 cup sauerkraut

2 quarts beef stock (if you're using boxed stock, make sure it's gluten-free)

1 small head green cabbage, thinly sliced

6 slices Swiss cheese

Prepare to make the soup. Preheat the oven to 425°F.

Sear the corned beef. Set a Dutch oven over medium-high heat. Pour in the oil. When the oil is hot, sear one piece of the corned beef. Cook until the bottom is browned, 3 to 4 minutes. Flip over the meat and brown the other side. Transfer the corned beef to a plate and repeat with the remaining pieces.

Cook the aromatics. Add the onions to the hot oil. Cook, stirring frequently, until the onions are deep brown and reduced in volume, about 15 minutes. Add the garlic and cook, stirring frequently, until the garlic is browned but not burned. Add the rosemary, thyme, mustard seeds, and caraway seeds and cook, stirring, until their scents are released, about 2 minutes. Pour in the reserved liquid and spices from the corned beef package and stir.

Deglaze with red wine. Pour the wine over the onions and spices and stir, scraping any crisp bits from the bottom of the pan. Cook until the wine has reduced in volume by half, 5 to 7 minutes.

Simmer the soup. Add the sauerkraut and cook, stirring, until it is fully incorporated and hot. Pour in beef stock. Bring it to a boil, then turn off the heat. Put the Dutch oven into the hot oven and cover it. Let the soup simmer until you can take a fork and gently shred the corned beef apart with ease, 2 to 3 hours. Take the soup pot out of the oven. Turn on the broiler.

Finish the soup. Add the sliced cabbage to the soup and stir. When the cabbage is wilted, spoon the soup into four oven-safe soup bowls. Top each bowl of soup with a slice of Swiss cheese. Put the soup bowls under the broiler and watch them closely. As soon as the cheese is melted and bubbly over the top of the soup, turn off the broiler and take out the soup. Serve immediately.

Feel like playing?

Of course, if you're dairy-free and can't do cheese, you can skip that last step and still enjoy this soup.

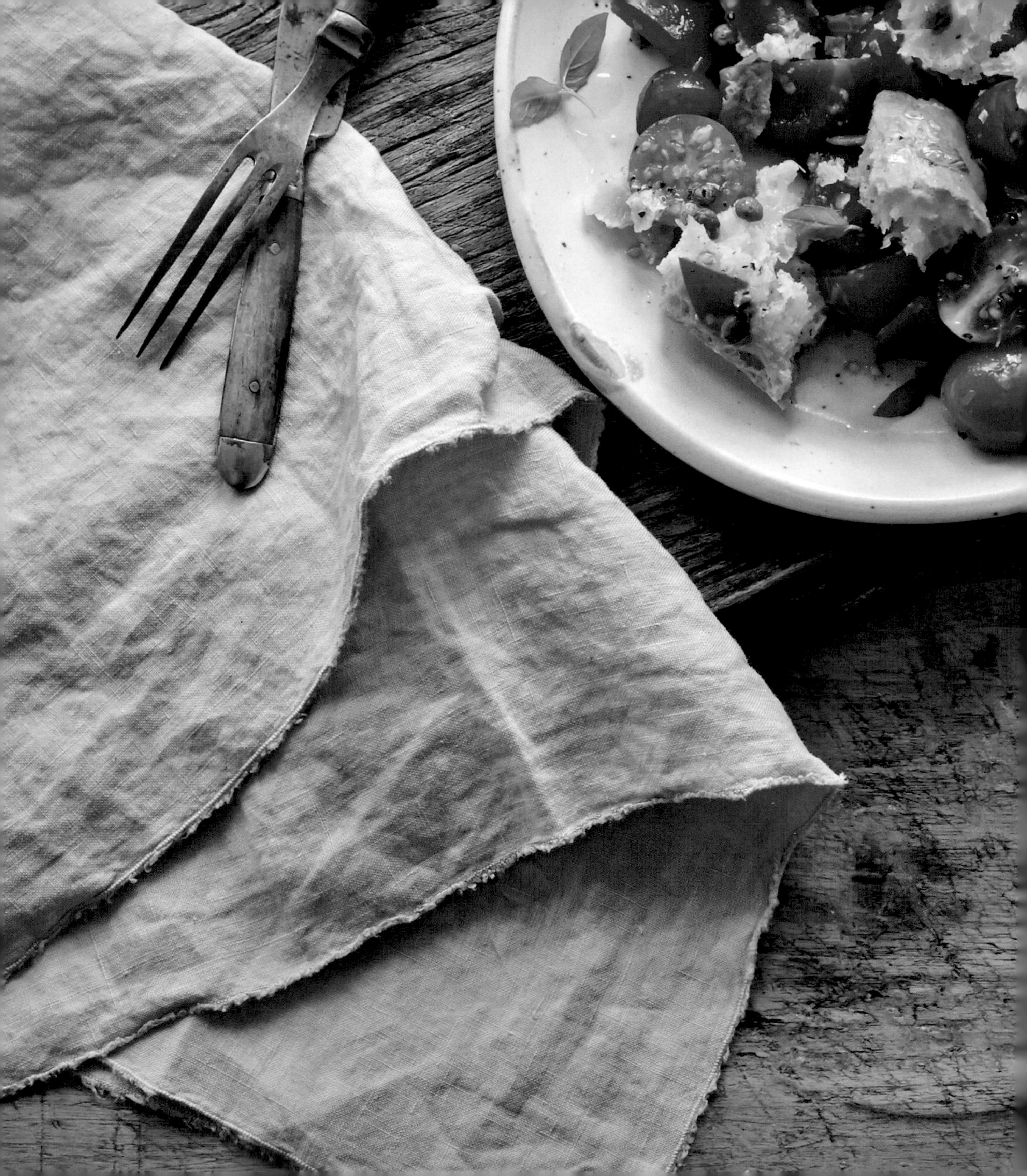

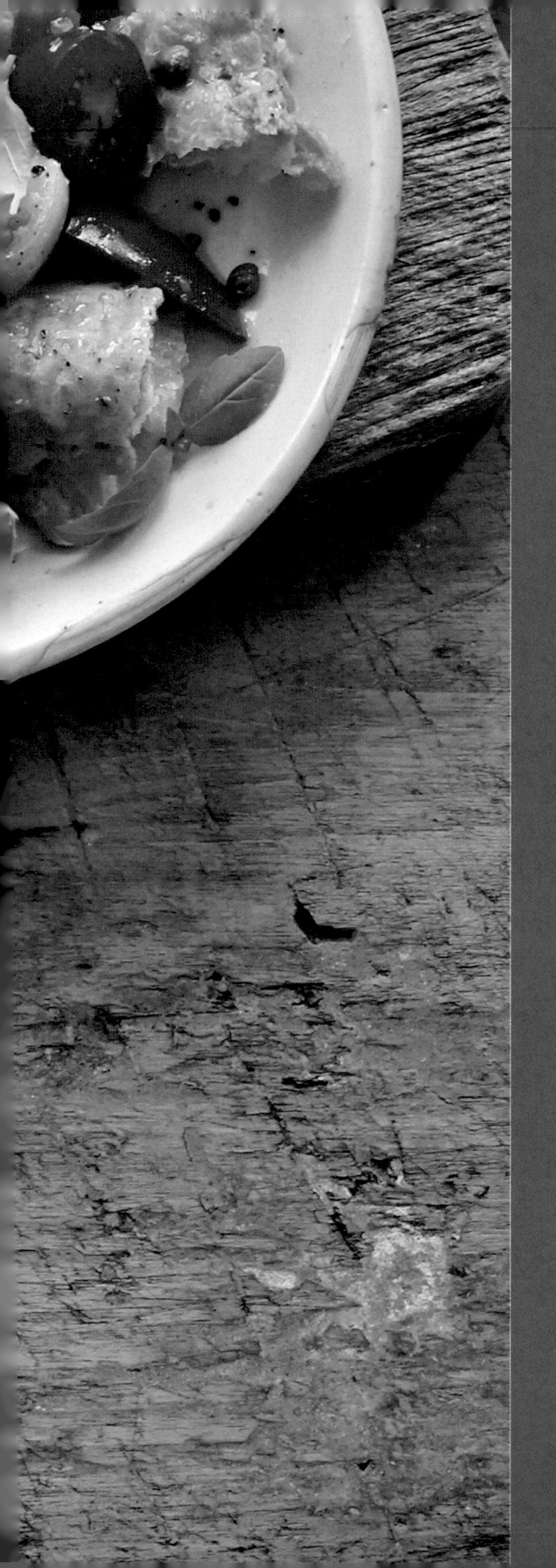

SIDES

CORNBREAD

The Civil War may have ended more than a century ago, but the war between the North and South endures through cornbread. In the north, cornbread is light and fluffy, almost like a cake, with flour and a sweetener. In the South, cornbread is dense, made only with cornmeal, and absolutely not sweet. In the name of peace, we offer you both variations here.

NORTHERN CORNBREAD

Feeds 8

This is northern cornbread, for sure. Having been raised on it, Danny and I both like a touch of sweetness in our cornbread. Since cornbread doesn't require the elastic qualities of gluten, our basic all-purpose flour blend works like a wonder here.

140 grams All-Purpose Gluten-Free Flour Blend (page 17)

2 tablespoons organic cane sugar

4 teaspoons baking powder

¾ teaspoon salt

¼ cup lard or vegetable shortening

2 large eggs, at room temperature

¾ cup whole milk (we use coconut milk)

2 tablespoons honey

1 cup (160 grams) stone-ground cornmeal (make sure it's gluten-free)

Prepare to cook. Preheat the oven to 425°F.

Mix the dry ingredients. In a large bowl, whisk together the flour, sugar, baking powder, and salt.

Cut in the shortening. Cut the shortening into the flours, the way you would when making a pie dough. You should end up with walnut-size pieces in a sandy flour.

Add the wet ingredients. In a small bowl, combine the eggs, milk, and honey. Make a well in the center of the dry ingredients and pour in the liquid. Stir with a rubber spatula until everything is combined.

Finish the batter. Stir in the cornmeal, whisking fast, until it is just combined. Do not overstir.

Bake the cornbread. Pour into a greased 9 x 9 x 2-inch pan. Slide it into the oven. Bake for 20 to 25 minutes, or until the sides of the cornbread are slightly shrinking from the pan and a toothpick comes out clean. Cool in the pan for 10 minutes, then serve warm.

SOUTHERN CORNBREAD

Feeds 8

If you want a traditional southern cornbread, life is easy for you. This recipe from John Thorne's brilliant book, Serious Pig, *needs no improvement. The book, which is a series of essays and recipes on the joys of regional American cuisine, has been a great gift for us in creating this cookbook as well.*

1 cup (160 grams) stone-ground cornmeal (make sure it's gluten-free)

½ teaspoon cream of tartar

½ teaspoon baking soda

½ teaspoon fine sea salt

1 large egg

¾ cup low-fat buttermilk

1 tablespoon lard

Prepare to cook. Preheat the oven to 425°F.

Whisk together the dry ingredients. In a large bowl, whisk together the cornmeal, cream of tartar, baking soda, and salt.

CONTINUED

Prepare the wet ingredients. Crack the egg into a small bowl. Beat it gently. Whisk in the buttermilk.

Prepare the pan. Put the lard into an 8-inch cast-iron skillet. Put it in the oven for 5 minutes.

Finish the batter. Make a well in the center of the dry ingredients and pour in the liquids. Using a rubber spatula, stir them together until they are thoroughly combined.

Bake the cornbread. Take the hot skillet out of the oven carefully. Swirl the fat around the skillet and up the sides. Pour in the batter, which will sizzle, and stir it around quickly with the whisk. Bake until the cornbread is golden brown and the top is firm, about 20 minutes.

Turn the cornbread upside down onto a wire rack to remove it from the skillet. Cut it into wedges and serve.

Feel like playing?

If you have access to corn flour for the Northern Cornbread, you'll have an even cornier cornbread. You could also add whole corn kernels. It's hard to make a grain-free cornbread, if you consider corn a grain. But we've made a lovely bread using only buckwheat flakes with this recipe.

MACARONI SALAD

Feeds 6

Look, we know the traditional macaroni salad is gloopy with mayonnaise and mustard, a kind of egg salad with macaroni instead. But after seeing too many macaroni salads wilting in deli cases, we have both lost our taste for that salad. This is a new twist, a sort of Mediterranean flavor to celebrate the summer. The key is this strong oregano vinaigrette, inspired by one we tried during our visit to Mozza in Los Angeles. It has a bite to it, a memorable taste that mingles with the feta and sun-dried tomatoes to taste a little fresher than that macaroni salad you have eaten for decades.

FOR THE OREGANO VINAIGRETTE

1 tablespoon red wine vinegar

1 tablespoon dried oregano

Freshly squeezed juice of 1 lemon

1 clove garlic, peeled and minced

Kosher salt and freshly ground black pepper

¾ cup extra-virgin olive oil

FOR THE SALAD

4 cups cooked gluten-free macaroni

2 large stalks celery

¼ cup sun-dried tomatoes, soaked and drained

1 ounce (¼ cup) crumbled feta cheese

¼ cup kalamata olives

½ small red onion, peeled and chopped

2 tablespoons chopped fresh Italian parsley

Freshly grated zest of 1 lemon

Kosher salt and freshly ground black pepper

Make the vinaigrette. Combine the vinegar, oregano, lemon juice, garlic, and salt and pepper in a mason jar. Shake them up to combine. Let the ingredients rest for 5 minutes to allow the oregano to hydrate. Slowly pour the olive oil into the jar and shake it all up. (If you want the vinaigrette to fully emulsify, do this in a blender instead.)

Make the salad. Combine the cooked macaroni, celery, sun-dried tomatoes, feta cheese, olives, onions, parsley, and lemon zest in a large bowl. Slowly, drizzle some of the vinaigrette around the edges of the bowl. Toss the salad thoroughly before adding more vinaigrette. You don't want to overdress this salad. And save some of that vinaigrette for later. Season with salt and pepper and serve immediately.

Feel like playing?

If you do want to make the traditional macaroni salad gluten-free, simply combine the macaroni with mayonnaise, mustard, celery, onion, parsley, and a few tablespoons of sour cream. I bet you can make a great one.

MACARONI AND CHEESE

Feeds 4

Macaroni and cheese has become ubiquitous in the American diet, particularly since that blue box of mac and cheese showed up in grocery stores in the 1930s. It's hard to name the region of the United States in which this originated, although New England claims it as macaroni pudding, a popular casserole at church suppers. There are some that claim Thomas Jefferson brought the idea for the dish home to Virginia after a trip to Italy. (I like that idea best, of one of our founding fathers also inventing our most popular dish.) Given this, there are as many ways to make macaroni and cheese as there are people who want to eat it. This is a quick method, intended for families who want to eat fast. Instead of making a roux and classic cheese sauce, we let the magic of pasta water thicken the cheese sauce. With this recipe, you can have macaroni and cheese on the table as quickly as you could if you bought that box.

1 pound gluten-free macaroni

4 ounces (1 cup) freshly grated Cheddar cheese

4 ounces soft chèvre

Kosher salt and freshly ground black pepper

Cook the pasta. Set a large pot of water over high heat. Add enough salt to make the water taste like the ocean. When the water comes to a boil, pour in the pasta. Stir continuously for the first minute. Cook until the pasta has softened but still has a good bite. The time will differ according to the brand of pasta you use, but start checking after about 8 minutes.

Make the sauce. Spread the Cheddar cheese on the bottom of a large bowl. Dot the top of the Cheddar with the chèvre. When the pasta is cooked al dente, drain, reserving a little more than ½ cup of the pasta water, and move the pasta over to the bowl, on top of the cheeses. Add ½ cup of the pasta water to the bowl as well. Do NOT stir. Let the pasta sit for 5 minutes.

After 5 minutes, stir up the cheeses and pasta. You should have a good, creamy sauce. If it's not quite creamy enough, add more pasta water 1 tablespoon at a time. Season with salt and pepper.

Feel like playing?

There's so much playing you could do here. If you don't have access to chèvre, try an equal weight of cream cheese. We like Gruyère or Parmesan in place of the Cheddar. We also like to add vegetables to this, like thin slices of sweet potato, handfuls of kale, or leaves of spinach. After the 5 minutes of sitting in the hot pasta, the vegetables wilt to become part of the dish. Smoked paprika, fennel seeds, or dried oregano add to the taste as well.

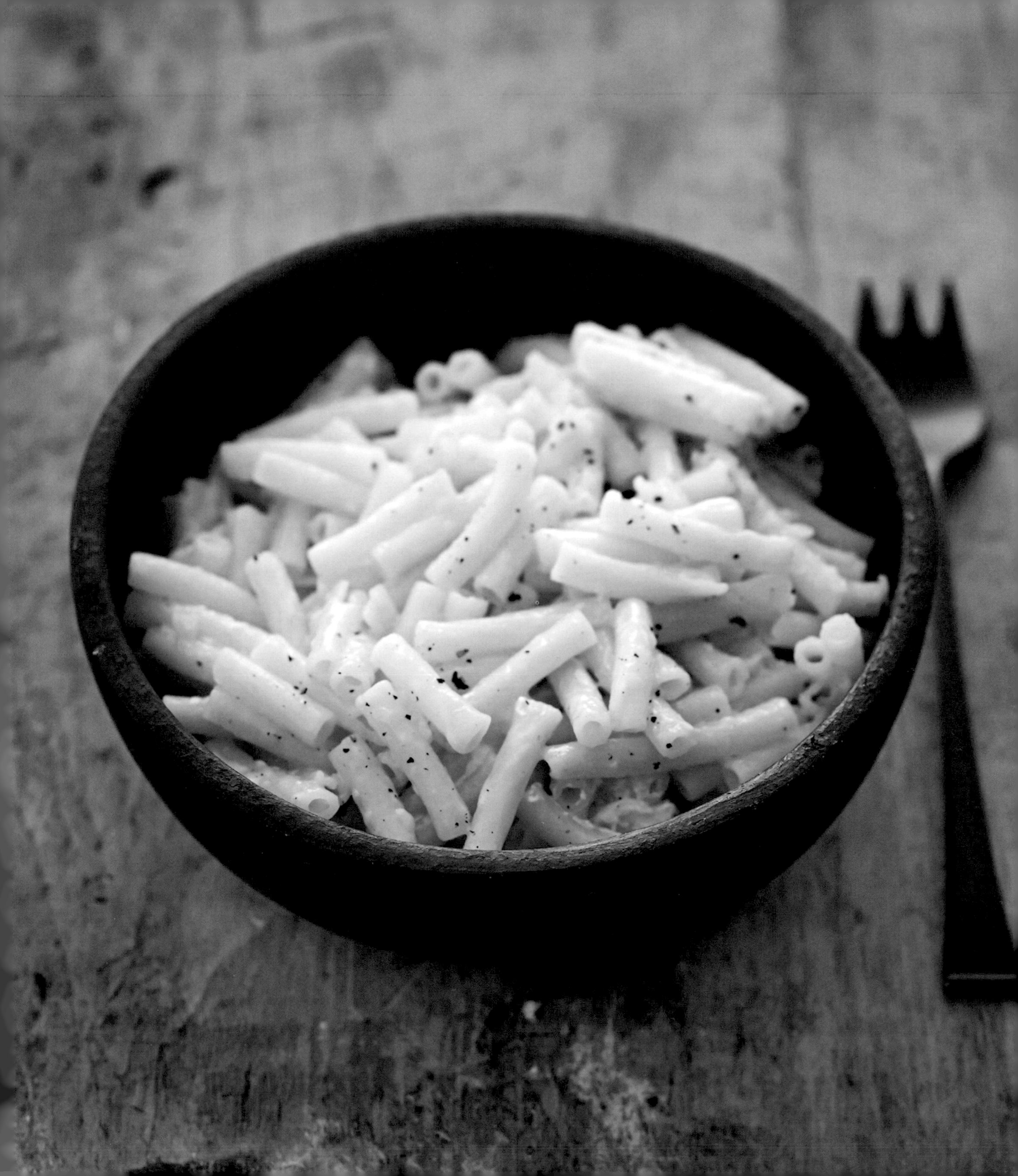

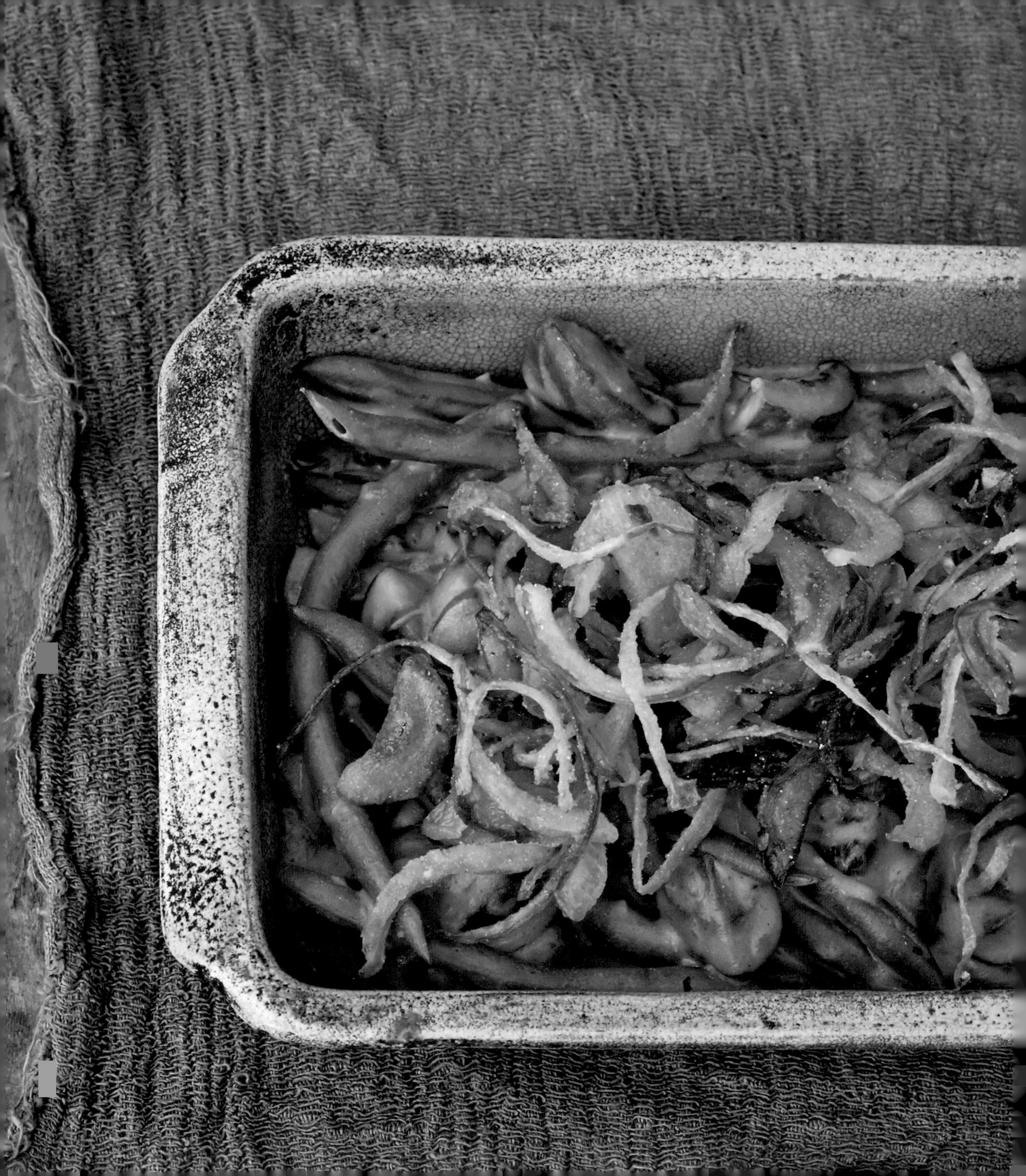

GREEN BEAN CASSEROLE

Feeds 6

This might be the ultimate American casserole. The traditional one uses canned green beans, canned cream of mushroom soup, and fried onions out of a can. This recipe, adapted from Alton Brown and Deb Perelman at Smitten Kitchen, requires only a few more steps to make a side dish for Thanksgiving dinner that everyone might love. It's a lot more memorable than the one out of a can.

1½ pounds green beans, trimmed and snapped in half

FOR THE CRISP ONIONS

70 grams All-Purpose Gluten-Free Flour Blend (page 17)

Kosher salt and freshly ground black pepper

2 medium yellow onions, peeled and thinly sliced

Peanut oil or lard for frying

FOR THE CASSEROLE

1½ cups chicken or vegetable stock (if you're using boxed stock, make sure it's gluten-free)

3 tablespoons unsalted butter

2 cups sliced cremini or white mushrooms

Kosher salt

2 cloves garlic, peeled and minced

35 grams All-Purpose Gluten-Free Flour Blend (page 17)

½ cup coconut milk

Freshly ground black pepper

Prepare to cook. Preheat the oven to 400°F.

Blanch the green beans. Set a large pot of salted water over high heat. Bring the water to a boil. Put a large bowl of ice water in the sink. Put the green beans in the boiling water and cook for 5 minutes. (If the beans are slender, cook for 3 minutes.) Plunge the hot green beans into the ice water. Let them sit for 1 minute, then immediately drain the water. Dry the beans with a towel and spread them out on a baking sheet to air-dry entirely.

Make the crisp onions. Put the flour and salt and pepper into a wide bowl. Toss the onions in the flour to coat entirely. Put enough fat into a large cast-iron skillet to make a depth of 1 inch. Set the skillet over medium-high heat. When you can flick a tip-of-your-finger-full of water into the fat and it sizzles, you are ready to fry. Lower a light layer of the sliced onions into the fat and fry until they are lightly golden. Remove them with a slotted spoon and transfer to a plate lined with paper towels. Repeat until all the onions are fried. Set them aside for later.

Make the mushroom sauce. Pour the stock into a large pot and bring to a boil over high heat. Turn the heat down to low and keep it at a simmer. Set a cast-iron skillet over medium-high heat. Put the butter in the skillet. When the butter has melted, add the mushrooms and season lightly with salt. Cook, stirring occasionally, until the mushrooms are hot and wilted, about 5 minutes. Add the garlic and cook, stirring, for 2 more minutes. Toss the flour over the tops of the mushrooms and stir until the mushrooms are fully coated. Pour ¼ cup of the hot stock into the skillet, stirring constantly. When the stock is incorporated into the mushrooms and bubbly hot, add another 1/4 cup. Continue this until all the stock is added and the sauce is thick. Add the coconut milk and keep stirring until the sauce is reduced and thickened, about 5 minutes.

Assemble the casserole. Put the green beans into a large baking dish. Pour in the mushroom sauce. Toss until everything is coated. Sprinkle a bit of pepper on top. Top with the crisp onions. Bake until the sauce is bubbly around the edges of the onions, about 15 minutes. Serve.

Feel like playing?

This makes a lot of crispy onions. You might not want to use them all for the casserole. Then again, you might. If you have leftovers, they're great in green salads. For an even thicker sauce, use 1 more tablespoon of butter and 2 more tablespoons of flour. If you don't want to use coconut milk, use cream in its place.

SCALLOPED POTATOES

Feeds 6

My mom always made scalloped potatoes from scratch for Easter dinner. We weren't terribly religious, but we ate these potatoes every year. Danny ate them only from the box, and he didn't care for them until he had some made by a French chef at one of the restaurants where he worked. There, he learned to beat eggs until stiff and dip the potato slices in them to thicken the sauce even more. I don't think you have to wait until Easter to eat these potatoes. That would be a shame.

- 2 large egg whites, at room temperature
- ¼ teaspoon cream of tartar
- 3 pounds russet potatoes, peeled and thinly sliced
- 3 cups whole milk
- 1 clove garlic, peeled
- 1 sprig fresh rosemary
- Few scrapes freshly grated nutmeg
- 3 tablespoons unsalted butter, softened
- 6 ounces (1½ cups) freshly grated Parmesan cheese (Gruyère or Swiss would be good too)
- 1 cup heavy cream
- Kosher salt and freshly ground black pepper

Prepare to cook. Preheat the oven to 375°F.

Beat the egg whites. Add the egg whites and cream of tartar to the bowl of a stand mixer. (Make sure the mixer is clean and dry.) Using the whisk attachment, beat the egg whites to stiff peaks. Set aside.

Simmer the potatoes. Set a Dutch oven over high heat. Add the potatoes, milk, garlic, rosemary, and nutmeg to the pot. Bring the milk to a boil, stir, and reduce the heat to low. Simmer until the potatoes are tender, about 4 minutes.

Drain the potatoes. Drain the potatoes into a colander set over the sink, with a bowl under it to keep the milk. The milk will be thick with the potato starch, which will help the texture of the final dish. Remove the rosemary and garlic and discard.

Assemble the casserole. Grease a 9 x 13-inch baking dish with the butter. Gently, toss the potato slices in the stiff egg whites. Arrange one layer of sliced potatoes in the greased dish. Top them with half of the cheese. Repeat with another layer of potatoes. Pour the reserved milk and the cream evenly over the dish. Season with salt and pepper. Top with the remaining cheese. Bake until the milk and cream have thickened and the cheese on top is bubbly brown, about 45 minutes. Serve immediately.

Feel like playing?

If you cannot eat dairy, you can use your favorite nondairy milk here. We've tried coconut milk in place of the cream, which lends a definite coconut taste to the dish. I like it just fine, actually. You might too.

CHEESY CORN CASSEROLE

Feeds 6

This is not a diet dish. Let's just state that right away. With bacon, butter, milk, and three kinds of cheeses, it can only nominally be called a vegetable side dish. But, this is an American classics book and some Americans love this kind of dairy-and-calorie bomb occasionally. (We would be some of those Americans.) Made famous as a barbecue side at Smokestack restaurant in Kansas City, this recipe came to us through a Saveur *feature on great barbecue places. Frankly, we wanted one of everything we saw, but this decadent, cheesy side—a little mac and cheese, a little Mornay sauce, a little bit heaven—stuck with us the longest. We cut the Velveeta and cream cheese and added Gruyère and chèvre instead. But really, it's just a darned fine side.*

Fat for greasing the baking dish

4 thick slices bacon, chopped

6 tablespoons unsalted butter

4 cloves garlic, peeled and minced

70 grams All-Purpose Gluten-Free Flour Blend (page 17)

3 cups whole milk (we'd use rice milk if you have to be dairy-free)

8 ounces (2 cups) freshly grated Cheddar cheese

4 ounces (1 cup) freshly grated Gruyère cheese

2 ounces soft chèvre

1 teaspoon smoked paprika

3 pounds corn kernels

Kosher salt and freshly ground black pepper

Prepare to cook. Preheat the oven to 375°F. Grease a 9 x 13-inch baking dish.

Cook the bacon. Set a Dutch oven over medium heat. Add the bacon. Cook, stirring frequently, until the bacon is browned and has released its fat, about 8 minutes.

Make the roux. Add the butter and garlic to the Dutch oven and cook, stirring, until the scent is released, about 1 minute. Add the flour to the mix and whisk it constantly until it begins to brown, about 1 minute.

Make the sauce. Whisk in the milk, a little at a time, stirring constantly. When all the milk has been added, bring it to a boil, being careful not to burn it. Cook until everything has thickened, about 2 minutes. Add all three cheeses and the smoked paprika. Cook, stirring frequently, until all the cheese has melted and the mixture is smooth. Turn off the heat. Add the corn and stir. Season with salt and pepper.

Bake the casserole. Pour the cheesy corn goodness into the prepared baking dish. Bake until the top is browned and bubbling, about 45 minutes. Let it cool just a bit before serving so you don't burn your mouth.

Feel like playing?

You could make this vegetarian by skipping the bacon and going right to the butter and garlic. Frankly, I wouldn't try to make this lower in calories or fat. Eat a small amount and enjoy it. The next day, have salad instead.

POTATO FILLING

Feeds 6

We were first introduced to potato filling in a church basement in Lancaster County, Pennsylvania. When the good folks who threw the potluck for us there pointed out the baking dish full of piping-hot potatoes and bread, Danny and I were confused. What was potato filling? "You've never heard of this?" they asked, amazed. "Oh, this is such a Dutchy dish!" (Dutchy *is the adjective for Pennsylvania Dutch.) Danny ate some, since they had brought the gluten version for him to try, and he was instantly won over. Take creamy mashed potatoes and bread stuffing for the Thanksgiving table, combine them in a baking dish, dot them with butter, and bake until everything is hot and bubbling. We make this for our Thanksgiving dinner now.*

Fat for greasing the baking dish

FOR THE MASHED POTATOES

4 large russet potatoes, peeled and chopped into similar-size cubes

4 tablespoons unsalted butter, softened

2 to 3 tablespoons extra-virgin olive oil

Kosher salt and freshly ground black pepper

FOR THE STUFFING

1 loaf gluten-free Sandwich Bread (page 53), diced into 1-inch cubes

4 tablespoons unsalted butter

1 large yellow onion, peeled and chopped

2 stalks celery, chopped

2 tablespoons chopped fresh sage

FOR THE FILLING

3 large eggs, at room temperature, beaten

½ cup heavy cream or coconut milk (optional)

4 tablespoons unsalted butter

Prepare to cook. Preheat the oven to 350°F. Grease the bottoms and sides of a 9 x 13-inch baking dish.

Cook the potatoes. Set a Dutch oven on the stove. Fill it three-quarters full with cold water and enough salt to make it taste like the ocean. Add the potatoes to the cold water. Bring the water to a boil over high heat, then reduce the heat to medium. Simmer until a knife slides right through one of the potatoes without any force, 10 to 15 minutes. Drain the potatoes into a colander in the sink. Let the potatoes steam there for about 5 minutes to allow them to dry.

Rice the potatoes. If you own a potato ricer or food mill, push the potatoes through it. Or, you could push the potatoes through a fine-mesh sieve with the back of a ramekin or wooden spoon.

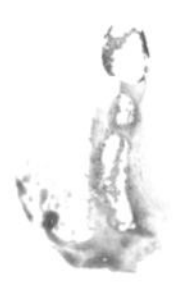

Mash the potatoes. Put the potatoes back in the Dutch oven. Stir the softened butter into the potatoes and fold it in with a rubber spatula. Pour in the oil and continue to fold until the potatoes are a smooth puree. Season with salt and pepper.

Toast the bread. Spread the bread cubes out on a baking sheet. Put the baking sheet in the oven and toast the bread. After 10 minutes or so, toss the bread cubes around to another side. When all sides are toasted, about 20 minutes, take the bread out of the oven.

Make the stuffing. Set a Dutch oven over medium heat. Add the butter. When the butter has melted, add the onions and celery. Cook until the onions are soft and translucent, stirring occasionally, about 7 minutes. Add the sage and cook, stirring, until the scent is released, about 1 minute. Stir in the bread cubes.

Make the filling. Put the mashed potatoes and stuffing together in a large bowl. Add the eggs and fold them all together. If you feel the filling is not quite creamy enough, you can add the cream or coconut milk. Pour the filling into the prepared baking dish. Dot the top with the butter. Bake until the top is bubbling golden brown, about 45 minutes.

Serve. Afterward, lie down.

Feel like playing?

Try another herb, like thyme, in place of the sage. You could easily use another fat in place of the butter. Choose the one that works best for your family.

SMOKY SWEET CORN FRITTERS

Feeds 6

In the middle of July and into August, there's nothing better than fresh corn. For the first few days of corn season, we eat corn on the cob with nearly every dinner. At first, that corn is slathered in butter and salt. Then we graduate to cotija cheese and a squeeze of lime juice. By the second or third week, we still crave corn but we want a different texture. Grilling the corn before cutting off the kernels, plus the sharp bite of aged Cheddar cheese and a shake of smoked paprika, makes these smoky sweet corn fritters a little unexpected and very much a hit at every summer party we have thrown.

6 ears sweet corn, husks and threads removed

3 tablespoons extra-virgin olive oil

2 large eggs, beaten

4 ounces (1 cup) freshly grated sharp Cheddar cheese (or soft chèvre)

4 scallions, finely sliced

⅓ cup chopped fresh basil leaves

45 grams All-Purpose Gluten-Free Flour Blend (page 17)

½ teaspoon smoked paprika (optional)

Kosher salt and freshly ground black pepper

Fat or oil of your choice for frying (we use olive oil or butter)

Prepare to cook. Fire up the grill. Make sure it's screaming hot.

Grill the corn. Coat the ears of corn in the olive oil. Put them on the grill. Let them get a bit of color on one side, about 2 minutes, then flip and grill until all the sides are smoky hot and almost charred. Remove the corn from the grill and allow to cool to room temperature.

Prepare the corn. Using a sharp knife, slice the kernels off the corn. Flip the knife around and use the back of the knife to push out as much of the milk from the kernels as possible. Put the kernels and milk into a large bowl.

Make the fritter batter. Mix the eggs, cheese, scallions, basil, flour, smoked paprika, and salt and pepper with the corn. Let the batter sit for a few moments for the liquids to absorb the flour.

Make a tester. Set a large skillet over medium heat. Add enough of the fat of your choice to make a generous puddle in the middle of the skillet. Make a small fritter with the corn batter and put it in the hot fat. Fry until the bottom is golden brown, about 2 minutes, then flip and fry it on the other side. Turn off the heat and take the fritter out of the skillet to cool. Taste the fritter. Need more salt and pepper? A little more smokiness? More cheese? Add to your own taste.

CONTINUED

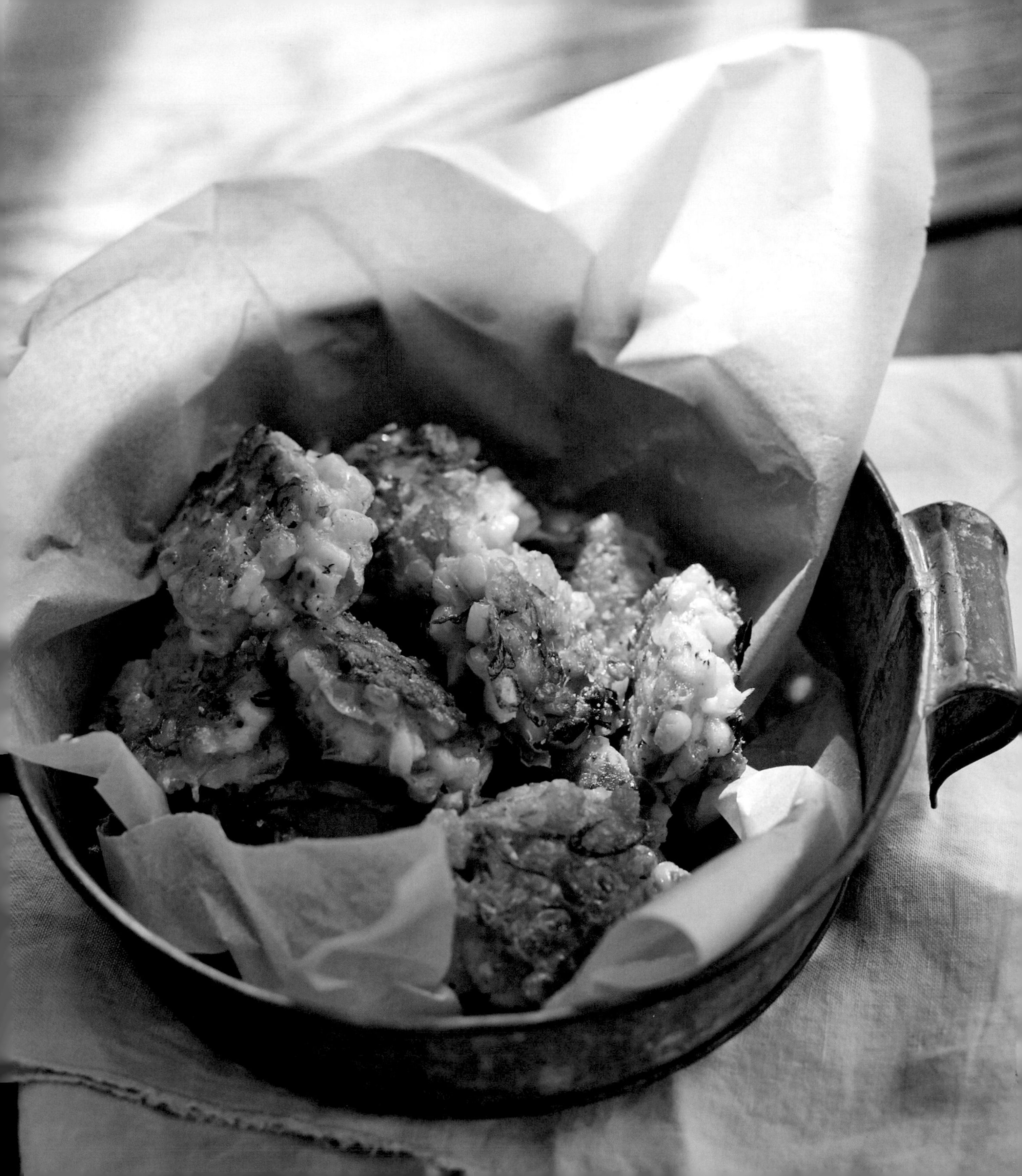

Make the fritters. Turn the heat on medium again. Add enough fat to cover the entire skillet. Fry the fritters in the same way you fried the tester. When both sides are golden brown, transfer the fritters to a serving platter.

Feel like playing?

We don't specify the fat for frying because each of you will have a preference here. But using melted butter or lard gives these fritters quite the savory taste. If you want a less smoky flavor in these fritters, simply omit the grilling step and the smoked paprika. If you need to be dairy-free as well as gluten-free, take out the cheese and add a bit more flour for bulk. Finally, we learned a trick for cutting corn from Saveur *magazine: balance the corncob on the center stem of a Bundt pan, then let the kernels and milk fall into the pan. This will make you cook corn fritters more often.*

CALIFORNIA ROLL SUSHI SALAD

Feeds 4

The first sushi I ever ate, back in the 1980s, was a California roll. That's not much of a surprise—this popular-in-America roll with avocado and crab contains no raw fish. Quickly, I graduated to spicy tuna rolls and the omakase *menu at good sushi restaurants. Sushi remains one of my favorite foods of all time. I stopped eating California rolls a while ago. Most California rolls use imitation crabmeat, which contains gluten. But the combination of crab, avocado, and cucumber still inspires me. Danny and I started playing with a sushi rice salad with those flavors and fell in love with this dish. We serve it as a side dish with salmon or as a main course on a hot day.*

FOR THE VINEGAR RICE

2 cups sushi rice

2 cups water

¼ cup rice wine vinegar

3 tablespoons organic cane sugar

1 teaspoon kosher salt

FOR THE SALAD

1 tablespoon gluten-free tamari

1 teaspoon wasabi powder

1 avocado, pitted, peeled, and cut into thin slices

1 large cucumber, peeled and cut into matchsticks

½ cup fresh lump crabmeat

1 tablespoon pickled ginger, cut into slices

Make the vinegar rice. Rinse the rice under cold water until the water runs clear, at least 10 minutes. This removes much of the starch, making the rice easier to cook. Set a small pot over high heat. Add the rice and water. Bring the water to a boil, then reduce the heat to low. Simmer the rice with the lid on the pot, which will steam the rice, for 15 minutes. Turn off the heat. Keep the lid on the pot and allow it to sit for 15 more minutes. Mix together the vinegar, sugar, and salt. Transfer the rice to a baking sheet, then drizzle the salty vinegar over it. Gently, fold the vinegar into the rice, being careful not to smoosh the rice. Spread out the rice and allow it to cool.

Make the toppings. Whisk together the tamari and wasabi powder. Put the avocado, cucumber, and crabmeat into a large bowl. Drizzle the tamari mixture over them and toss lightly.

Finish the salad. Add the cooled rice and the pickled ginger to the bowl. Toss gently. Serve.

Feel like playing?

As much as we love white rice, sometimes we prefer this salad with cucumber as the base. If you have a spiralizer or mandoline, cut the cucumber into long noodles. Serve the crab-avocado mixture over the cucumber, dressing with the wasabi and tamari mixture.

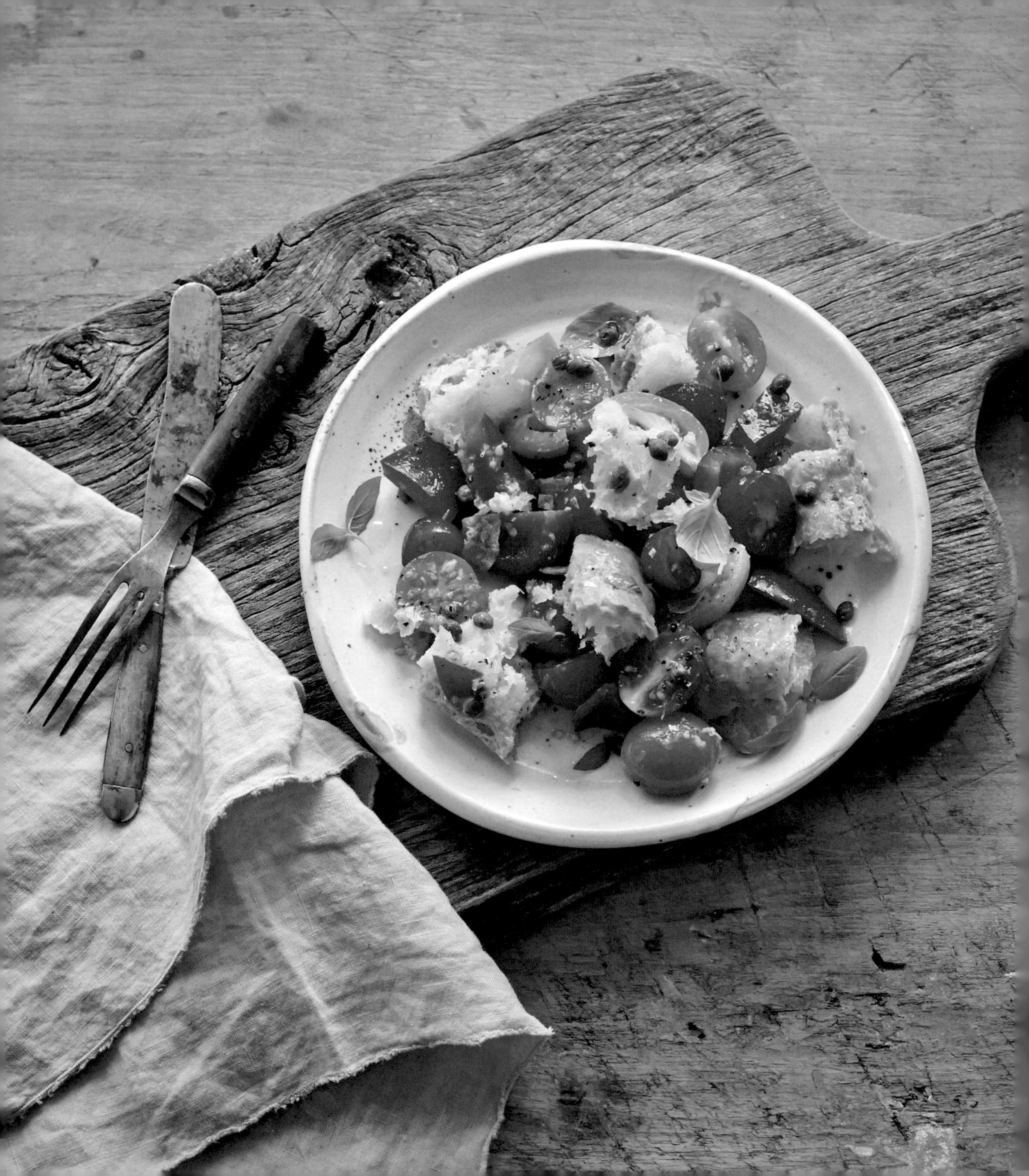

PANZANELLA

Feeds 6

This Tuscan-inspired salad is a classic make-do dish when you don't have much money. You have stale bread (that's easy with gluten-free!), some ripe tomatoes, some other vegetables, and some leftover vinaigrette. Go. It's funny that it has been elevated to some sort of gourmet dish. Really, you just tear apart bread with your hands, soak it in a vinaigrette with a strong acid kick, and throw in what you have. Summertime, late evening, this is one of my favorite meals in the world.

FOR THE VINAIGRETTE

1 tablespoon red wine vinegar

1 tablespoon fresh basil leaves

Freshly grated zest and freshly squeezed juice of 1 lemon

3 anchovies

¾ cup extra-virgin olive oil

Kosher salt and freshly ground black pepper

FOR THE SALAD

½ gluten-free Sourdough Bread baguette or boule (page 50), torn into pieces

2 pounds ripe tomatoes, chopped

2 large red bell peppers, diced

1 cup fresh basil leaves, torn into pieces

¼ cup drained capers

Make the vinaigrette. Add the vinegar, basil, lemon zest and juice, and anchovies to a blender. Puree everything together. With the blender running on low, slowly drizzle in the olive oil until the vinaigrette is smooth and emulsified. Taste. Season with salt and pepper, but remember that the anchovies are salty and the capers in the salad will also add salt.

Soak the bread. Put the bread in a large bowl. Pour half the vinaigrette onto the bread and toss it to coat evenly. Set aside the bowl for 10 minutes.

Dress the vegetables. Put the tomatoes, peppers, basil, and capers into another bowl. Toss them with enough vinaigrette to coat but not enough to drown the vegetables. (You probably won't use all of it yet.) Let the vegetables sit for 10 minutes.

Finish the salad. Combine the soaked bread and dressed vegetables. Toss together. If you feel you need to add more vinaigrette, do so here. Let the salad sit for 15 minutes before serving.

Feel like playing?

This recipe is meant for playing. These are only suggestions, after all. Once you have this basic template, you can use whatever you want in this salad. Cucumbers? Sure. Red onions? Why not? Yellow peppers and jalapeños? Go. Just remember—this is nothing more than a delicious way to use up stale bread.

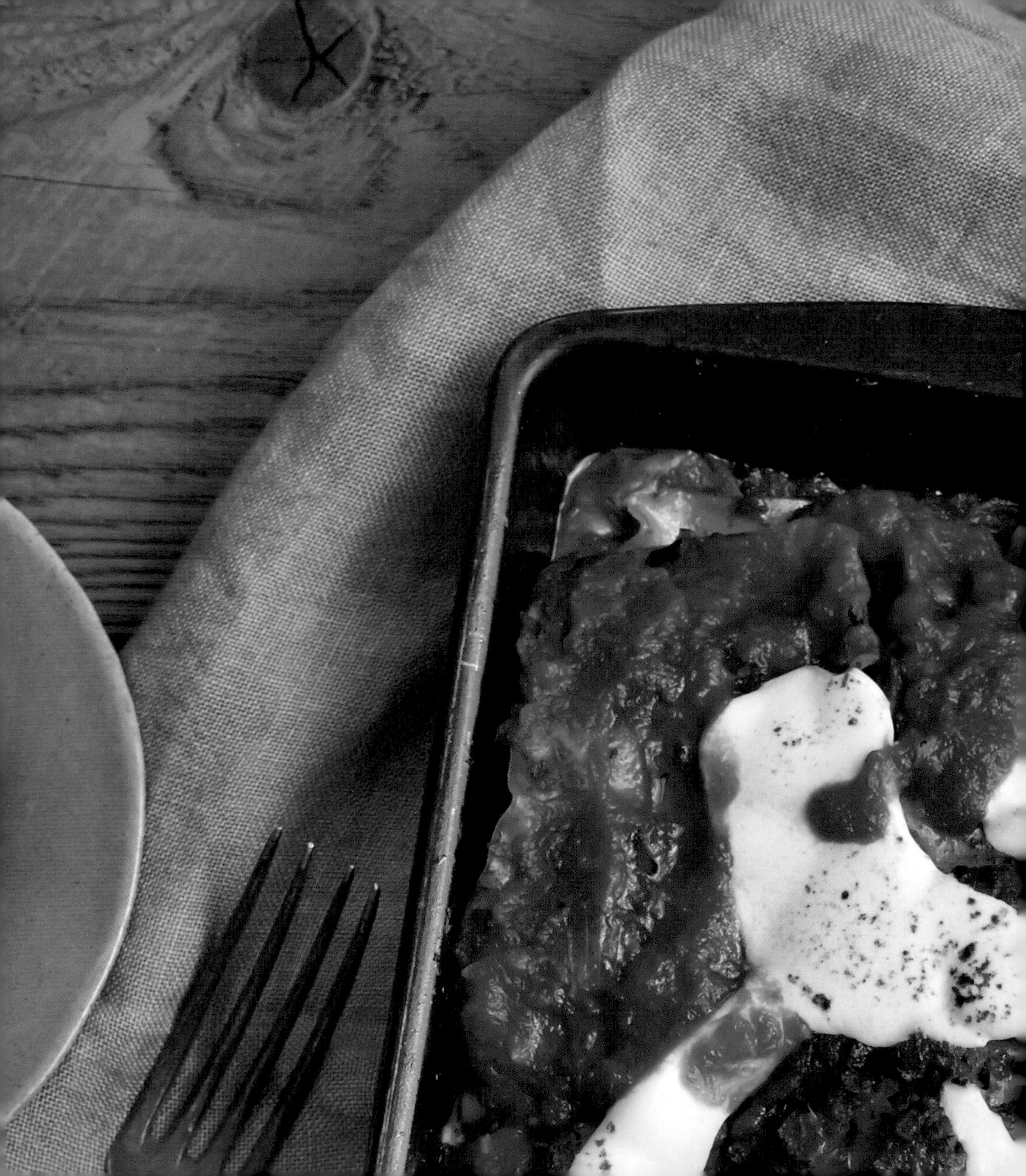

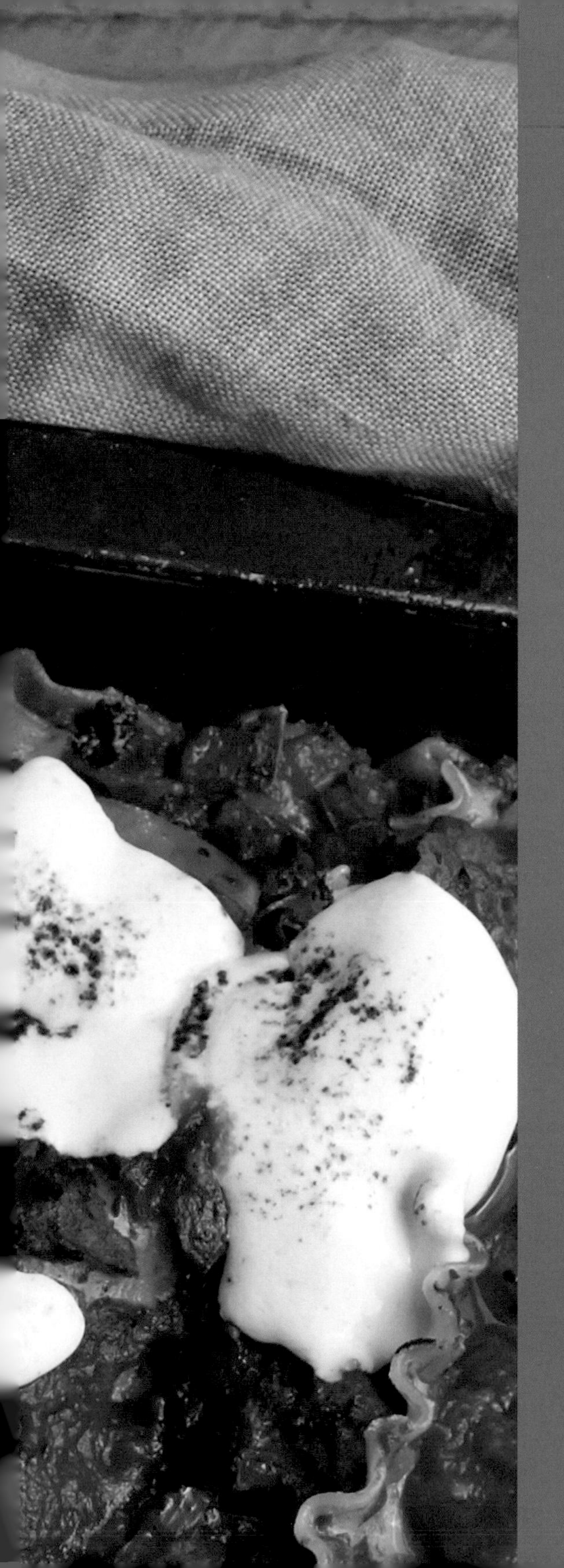

MEAT MAIN DISHES

CHICKEN-FRIED STEAK

Feeds 4

It's not clear where chicken-fried steak started (some call it country-fried steak). Texans claim the recipe as theirs, saying a tired short-order cook mixed up a fried chicken recipe and a steak recipe and invented this delicious breaded beef dish. However, there are recipes for it in the Los Angeles Times *in 1924 and in a cookbook published in Topeka, Kansas in the 1940s. Clearly, chicken-fried steak belongs to all of us. Danny and I did a methodical taste test one day, making chicken-fried steak with every possible cut of beef we could think of. The good news? The absolutely best chicken-fried steak was made with cube steak, the cheapest cut of beef! Even after a day of eating bits of chicken-fried steak all day, we still love this dish.*

2 pounds cube steak, cut into 4 pieces

Kosher salt and freshly ground black pepper

140 grams All-Purpose Gluten-Free Flour Blend (page 17)

½ teaspoon garlic powder

½ teaspoon onion powder

½ teaspoon finely chopped fresh rosemary

3 large eggs, beaten

Fat or oil of your choice for frying (we use peanut oil or lard)

2½ cups whole milk

Prepare to cook. Using a meat mallet, pound each cube steak to a ¼-inch thickness. Season the cube steak with salt and pepper on both sides.

Season the flour. In a wide bowl, combine the flour with the garlic powder, onion powder, and rosemary. Add the eggs to another wide bowl next to the flour.

Dredge the steaks. Dredge a cube steak on both sides in the flour. Dredge it in the eggs, then in the flour again. Put the cube steak on a wire rack. Finish the rest of the steaks in the same way. Let the steaks sit for 15 minutes before cooking.

Cook the chicken-fried steaks. Set a large cast-iron skillet over medium-high heat. Add enough fat to the skillet to generously cover the bottom of the skillet. When the fat is hot, add 2 of the steaks to the pan. Cook until the bottom is brown and crisp, about 4 minutes. Flip the steaks and cook until the other side is golden brown, about 4 minutes more. Move the steaks to a plate and repeat with the remaining steaks.

At this point, if you wish, you can put the chicken-fried steaks in an oven set to 300°F to keep them warm while you make the gravy.

Make the gravy. Scrape up all the golden brown bits from the bottom of the skillet. Turn the heat to medium-low. Add 3 tablespoons of the flour remaining in the dredging bowl to the skillet and whisk

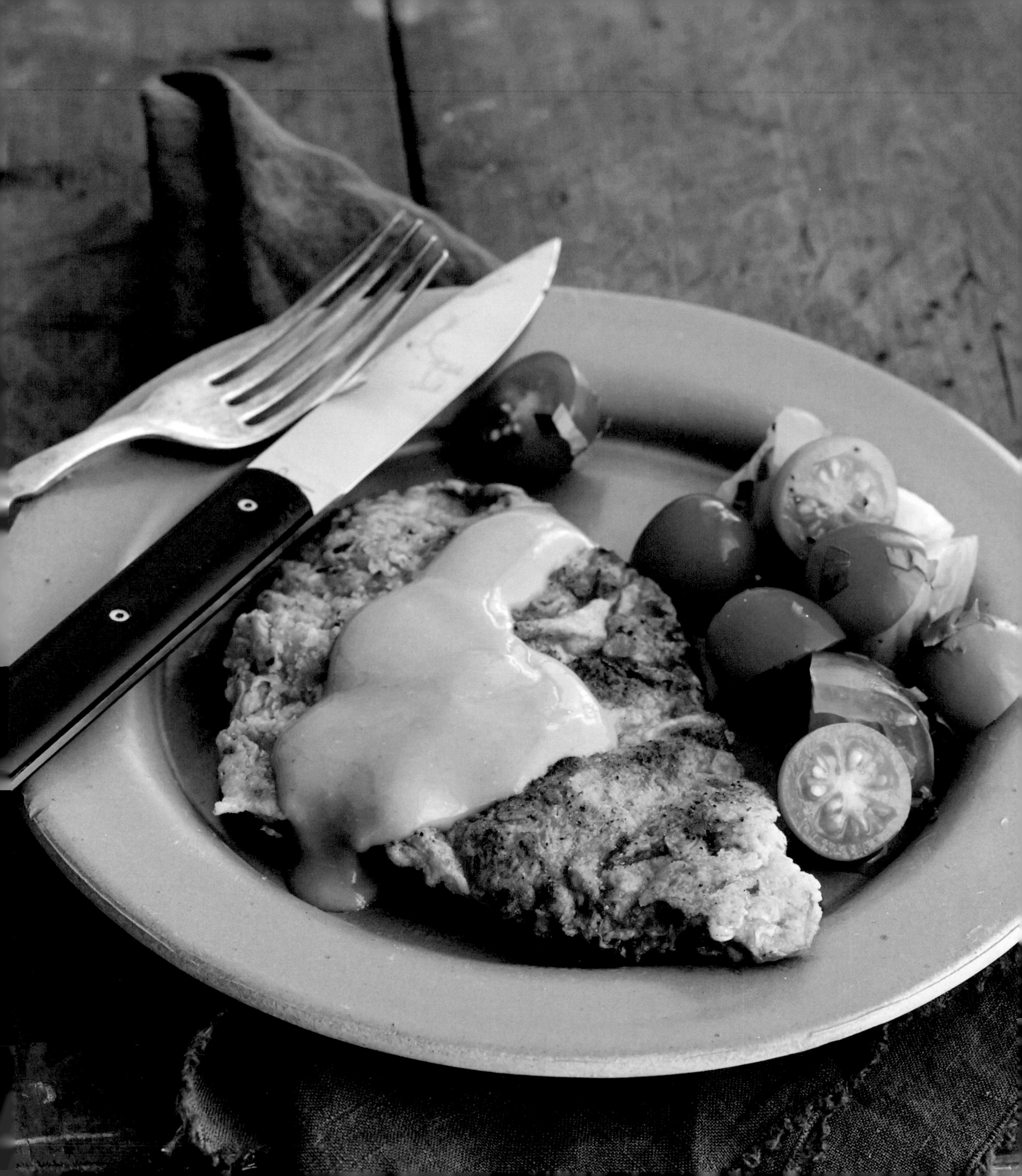

it into the hot fat, stirring constantly. When the flour releases a warm scent, after about 3 minutes, add ½ cup of the milk at a time, whisking constantly. Keep adding milk and whisking until the gravy thickens. When the gravy is thick enough to coat the back of a spoon, after 5 to 10 minutes, season it with salt and pepper.

Serve the chicken-fried steaks with gravy generously poured over them.

Feel like playing?

Milk gravy is the traditional pan gravy here. However, if you would like a less milky gravy, and more of a chicken taste, use 2 cups of chicken broth to ½ cup of milk, or no milk at all!

TERIYAKI CHICKEN

Feeds 4

The flavors of teriyaki are certainly Japanese in nature. However, teriyaki chicken—the dish popular with kids in sushi restaurants and adults all over America—is not traditionally Japanese. Instead, Japanese settlers in Hawaii combined traditional ingredients like soy sauce with local flavors such as pineapple juice and came up with a marinade for chicken. Teriyaki shops are all over Seattle, super cheap and generally great, and I can never have anything from them due to the wheat in soy sauce. But this one? Well, we can have this teriyaki chicken any time we feel like it.

½ cup gluten-free tamari

¼ cup white wine

¼ cup mirin

¼ cup pineapple juice

¼ cup honey

1 ounce fresh ginger, peeled and sliced

2 tablespoons sesame oil

1 clove garlic, peeled and chopped

4 chicken thighs, skin on

4 chicken drumsticks, skin on

Make the marinade. Add the tamari, white wine, mirin, pineapple juice, honey, ginger, sesame oil, and garlic to a blender. Blend until everything is well combined.

Marinate the chicken. Pour the teriyaki marinade over the chicken thighs and drumsticks in a large bowl. Make sure the chicken is completely covered. Marinate for at least 1 hour and as long as 12 hours.

Prepare to cook. Turn on the grill. Crank the heat up as high as possible. Pull the chicken out of the marinade, place onto the grill, and cook, turning occasionally, until the chicken has reached an internal temperature of 180°F, 10 to 12 minutes.

Or, if you don't want to use the grill, preheat the oven to 425°F. Pull the chicken out of the marinade and arrange in a baking pan. Bake until the chicken has reached an internal temperature of 180°F, about 20 minutes. Serve immediately.

Feel like playing?

You could use this same marinade for pork loin, salmon, or tofu.

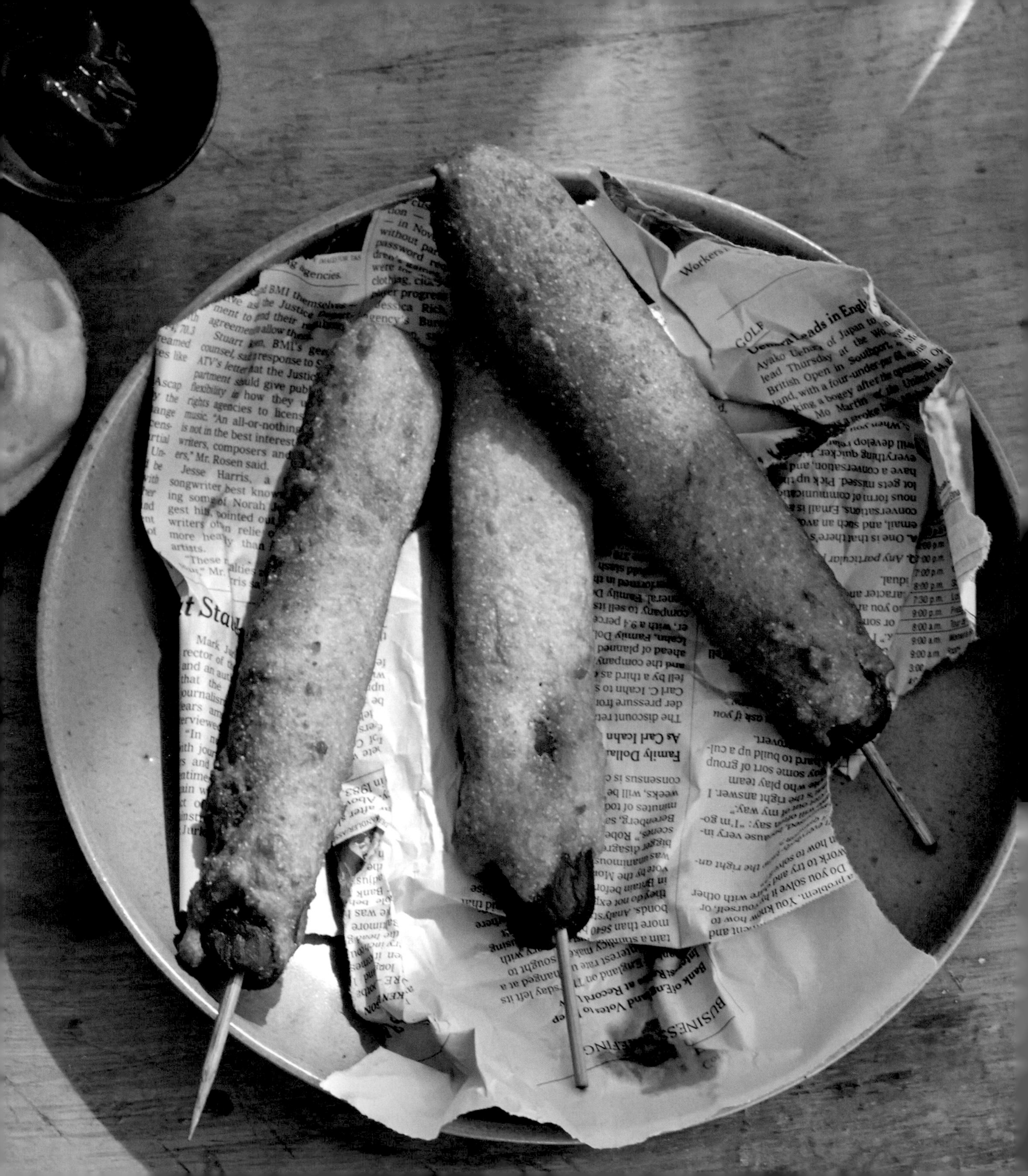

Jesse Harris, a
rights agencies to licens
writers, composers and
ers," Mr. Rosen said.
Ayako Uehara of Japan to
lead Thursday at the
British Open in Southport,
As Carl Icahn
The discount
Bank of England Votes to
BUSINESS

CORN DOGS

Feeds 4

Corn dogs: the food of fairs, amusement parks, and elementary school lunchrooms. I ate my fair share of these as a kid, and then I went years and years without them. Once I learned what was in most hot dogs, I couldn't stomach the thought of coating them in batter and frying them in oil. Luckily, now there are good-quality hot dogs on the market, ones made without nitrites, weird chemicals, or gluten. Imagine hot dogs where we can recognize every ingredient on the package as food! Of course, these shouldn't be everyday food. But on the Fourth of July, eating with friends on a hot day, a gluten-free corn dog is a lovely treat.

¾ cup (120 grams) cornmeal (make sure it's truly gluten-free)

120 grams All-Purpose Gluten-Free Flour Blend (page 17)

1 teaspoon kosher salt

½ teaspoon baking powder

¼ teaspoon baking soda

¾ cup milk (any kind you like)

1 large egg, at room temperature

4 jumbo hot dogs

4 cups fat or oil of your choice for frying (we like rice bran oil for this)

Make the batter. In a bowl, whisk together the cornmeal, flour, salt, baking powder, and baking soda. Make a well in the center of the dry ingredients. Add the milk and egg. Whisk them all together until the batter is smooth. Pour the batter into a tall glass and let it sit for 20 minutes.

Put the hot dogs on wooden skewers.

Heat the oil. Set a Dutch oven over medium-high heat and add the fat. Heat the fat to 360°F, measuring with an instant-read thermometer.

Fry the corn dogs. Dip each hot dog into the batter. Swirl the dog around in the batter until it is fully and evenly coated in batter. Gently, submerge the entire hot dog in the oil. Repeat with another hot dog. Fry the corn dogs until the coating is brown and firm, 4 to 5 minutes. Transfer the corn dogs to a paper towel–lined plate. Let the oil come back up to the proper temperature and fry the remaining corn dogs. Serve immediately.

Feel like playing?

This one is pretty straightforward, so there's not much you can do here. However, if you have access to corn flour (not cornstarch), like the one made by Bob's Red Mill, you could use that as a substitute for the flour blend and have an even cornier-tasting corn dog.

CLASSIC AMERICAN MEAT LOAF (WITH A TWIST)

Feeds 8

Some days, there's really no better meal than meat loaf. Deeply satisfying and meaty, full of flavor, and a great leftover, this is a classic American dish anyone can make. (Okay, vegetarians aren't crazy about this dish.) Of course, Americans didn't invent meat loaf. There were recipes for it in Roman cookbooks and in French cookbooks from the seventeenth century. The idea of mixing meat with spices, eggs, and some form of bread is a human idea of thrift and needing to get dinner on the table. But meat loaf is here to stay in the United States. For all his formal French culinary training and playing with food, Danny still prefers meat loaf to almost any other meal. This one, with milk-soaked gluten-free breadcrumbs and the unexpected savory ingredient of fish sauce (it doesn't make the meat loaf taste like fish, it just makes it delicious), is the one we cook in our kitchen.

Fat for greasing the pan

1½ cups gluten-free breadcrumbs

½ cup whole milk

1 tablespoon extra-virgin olive oil

1 large yellow onion, peeled and chopped

2 cloves garlic, peeled and chopped

½ cup chopped fresh Italian parsley

3 tablespoons chopped fresh basil

1 pound ground pork

1 pound ground beef

3 large eggs, beaten

1 tablespoon fish sauce (make sure it's gluten-free)

1 tablespoon Dijon mustard

1 teaspoon kosher salt

⅓ cup ketchup

Prepare to bake. Preheat the oven to 425°F. Grease a 9 x 5-inch loaf pan. Soak the breadcrumbs in the milk as you make the rest of the meat loaf.

Cook the aromatics. Set a large skillet over medium-high heat. Add the olive oil. When the oil is hot, add the onions and garlic. Cook, stirring occasionally, until the onions are soft and translucent, about 7 minutes. Add the parsley and basil and cook, stirring, until the scent is released, about 1 minute. Take off the heat and let cool.

Make the meat loaf. Put the pork and beef into a large bowl, gently breaking the meat into smaller parts. Add the milk-soaked breadcrumbs, the onion mixture, eggs, fish sauce, mustard, and salt. Mix everything together gently. If you mix the meat loaf too hard, and too thoroughly, it will be tough. Mix only until all the ingredients are mixed together and then stop. Turn over the meat loaf mixture to make sure there aren't ingredients hiding at the bottom and if there are, mix them in. Put the mixture into the loaf pan. Brush the top of the meat loaf with the ketchup.

Bake the meat loaf. Bake until the meat loaf has reached an internal temperature of 155°F, 45 minutes to 1 hour. Cool for 15 minutes before serving.

Feel like playing?

If you can't do the fish sauce, try Worcestershire sauce instead. The best meat loaf we make uses veal along with the pork and the beef, but we only make it when we can find humanely raised veal. Need I mention that this makes a mighty fine cold meat loaf sandwich the next day?

SAUSAGE LASAGNA WITH SLOW TOMATO SAUCE

Feeds 8 to 10

Since I was a kid, I've loved the sound of a big pot of tomato sauce simmering on the back burner all Sunday afternoon. I'm pretty sure I can trace it to the scene in The Godfather *when Clemenza hovers over his sauce, explaining to Michael Corleone how to do this right. Before there were bottled jars of tomato sauce—the only kind I ate as a kid—there were Italian-American grandmothers and uncles making slow tomato sauce. Believe us when we say that your homemade lasagna is worth the 4 or so hours of simmering that this sauce requires. No one will ever complain that this dish is gluten-free.*

FOR THE SAUCE

Two 28-ounce cans Italian tomatoes (San Marzano tomatoes are best)

½ cup extra-virgin olive oil

1 large yellow onion, peeled and chopped

4 cloves garlic, peeled and chopped

Pinch red pepper flakes

Kosher salt

FOR THE LASAGNA

2 tablespoons extra-virgin olive oil

2 pounds sweet Italian sausage, sliced

1 pound cremini mushrooms, sliced

1 large red bell pepper, chopped

3 tablespoons finely chopped fresh basil

1 tablespoon finely chopped fresh oregano

1 package gluten-free lasagna noodles

1 cup ricotta cheese

8 ounces (2 cups) shredded fresh mozzarella cheese

4 ounces (1 cup) freshly grated Parmesan cheese

Prep the tomatoes. Open the cans of tomatoes and pour them into a large bowl. Crush up the tomatoes with your hands, pulling them apart into fine shreds. Sometimes the tops of the tomatoes are tough. If so, take those out. You want soft tomato shreds in juice here.

Make the sauce. Set a Dutch oven over medium-low heat. Pour in ½ cup of the olive oil. When the oil is hot, add the onions and garlic. Cook until the onions and garlic are both browned and fragrant, about 10 minutes. Don't burn them, or the entire sauce will taste disgustoso. Instead, watch the onions and garlic closely. If they start to grow too brown, pull the pot off the heat, reduce the heat,

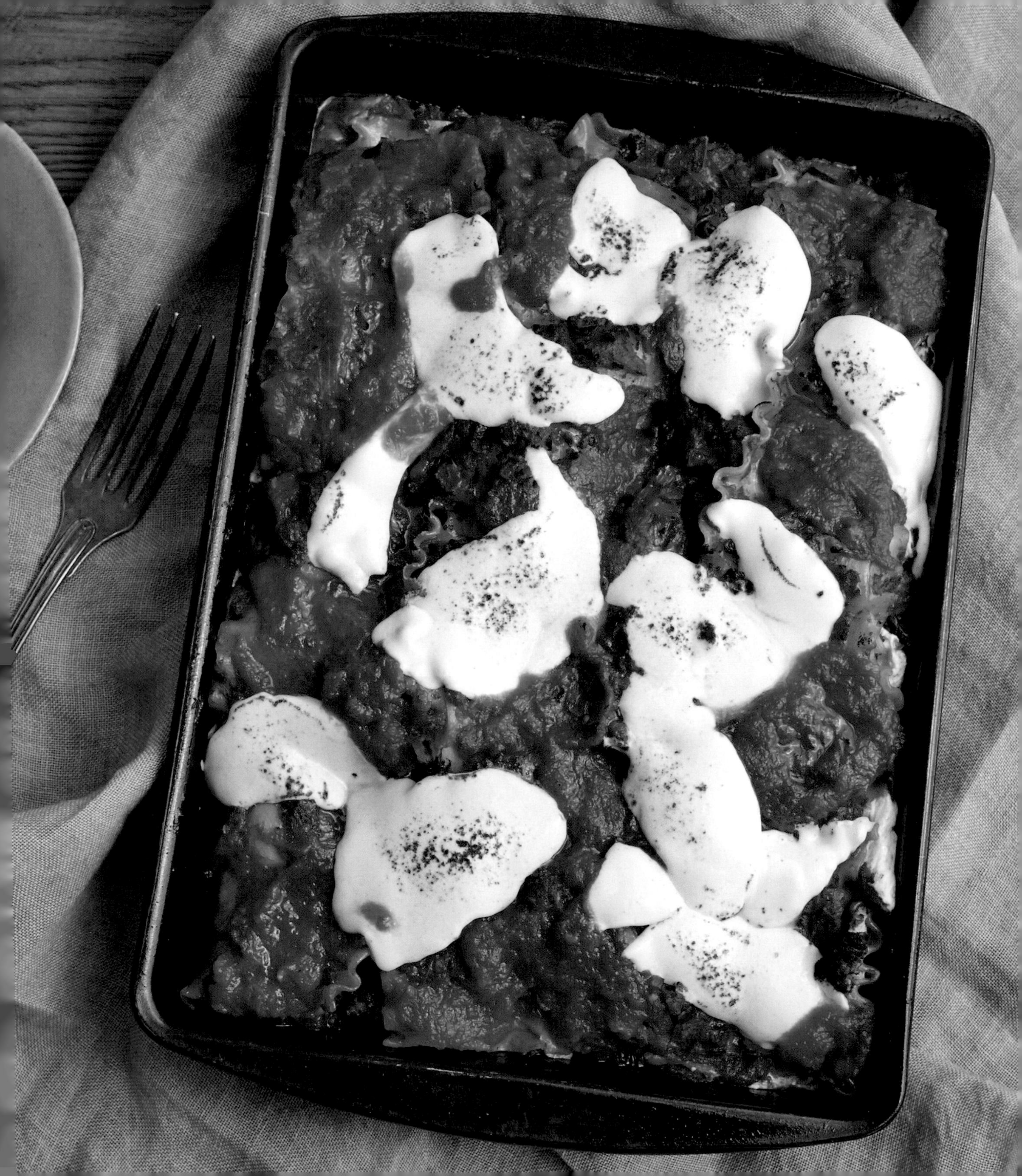

and continue cooking on a lower heat. Pinch in the red pepper flakes and cook for 30 seconds, stirring. Add the tomatoes and stir it all up. Turn the heat down to low and let the tomato sauce simmer, just barely bubbling at the surface, for hours. We mean it—hours. Go watch a movie and get up every 20 minutes or so to give the sauce a stir. Do the laundry. Make lunch. Just watch that sauce and simmer it slowly until it is reduced and smells so good you can't take it anymore. That's usually about 4 hours around here. Season with salt.

Cook the sausage filling. Set a large cast-iron skillet over medium-high heat. Pour in the remaining 2 tablespoons of olive oil. Add the sausage and cook, stirring occasionally, until is browned. Remove the sausage from the pan. Add the mushrooms and bell pepper and cook, stirring occasionally, until the mushrooms are wilted and the pepper is softened, about 5 minutes. Add the basil and oregano and cook, stirring, until the scent is released, about 1 minute. Add the sausage back in and cook, stirring, until heated through.

Prepare to bake. Preheat the oven to 450°F.

Make the lasagna. Put 2 sheets of the pasta, side by side, to cover the bottom of a 9 x 13-inch baking dish. Add enough of the sausage filling to lightly cover the pasta, followed by a scoop of the tomato sauce, some ricotta, some of the mozzarella, and some of the Parmesan. Repeat until the entire baking dish is filled, finishing with a layer of pasta, then tomato sauce, then a thick layer of the mozzarella and Parmesan.

Bake the lasagna. Cover the dish with aluminum foil, making a loose tent to protect that top layer of cheese, and slide it into the oven. Bake for 20 minutes. Remove the aluminum foil and bake until the cheese is browned and bubbly, about 10 minutes. Cool for 10 minutes, or until you can't wait one more minute, then serve.

Note: Our favorite gluten-free lasagna noodles are made by Jovial, from Italy.

Feel like playing?

You can easily make this a vegetarian lasagna by removing the sausage. Vegan? Well, you could use dairy-free cheese. And if you are avoiding grains, we've done a variation on this with long strips of zucchini as the lasagna noodles! Also, you'll probably have tomato sauce left over. What a shame! You'll have to make pasta or dishes all week long with homemade tomato sauce instead of picking up another jar from the store.

BREADED PORK CHOPS

Feeds 4

Many of us grew up eating breaded pork chops with breading that came from a box. You might have eaten this too—remember watching your mom or dad shake the pork chop in the supplied bag full of spices and flour, then baked them in the oven? Well, there's no need to buy that box, especially because it's full of gluten. Take a few minutes to make your own breading and you'll have a far fresher meal than the one from the box could ever provide.

- Four 12-ounce bone-in pork chops
- Kosher salt and freshly ground black pepper
- ½ cup cornmeal (make sure it's gluten-free)
- ½ cup gluten-free breadcrumbs
- 1 tablespoon smoked paprika
- 1 teaspoon ground fennel seeds
- 1 teaspoon dried oregano
- ½ teaspoon onion powder
- ½ teaspoon garlic powder
- 5 tablespoons Dijon mustard

Prepare to bake. Preheat the oven to 400°F. Line a baking sheet with parchment paper. Put a wire rack on top of the parchment paper. Season the pork chops with salt and pepper on both sides.

Make the breading. Put the cornmeal, breadcrumbs, smoked paprika, fennel seeds, oregano, onion powder, and garlic powder into a large plastic bag and shake until they are all combined.

Bread the pork chops. Coat each pork chop in the mustard. Put one pork chop at a time into the bag of breading. Shake it all around until it's evenly coated. Put it on the rack on the baking sheet. Repeat with the rest of the chops.

Bake the pork chops. Bake the pork chops until they are golden brown and have reached an internal temperature of 155°F, about 20 minutes. Serve immediately.

Feel like playing?

Feel like making chicken instead? This would be a great breading for chicken thighs, drumsticks, or breasts. This technique and breading would work really well with fish as well, especially snapper or salmon. Just brush the fish fillets with oil, skip the mustard, and dredge the fish lightly into the breading, rather than shaking it in a bag. It will probably take 10 to 15 minutes to bake.

CHICKEN ENCHILADAS WITH RED CHILE SAUCE

Feeds 6

There's going to be disagreement here. This classic Tex-Mex red sauce, delicious and thick with red chiles and great spices, is fantastic slathered over chicken enchiladas. Most everyone agrees on that. The disagreement comes from what to call it. In New Mexico and the Southwest, it's red chile sauce, except in Colorado, where it's chile Colorado. In Texas, it's red chile gravy. Of course, all of those have tiny variations by region. We call it red chile sauce, because that's what we saw most often in our travels. But, to quote a cheesy old joke, we don't care what you call it, as long as you don't call us late for dinner.

FOR THE RED CHILE SAUCE

6 whole dried red chiles (we use guajillo chiles)

¼ cup lard or other fat

35 grams All-Purpose Gluten-Free Flour Blend (page 17)

2 cloves garlic, peeled and minced

1 teaspoon chili powder

½ teaspoon ground cumin

½ teaspoon smoked paprika

¼ teaspoon dried oregano

¼ teaspoon chipotle chile powder

1 tablespoon tomato paste

2 cups chicken stock (if you're using boxed stock, make sure it's gluten-free)

Kosher salt and freshly ground black pepper

1 tablespoon honey

FOR THE ENCHILADAS

2 tablespoons extra-virgin olive oil

1 large yellow onion, peeled and chopped

2 small red bell peppers, chopped

2 cloves garlic, peeled and sliced

2 tablespoons chili powder

1 tablespoon smoked paprika

1 tablespoon dried Mexican oregano

1 teaspoon ground cumin

Pinch red pepper flakes

One 14-ounce can diced tomatoes, drained

1 canned chipotle pepper in adobo sauce (make sure it's gluten-free)

3 cups chopped roasted chicken

2 cups chicken stock (if you're using boxed stock, make sure it's gluten-free)

16 gluten-free tortillas (see page 109)

1 pound (4 cups) freshly grated Monterey Jack cheese

Hydrate the chiles. Pour 4 cups of boiling water over the chiles in a large bowl. Let them sit for 30 minutes. Take them out of the water, and remove the stems and as many seeds as you want. (The more seeds left in, the more heat will be in the final sauce.) Chop the chiles.

Make the red chile sauce. Set a Dutch oven over medium heat. Add the lard. When the lard is melted, add the flour. Cook, stirring frequently, until the flour releases a warm scent, about 3 minutes. Add the garlic and cook, stirring frequently, until the garlic's scent is released, about 2 minutes. Add the chili powder, cumin, smoked paprika, oregano, and chipotle chile powder and cook, stirring, for 1 minute. Add the tomato paste and stir until everything is evenly coated. Pour in the stock and whisk everything together well until every ingredient is incorporated. Add the chopped chiles and bring the liquid to a boil, stir, then turn down the heat to low. Let the sauce simmer for 30 minutes. Pour half the sauce into a blender and puree it. Pour that into a large bowl and puree the rest of the sauce. Return the sauce to the pot and turn the heat to medium. Bring the sauce to a low boil, then turn down the heat to low. Season with salt and pepper and add the honey. Set aside.

Prepare to bake. Preheat the oven to 400°F.

Make the chicken filling. Clean the Dutch oven and set it over medium-high heat. Pour the olive oil into the Dutch oven. When the oil is hot, add the onions, bell peppers, and garlic and cook, stirring occasionally, until the onions are soft and translucent, about 7 minutes. Stir in the chili powder, smoked paprika, oregano, cumin, and red pepper flakes and stir until the scent is released, about 1 minute. Add the tomatoes and chipotle pepper and cook, stirring, until they are heated through, about 2 minutes. Add the roasted chicken and stir to coat, then pour in the stock. Bring the liquid to a boil, then turn down the heat to medium-low and cook for 15 minutes.

Make the enchiladas. Set a cast-iron skillet over high heat. Put a tortilla onto the skillet. Cook until the tortilla is softened and a bit charred, about 1 minute. Flip the tortilla and cook for 1 minute more. Remove the tortilla and fill it with enough chicken filling that you can still roll it up (about 3 tablespoons, depending on the size of your tortillas). Put the filled tortilla into a 9 x 13-inch baking dish, seam side down. Repeat with the remaining tortillas and filling.

CONTINUED

Bake the enchiladas. Pour the red chile sauce over the filled enchiladas, and sprinkle the cheese over the top. Bake until the cheese is melted, bubbling, and starting to brown, about 30 minutes. Serve immediately.

Feel like playing?

There's no need to keep this red chile sauce just for enchiladas. It works well with eggs for a huevos rancheros recipe. Try it as a sauce for roasted chicken or fish. I like it tangled up in zucchini noodles too.

TATER TOT HOT POT

Feeds 6 to 8

Of all the Midwestern casseroles we were requested to make for this book, the one with the most interesting name also had the most votes. Tater Tot Hot Pot, also known as Tater Tot hot dish or Tater Tot casserole, must be the most beloved of all Midwestern dishes. And why not? Tater Tots, those little nuggets of crispy fried potatoes, balanced on top of beef, cheese, green beans, and cream of something soup (see the Cream of Mushroom Soup recipe on page 126)—this is a one-pot wonder. Most commercial tots contain wheat flour, although there are a few brands without it. So if you don't feel like making your own—even though we suggest you try—you could make this dish quickly for dinner. As they say in Napoleon Dynamite, *"Hey, give me some of your tots!"*

FOR THE TOTS

3 pounds russet potatoes, peeled and cut into 1-inch chunks

2 quarts fat or oil of your choice for frying (peanut oil is particularly tasty here)

1 tablespoon potato starch

2 teaspoons kosher salt

Pinch freshly ground black pepper

FOR THE CASSEROLE

1 pound green beans

2 tablespoons extra-virgin olive oil

1½ pounds ground beef

3½ cups Cream of Mushroom Soup (page 126)

Kosher salt and freshly ground black pepper

12 ounces (3 cups) freshly grated Cheddar cheese

Fry the potatoes. Put the potato chunks in a bowl of cold water and shake it all around for 10 seconds. Drain through a fine-mesh sieve and let the potatoes sit there for 5 minutes. Set a large wok or Dutch oven over high heat. Add the oil and heat until it has reached 350°F on an instant-read thermometer. Lower half of the potato chunks into the hot oil with a Chinese spider or slotted spoon. Stir them, very gently, once in a while, frying until they are light golden brown and tender, about 4 minutes. (Be sure to keep checking the temperature of the oil. If it grows too hot, turn down the heat.) Transfer the potatoes to a paper towel–lined plate and let cool. Return the oil to 350°F and fry the rest of the potatoes. Turn off the heat but leave the wok on the stove.

Make the tots. Transfer one-quarter of the cooled potatoes to the bowl of a food processor. Pulse until the potatoes are broken down to roughly ⅛-inch pieces, about 8 pulses. Move the potatoes to a large bowl and continue until you have finished all the potatoes. Sprinkle the potato starch, salt, and pepper over the broken-down potatoes. Gently, form the potato mixture into tots—about ¾ inch wide and 1 inch long.

CONTINUED

Fry the tots. Turn the heat under the wok to high again and reheat the oil to 350°F. Gently lower the tots into the hot oil. Fry for 1 minute, then break apart the tots gently with a Chinese spider. Fry until they are golden brown and super crisp, about 4 minutes. Transfer the tots to a paper towel–lined plate. Season with salt immediately. (You can eat a few here. In fact, feel free to stop here. The best part about this dish is the tots. But, if you want to make a casserole, stop eating.)

Prepare to bake. Preheat the oven to 425°F.

Blanch the beans. Set a large pot of salted water over high heat. Take the ends off the green beans and snap them in half. When the water is boiling, put the green beans in the pot. Blanch them for 1 minute and then immediately transfer to a bowl of ice water in the sink. When the green beans are cool to the touch, drain them.

Brown the beef. Set a Dutch oven over medium-high heat. Pour in the oil. When the oil is hot, add the ground beef. Cook, stirring occasionally, until the beef is entirely browned, about 5 minutes. Remove the beef with a slotted spoon and discard the oil. Add the cream of mushroom soup to the pot. When it is fully heated, add the ground beef and blanched green beans, and stir. Season with salt and pepper.

Bake the casserole. Pour the beef and soup mixture into a 9 x 13-inch baking dish. Sprinkle the cheese over the top evenly. Place the tots in rows across the baking dish. Bake until the cheese has melted into the casserole and everything is bubbling and browned, about 25 minutes. Serve immediately.

Feel like playing?

We've made the tots with sweet potatoes and they were mighty fine. You could make this with ground pork as well, or with another kind of cheese. This recipe is really just a template for the casserole you want to make in your kitchen.

SAVORY PIECRUST

Makes enough for 1 double crust

The pie dough recipe (on page 226) is great for fruit pies and chocolate pies. But a savory meat or seafood pie needs a heartier dough. Adding the mashed potato and egg yolk to the dough gives you a dough sturdy enough to stand up to elk or salmon.

1 potato (150 grams), peeled and coarsely chopped

365 grams All-Purpose Gluten-Free Flour Blend (page 17)

½ teaspoon fine sea salt

9 tablespoons (125 grams) cold unsalted butter, cut into 1-inch cubes

1 large egg yolk

Cook the potato. Set a small pot over high heat. Fill it three-quarters full with cold water and enough salt to make the water taste like the ocean, plus the chopped potato. Bring the water to a boil, then turn down the heat to low to simmer the water. Cook the potato until a knife runs through it easily, about 15 minutes. Push the soft potato through a ricer or fine-mesh sieve. Set it aside to cool.

Make the dough. Put the flour and salt into the bowl of a food processor and whirl them up. Add the cold butter chunks and pulse the food processor until the flour is sandy and the butter is the size of lima beans. Add the egg yolk and cooled potato and pulse until the dough is well combined. Dump the dough onto a clean, cool surface. Gently, move the dough around with your hands until it comes together into a ball. Form it into a disk. Wrap in plastic wrap and refrigerate for 30 minutes.

ELK AND MOREL MUSHROOM POT PIE

Feeds 8

There are still plenty of places in this country where a meat dish means something other than chicken, beef, or pork from the grocery store. In many places in the South and in wilderness areas like Alaska, folks hunt their meals and fill their freezers full of meat ready for the winter. We're inspired by the big game dishes of the Rocky Mountain areas, such as Colorado, Utah, Wyoming, and Montana, where an elk and morel mushroom pot pie doesn't sound like an exotic gourmet dish but more like tonight's dinner.

One 4-ounce package dried morel mushrooms

4 thick slices bacon, chopped

27 grams All-Purpose Gluten-Free Flour Blend (page 17)

Kosher salt and freshly ground black pepper

3 pounds elk meat, cut into 1-inch chunks

1 large yellow onion, peeled and chopped

2 cloves garlic, peeled and chopped

2 teaspoons chopped fresh rosemary

2 tablespoons tomato paste

1 cup full-bodied red wine (such as Cabernet Sauvignon)

3 cups beef stock (if you're using boxed stock, make sure it's gluten-free)

1 large russet potato, peeled and chopped

1 batch Savory Piecrust (page 183)

Prepare to cook. Preheat the oven to 350°F. Pour 1¼ cups of hot water over the morels in a large bowl. Allow the morels to soak while you prepare the filling.

Cook the bacon. Set a Dutch oven over medium heat. Put the bacon in the pot and cook, stirring occasionally, until the bacon is browned and has released its fat, about 10 minutes. Remove and set aside the bacon and turn off the heat.

Season the elk. Put the flour and salt and pepper into a plastic bag. Put half the elk meat cubes into the bag and shake until the meat is evenly coated. Remove the meat and continue with the rest of the meat.

Sear the meat. Turn the heat under the Dutch oven to medium-high. When the bacon grease is hot, add the elk meat (in batches). Sear the meat until the bottoms of the meat pieces are brown, about 3 minutes. Flip the meat and sear on all sides. Remove from the pot and sear the rest of the meat. Remove the meat from the pot.

Cook the aromatics. Add the onions and garlic to the pot. Cook, stirring occasionally, until the onions are soft and translucent, about 7 minutes. Add the rosemary and cook and stir until the scent is released, about 1 minute. Add the morels to the pot, reserving the soaking water, and cook for 1 minute. Add the tomato paste and stir it into the onions. Cook for 2 minutes.

Deglaze the pan. Pour the wine into the pan and stir everything up, being sure to scrape up all the goodness at the bottom of the pan. Cook until the wine has reduced by half its volume, about 4 minutes. Add the stock, the potato, and the reserved water from the mushrooms and stir them together. Put the meat back into the Dutch oven and cover it. Put the stew into the oven and cook until the meat is entirely tender to the fork. Start checking the meat after 3 hours. Take the Dutch oven out of the oven and let the stew cool to room temperature.

Form the pie. Roll out half of the piecrust and put it in a pie pan. Fill the crust with the elk stew. (If you have some leftover stew, go ahead and enjoy that here.) Roll out the remaining piecrust, arrange on top of the stew, and crimp the edges to seal. Make two small slits in the top crust to allow the steam to escape and put the pie in the oven. Bake until the top crust is golden brown and flaky, about 1 hour.

Allow the pie to cool to room temperature. Slice it up and serve.

Feel like playing?

You could use beef or bison here in place of the elk, if you don't have access to it.

CHICAGO DEEP-DISH SAUSAGE PIZZA PIE

Feeds 8 or more

Pizza lovers in most of the United States like thin crust, blistered and filled with air pockets, like the ones made in wood-fired ovens in Brooklyn. But pizza lovers in Chicago? They want nothing to do with that pizza. It's only thick-crust, deep-dish pizza pie for Chicago pizza aficionados. Is that even possible without gluten? You bet. Here it is.

4 tablespoons extra-virgin olive oil

1 batch gluten-free Pizza Dough (page 57)

4 cloves garlic, peeled and minced

1 teaspoon dried oregano

1 teaspoon dried basil

1 teaspoon dried rosemary

One 28-ounce can tomatoes (we prefer San Marzano), crushed

1 pound fresh mozzarella cheese, sliced

1 pound cooked sweet Italian sausage, sliced

8 ounces (2 cups) freshly grated Parmesan cheese

Prepare to prebake. Grease a 12-inch cast-iron skillet with 2 tablespoons of the olive oil. Preheat the oven to 400°F.

Prebake the crust. Put the dough into the bottom of the skillet, then gently press the dough up the sides of the skillet. Grease a piece of luminum foil large enough to reach to the edges of the dough and put it gently onto the top of the dough, greased side down. Fill the bottom of the dough with dried beans. Bake until the dough is starting to set and get firm, about 15 minutes. Let the dough cool to room temperature, then take the beans and aluminum foil off.

Make the sauce. Set a large skillet over medium-high heat. Pour in the remaining 2 tablespoons of olive oil. Add the garlic to the hot oil and cook, stirring frequently, until the scent is released, about 2 minutes. Add the dried oregano, basil, and rosemary and cook and stir until the scent is released, about 1 minute. Add the tomatoes and cook until the tomatoes are simmering and reduced, about 30 minutes. Stir occasionally. Take the sauce off the heat.

Prepare to bake. Turn the oven temperature up to 475°F.

Make the pie. Fill the crust with the mozzarella, reaching to the edges of the crust, even layering a bit to use it all up. Make the next layer with the sausage slices. Pour in the tomato sauce next, followed by the Parmesan on top.

Bake the pie. Bake the pie until the entire pie is bubbly and the top is golden brown, about 30 minutes. Let it cool for at least 20 minutes before slicing it up and serving it.

Feel like playing?

You can fill the pie any way you like, with vegetables like mushrooms and zucchini if you are vegetarian. If you have leftover tomato sauce from making the lasagna on page 174, use that here instead. I'm not sure making this with dairy-free cheese would be very satisfying, to tell you the truth. But you can figure that out. Also, cold leftover pizza pie is a great breakfast.

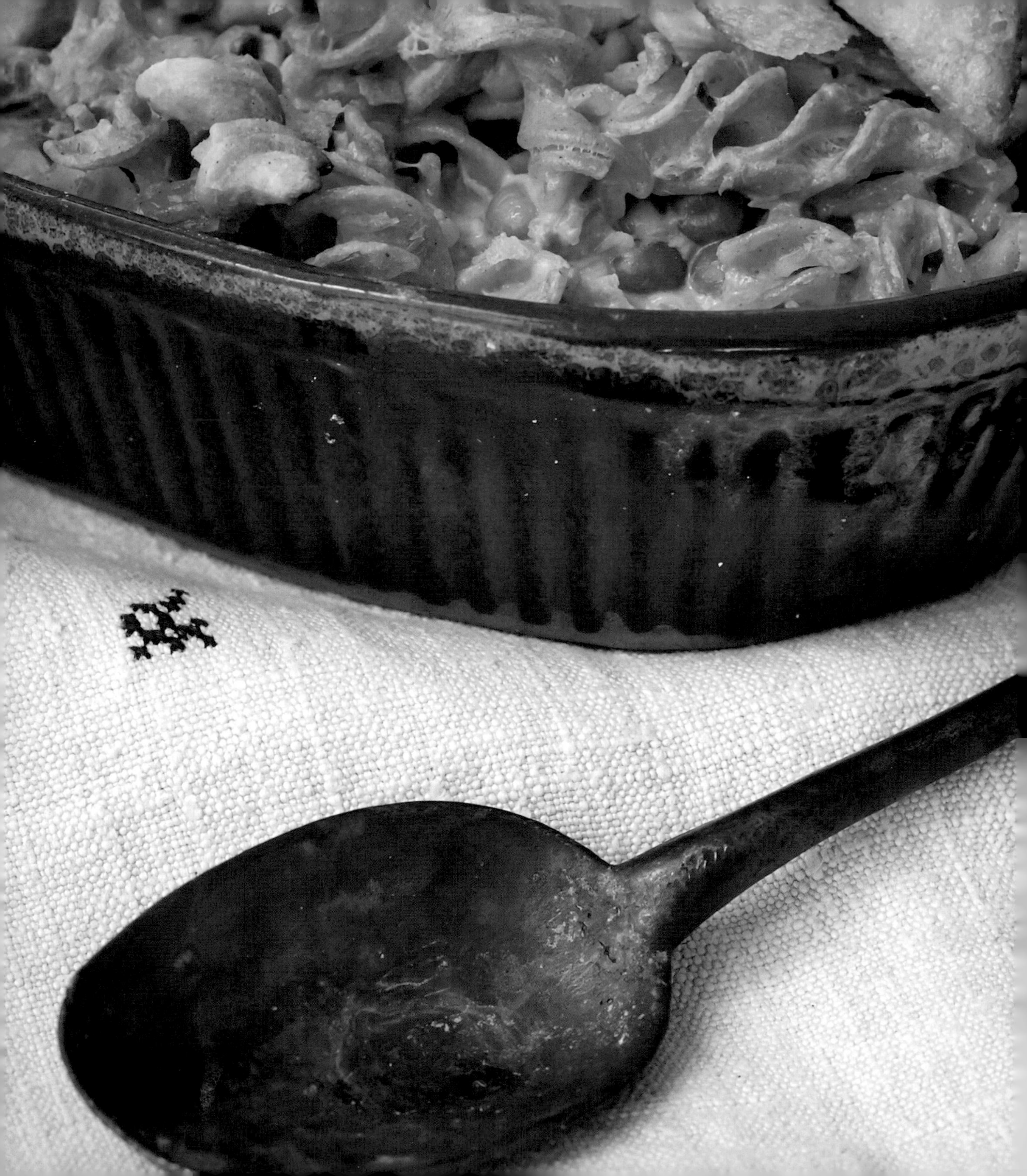

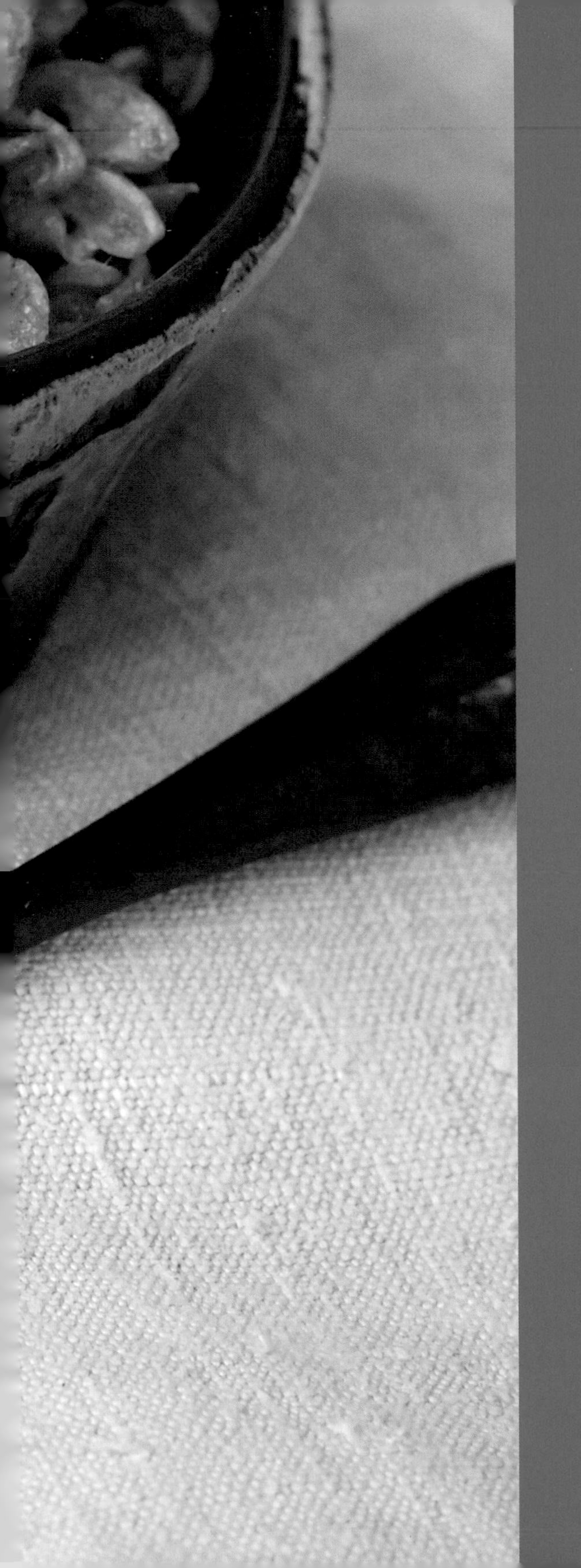

SEAFOOD MAIN DISHES

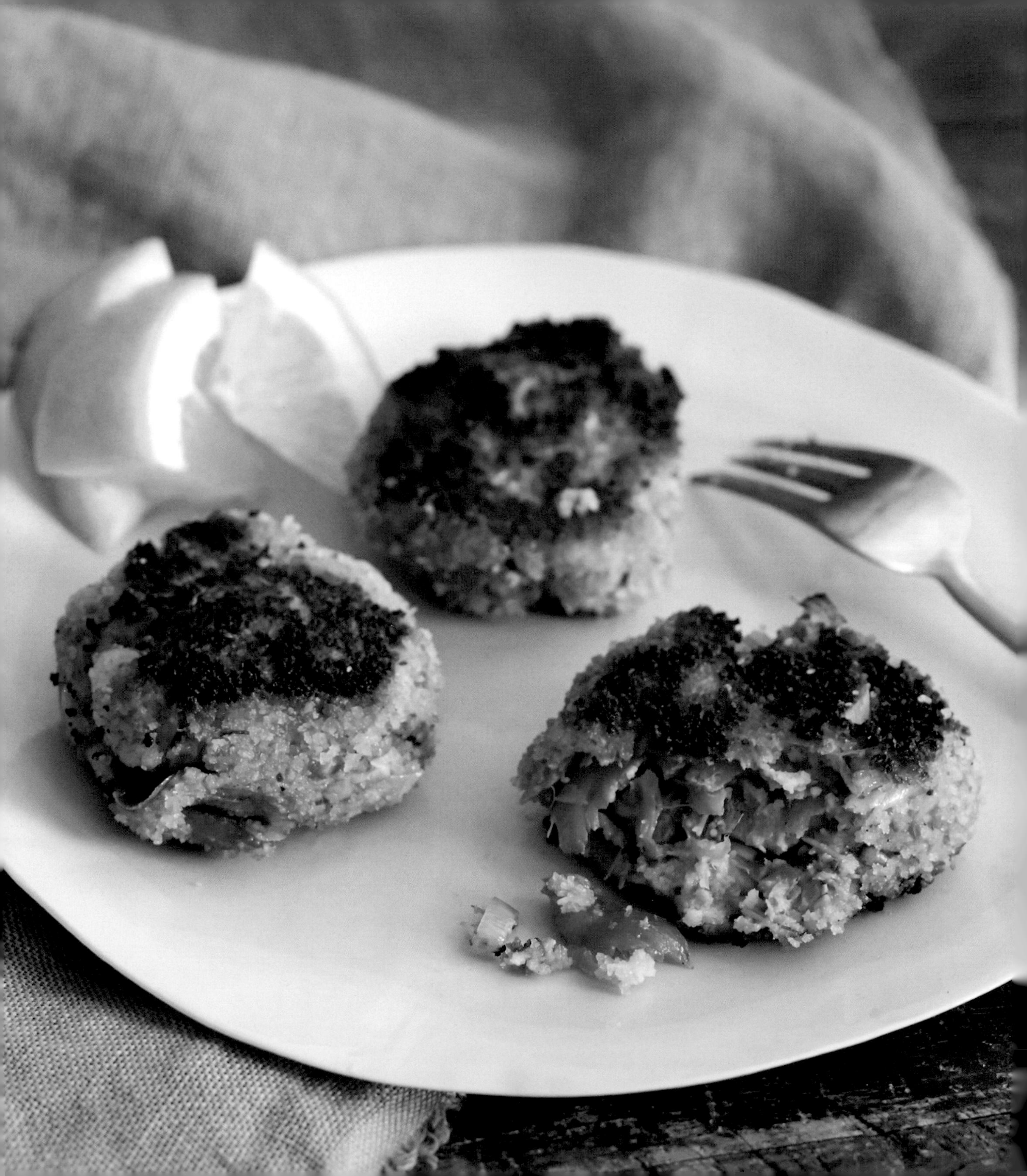

SALMON CROQUETTES

Feeds 4

Only by doing research for this book did Danny and I discover that salmon croquettes are a much-loved Southern tradition. Here in the Pacific Northwest, we feast on salmon as often as we can, especially the wild salmon from Alaska, so I thought they were invented here. We decided to play with this simple template by mixing salmon fillet and smoked salmon. The smoked salmon is already salted, so you won't need to salt these patties before you cook them. These, with a dollop of fresh aioli, a big green salad, and a table surrounded by people I love, is all the dinner I need.

6 ounces high-quality canned salmon

6 ounces high-quality smoked salmon

4 scallions, finely chopped

1 tablespoon chopped fresh dill

2 large eggs, beaten

½ cup gluten-free breadcrumbs

3 tablespoons extra-virgin olive oil

Make the croquettes. Flake the canned and smoked salmon into a large bowl. Break them apart with your fingers. You don't want giant chunks here. Add the scallions and dill and toss. Add the beaten eggs and half of the breadcrumbs. Stir gently until just combined. Form into 8 patties. Press both sides of each patty into the remaining breadcrumbs. Put the croquettes on a plate.

Fry the croquettes. Set a large cast-iron skillet over medium heat. Add the olive oil. Put the croquettes in the hot oil. Cook until the bottom of the croquettes are browned, about 4 minutes. Carefully flip them to the other side and cook until they are browned too. Serve immediately.

Feel like playing?

This isn't a fancy recipe. You could use any salmon you have, especially leftover cooked salmon from the night before. You could also do this with flaked tuna for a quick dinner. The quality of the salmon matters, however. We love salmon from Loki Fish Company, a family-owned business here in Seattle that uses good practices to catch fish without endangering the environment. You can buy their salmon online.

TUNA NOODLE CASSEROLE

Feeds 4 to 6

When we were researching this book, we quickly came to feel that there is no more distinctly American food of the late twentieth century than tuna noodle casserole. And we say: hurrah! There's a reason this dish has shown up at many a potluck and family gathering. We made a very fancy tuna noodle casserole for our first cookbook, with homemade fish stock, leeks, thyme, and cremini mushrooms. It's delicious. But honestly, I'd choose this dump-and-stir casserole, with gluten-free pasta and homemade cream of mushroom soup, every time over that fancy one now. Oh, and there's some bubbly Parmesan and crushed potato chips too.

Fat for greasing the baking dish

1 pound gluten-free fusilli

12 ounces canned tuna, drained and flaked

2½ cups (20 ounces) Cream of Mushroom Soup (page 126)

2 cups frozen peas

4 ounces (1 cup) freshly grated Parmesan cheese

1 cup crushed potato chips (make sure they are gluten-free)

Prepare to cook. Preheat the oven to 425°F. Grease a 9 x 13-inch baking dish.

Cook the pasta. Set a large pot of water over high heat. Add enough salt to make it taste like the ocean. When the water comes to a boil, add the fusilli. Cook until the pasta is tender but still has a bite, 7 to 10 minutes, depending on the brand you are using. Drain.

Make the casserole. Stir together the tuna, soup, and peas in a large bowl. Add the pasta and stir them up. Put the mixture into the prepared baking dish.

Bake the casserole. Bake the casserole until the soup starts to bubble around the pasta. Put the Parmesan and crushed potato chips on top. Bake until the potato chips are browned, about 5 minutes. Serve immediately.

Feel like playing?

Once you have the basic template down here, there's nothing wrong with gussying it up on your own. Fresh herbs, sautéed onions and leeks, butter-covered breadcrumbs instead of the chips—they're all great ideas. But don't be surprised if your guests aren't a little disappointed to not have their childhood favorites the way they expect them.

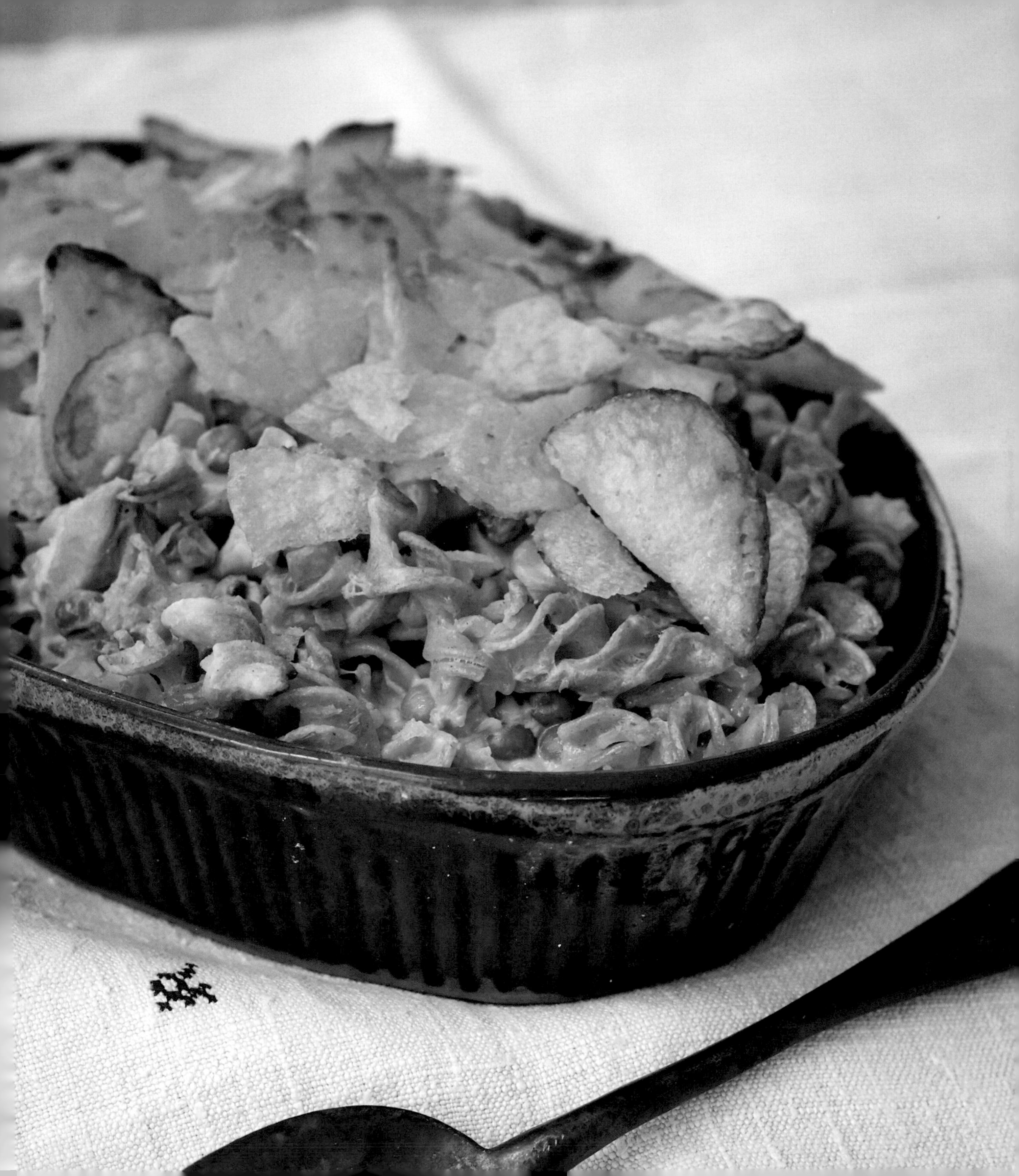

GREAT PAN-FRIED BREADED FISH

Feeds 4

This is not so much a specific recipe as a basic template for making your own great breaded fish at home. Maybe you have bass or snapper, tilapia or catfish, fresh fish from a lake in the Midwest or Pacific cod. Any of these fish do well with this treatment. It's also an easy weeknight dinner in any region of this country.

2 large eggs, at room temperature

¼ cup whole milk (you can use almond or rice milk if you can't eat dairy)

280 grams All-Purpose Gluten-Free Flour Blend (page 17)

2 cups gluten-free breadcrumbs

Four 8-ounce fish fillets (no thicker than ¾ inch thick)

Kosher salt and freshly ground black pepper

Fat or oil of your choice for frying (we like olive oil)

Lemon wedges for serving

Make the batter. In a wide bowl, beat the eggs and milk together. Spread the flour blend out in one wide bowl and the breadcrumbs in another. Line up the bowls: flour, then eggs and milk, then breadcrumbs.

Prepare to fry. Season the fish fillets with salt and pepper. Put one fish fillet in the flour, then turn it over and cover the other side in flour. (This is called dredging.) Shake the fish a bit to get rid of excess flour, then dunk the fish in the egg and milk mixture. Lift it up and let it drip for a moment, then press the fish into the breadcrumbs, coating both sides. Move the coated fish to a plate or wire rack. Repeat until you have coated all the fish fillets.

Cook the fish. Put a large cast-iron skillet over medium-high heat. Let the skillet heat up for a few moments. Add about 6 tablespoons of fat to the skillet. Let the fat heat up. Just before it starts to smoke, put the fish into the hot pan, laying the end closest to you down first and letting the fat splutter away from you. When the breadcrumbs begin to brown, turn down the heat to medium. When the bottoms are evenly golden brown, after 3 to 4 minutes, flip the fish. Cook until the other side is golden brown.

Serve the fish with a squeeze of lemon juice.

Feel like playing?

We like our fish with a mayonnaise sauce. Make a fresh remoulade: mayonnaise with cornichons, capers, tarragon, parsley, and mustard. That's one good meal.

FISH STICKS

Feeds 4

First invented in the twentieth century in Great Britain, where they are called the much more interesting fish fingers, fish sticks have been a favorite kid snack for decades. We make our own panko-like crumbs with stale tortilla chips. Believe us. It works. Anytime you have a leftover bag of tortilla chips that are going a little stale? Pulse up those chips and keep them in a jar. They'll keep as crumbs for quite a long time, so you can make these or anything you want to give a crisp crust.

2 cups stale corn tortilla chips

140 grams All-Purpose Gluten-Free Flour Blend (page 17)

3 large eggs, at room temperature

1 pound firm-fleshed fish, such as halibut or cod

Kosher salt and freshly ground black pepper

2 cups fat or oil of your choice for frying (we like peanut oil)

Pulse the chips. In the bowl of a food processor, pulse the tortilla chips until they become fine crumbs, about 5 minutes. Pour them into a wide bowl, and then put the flour blend into another wide bowl. Beat the eggs in another wide bowl and set all the bowls next to each other: flour, then eggs, then chips.

Prepare the fish. Cut the fish into strips about 1 inch thick and 3 inches long. Make sure the fish pieces are about the same size to ensure that each one is cooked evenly. Season the fish with salt and pepper.

Dredge the fish. Coat each fish stick on both sides in the flour, then the eggs, then the tortilla chip crumbs. Put the coated fish sticks on a wire rack and let them rest for at least 15 minutes and up to 1 hour.

Cook the fish. Set a large cast-iron skillet over medium heat. Pour in oil to a depth of 1 to 2 inches. Heat the oil until it hits 350°F on an instant-read thermometer. Carefully add 5 or 6 fish sticks to the hot oil. (You'll probably have to cook these in batches.) The oil will sizzle and bubble immediately. That's how you'll know the oil is hot enough, besides the thermometer. Cook until the coating on the fish is golden brown and crisp, 4 to 5 minutes. Remove the fish sticks from the oil and put them on a paper towel–lined plate to drain.

Repeat with the remaining fish sticks. Serve immediately.

Feel like playing?

If you want to make chicken strips for dinner, use strips of chicken breast instead of fish. Other than that, it's the same recipe.

SHRIMP AND GRITS CAKES

Feeds 4

Much of the great food of New Orleans in particular, and the South in general, is dipped and fried in wheat flour or built on bread. But the dish of creamy cheese grits and shrimp I swooned over at one of Emeril Lagasse's restaurants in New Orleans inspired me to come up with this dish with Danny after I returned home.

FOR THE GRITS

1 cup stone-ground corn grits (see Note)

1 teaspoon fine sea salt

3½ cups whole milk (try goat's milk, if you have access to it)

1 cup chicken stock (if you're using boxed stock, make sure it's gluten-free)

3 tablespoons extra-virgin olive oil, plus more for brushing

2 cloves garlic, peeled and chopped

4 ounces (1 cup) freshly grated aged white Cheddar cheese

2 tablespoons finely chopped fresh Italian parsley

1 teaspoon smoked paprika

FOR THE SHRIMP

1 pound collard greens, stems and center ribs discarded

5 thick slices bacon, chopped

2 cloves garlic, peeled and sliced

2 tablespoons unsalted butter

16 large shrimp (about 1 pound), peeled and deveined

½ cup chicken stock (if you're using boxed stock, make sure it's gluten-free)

Prepare to cook. In a small bowl, stir together the grits and salt.

Simmer the liquids. Set a small pot over medium heat. Pour in the milk and stock and whisk to combine. Bring the liquids to a boil, then reduce the heat to low and keep the liquids simmering, stirring occasionally.

Sauté the garlic. Set a Dutch oven over medium heat. Pour in 1 tablespoon of the olive oil. When the oil is hot, toss in the garlic. Cook, stirring frequently, until the garlic releases its scent, about 2 minutes. Please don't burn the garlic.

Cook the grits. Pour the grits and salt onto the garlic. Whisk them up. Slowly, pour in some of the hot liquid, whisking the entire time. Keep whisking, as this will help release the starches from the grits, making the final result creamy. Pour in more liquid and keep whisking. When all the liquid is incorporated into the grits, keep occasionally whisking and stirring and cooking the grits until they are wonderfully creamy, about 45 minutes. Turn off the heat.

Finish the grits. Add the cheese, parsley, and smoked paprika to the grits. Stir well to combine.

Mold the grits cakes. Use the remaining 2 tablespoons of olive oil to brush the insides of a standard-size muffin tin. Fill each muffin cup halfway with the grits. (If you have some left over, you could eat those creamy grits right away.) Chill the muffin tin in the refrigerator for at least 30 minutes, and preferably 2 hours.

Prepare the collards. Roll each leaf of collard greens into a long cigar shape. Cut the collard leaf into thin slices, leaving you with ribbons of collards.

Heat the grits cakes. Turn the oven onto broil. Unmold the grits cakes and put them in a couple of skillets. Brush them with olive oil and put them under the broiler. Heat until they are golden and piping-hot, about 3 minutes.

Cook the shrimp. Set a large skillet over medium-high heat. Put in the bacon and cook, stirring, until the bacon pieces are crisp and browned, about 5 minutes. Remove and set aside the bacon and keep the fat in the skillet.

Cook the garlic in the hot bacon grease until its scent is released, about 2 minutes. Add the butter. When the butter is melted, add the shrimp and pour in the stock. Stir and cook until the stock has reduced and the shrimp has cooked through, about 2 minutes. Take out the shrimp and add the collards to the skillet. Cook, stirring occasionally, until the collard ribbons are wilted and have turned darker green, about 5 minutes.

Combine the bacon, cooked shrimp, collards, and all the goodness from the skillet together.

Serve by giving each person 2 hot grits cakes, with the shrimp and collards mixture tumbled over the top.

Note: Stone-ground grits are well worth seeking out or buying online. I love the grits from Anson Mills, which grows and mills heirloom grains from the South. They do have gluten in the factory but seem to take great care to avoid cross-contamination. I've never grown sick from eating their grits.

Feel like playing?

Cooking collards with shrimp isn't one bit traditional, so you can keep it simpler by cooking the bacon and shrimp together. But it's nice to have a few vegetables in your dinner. If you're in a hurry, you can use quick-cooking grits for this dish, which will take about 5 minutes to cook. But they will never yield the same true corn taste and creaminess that come from taking your time.

CORDOVA SALMON

Feeds 4

During salmon season in September, Danny, Lucy, and I were lucky enough to travel to Cordova, Alaska, under the auspices of the Copper River Marketing Association. They wanted us to see where the most delicious salmon in the world are raised and fished. We were astonished by three things in Cordova: 1) how gorgeous that area of the earth is; 2) how the fishermen, scientists, and governmental officials work together harmoniously there for the sustainability of the fish; and 3) how often the people who live there eat salmon. After the third potluck we attended with at least twelve dishes made with my favorite fish, I asked someone there. "So, do you ever get tired of salmon?" She looked astonished and answered immediately: "Of course not." We think the citizens of Cordova would approve of this quick Asian-inspired broiled salmon.

1 pound salmon fillets, skin off and pin bones removed (we prefer wild Alaskan salmon)

2 tablespoons peeled and grated fresh ginger

2 tablespoons chopped fresh cilantro

2 tablespoons extra-virgin olive oil

1 tablespoon sesame oil

1 tablespoon gluten-free tamari

2 teaspoons fish sauce (make sure it's gluten-free; we prefer Red Boat)

1 clove garlic, peeled and minced

Freshly grated zest and freshly squeezed juice of 1 lime

Prepare the fish. Slice the fish into 2-ounce pieces, in the shape of fingers.

Make the marinade. In a large bowl, mix all the remaining ingredients together.

Marinate the fish. Put the salmon in the marinade and let it sit for 1 hour.

Prepare to cook. Preheat the broiler thoroughly. You want it to be really hot.

Broil the fish. Remove the fish from the marinade and place in a large cast-iron skillet. Put the skillet under the broiler. Cook until the fish has reached an internal temperature of 120°F, or about 1 minute. Serve immediately.

Feel like playing?

You could use any thick, fatty fish you want for this. Also, if you don't want to marinate fish in this sauce, it's a heck of a good marinade for chicken or tofu as well.

MACADAMIA-ENCRUSTED MAHI MAHI

Feeds 4

Since our daughter first saw photographs of Hawaii, she has been obsessed with the idea of visiting the fiftieth state. She's only five, but that girl is smart. We would love to visit Hawaii someday too. Until we can afford that vacation for the entire family, we'll have to enjoy the flavors of Hawaii in this dish instead.

1 cup chopped macadamia nuts

Freshly grated zest of 1 large orange

2 tablespoons shredded unsweetened coconut

1 clove garlic, peeled and minced

1 teaspoon olive oil

½ teaspoon ground ginger

70 grams All-Purpose Gluten-Free Flour Blend (page 17)

2 large eggs, beaten

Four 6-ounce-thick fillets mahi mahi

Kosher salt and freshly ground black pepper

2 tablespoons coconut oil, melted

Prepare to cook. Preheat the oven to 425°F.

Make the nut crust. In the bowl of a food processor, whirl up the macadamia nuts to a rough meal. Add the orange zest, coconut, garlic, olive oil, and ginger. Pulse until they are well combined. Put the nut meal in a wide bowl.

Dredge the fish. Put the flour blend in a wide bowl and the beaten eggs in another wide bowl. Season the mahi mahi fillets with salt and pepper. Dredge both sides of one fillet with flour, then the egg, then the nut meal. Put the dredged fish on a plate and repeat with the remaining fillets.

Cook the fish. Set a large cast-iron skillet over medium-high heat. Add the coconut oil. As soon as the coconut oil is melted, add the fish fillets, gently, to the hot fat. Cook until the bottom is browned, about 3 minutes, taking care to not burn the nuts. Flip the fish and put the skillet in the oven. Cook until the fish reaches an internal temperature of 120°F, about 7 minutes. Take the fish out of the oven and serve immediately.

Feel like playing?

This recipe would work well with any meaty white fish, such as halibut, sturgeon, or cod.

MEDITERRANEAN HALIBUT CHEEKS

Feeds 4 to 6

Fresh halibut fillets will substitute nicely here if you can't source the cheeks. (And yes, these are the cheeks of the halibut, which is a very large fish.) This dish was inspired by looking at a battered copy of a well-loved cookbook from The Fiddlehead Café, a hippie café in Juneau, Alaska, where our friend Adrienne ate many times. Alaskans know how to do great things with fresh fish and simple pantry items, since it's hard to grow much produce there for longer than a couple of months. Adrienne told us she always loved this simple halibut dish. So here's a bit of the Mediterranean, via Alaska, from our home on Vashon Island in Washington.

- Fat for greasing the baking dish
- 3 pounds halibut cheeks
- Kosher salt and freshly ground black pepper
- 70 grams All-Purpose Gluten-Free Flour Blend (page 17)
- 3 tablespoons extra-virgin olive oil
- ⅔ cup dry white wine (such as Sauvignon Blanc)
- 3 cups chopped tomatoes (canned are fine)
- 4 large cloves garlic, peeled and minced
- 3 tablespoons chopped fresh basil
- ¾ cup kalamata olives

Prepare to cook. Preheat the oven to 350°F. Grease a 9 x 13-inch baking dish.

Flour the fish. Season the halibut cheeks with salt and pepper. Lightly dredge each halibut cheek in the flour blend.

Sear the fish. Set a large cast-iron skillet over medium-high heat. Pour in 2 tablespoons of the oil. When the oil is hot, put the floured halibut cheeks into the skillet. Cook until the bottom is browned, about 1 minute, then flip and cook the other side, another minute. Remove the halibut cheeks and put them in the baking dish. (You might have to brown the fish in batches.)

Prepare the sauce. Pour the white wine into the skillet, scraping up the goodness from the bottom of the pan and incorporating it into the wine. Let the wine reduce by half its volume, about 3 minutes. Add the tomatoes, garlic, and basil and stir together. Bring the liquid to a boil, then turn down the heat to a simmer. Season with salt and pepper and the remaining 1 tablespoon of oil. Pour the sauce over the halibut cheeks and toss the kalamata olives on top.

Finish the fish. Cook the fish in the oven until the halibut cheeks flake easily and the sauce is bubbling hot, 5 to 10 minutes. Serve immediately.

Feel like playing?

Have fun with this. It's an easy dish and you'll master it quickly.

SEAFOOD POT PIE

Feeds 8

Those of us who live on the coasts are so darned lucky to have such extraordinary seafood so easily available. Sometimes, all we need is a piece of seared salmon to make a great dinner. But sometimes, on a winter night, it's nice to gather all our favorite seafood together with mushrooms, onions, and a savory pastry dough to make a seafood pie. Leftovers the next day are even better.

3 tablespoons unsalted butter

½ medium yellow onion, peeled and chopped

1 cup quartered white mushrooms

1 cup artichoke hearts, chopped

1 clove garlic, peeled and chopped

1 tablespoon chopped fresh tarragon

13 ounces canned clams, juice reserved

8 ounces salmon fillet, skin off and cut into large cubes

8 ounces bay shrimp

8 ounces cod (or other white fish), skin off and cut into large cubes

1 cup clam juice

1 batch Savory Piecrust (page 183)

Prepare to bake. Preheat the oven to 425°F.

Cook the aromatics. Set a Dutch oven over medium-high heat. Add the butter. As soon as the butter has melted, add the onions and mushrooms. Cook, stirring frequently, until the onions are soft and translucent and the mushrooms are wilted, about 7 minutes. Add the artichoke hearts and cook, stirring, for another minute. Add the garlic and tarragon, stir together, and cook until the scent is released, about 1 minute.

Finish the filling. Add the clams, salmon, shrimp, and cod to the pot. Pour in the reserved clam juice from the cans and the additional clam juice. Gently, stir everything together.

Make the pie. Roll out half of the pie dough. Put it into a 9-inch pie pan. Spoon the seafood filling into the pie pan. Roll out the second half of the dough, a little bigger than the first half. Put it on top of the filling and crimp the edges. Make two small slits in the top to allow the steam to escape. Bake the pie for 15 minutes, then turn down the oven to 375°F. Bake until the top of the pie is golden brown and the filling is bubbling in the slits on the top, about 45 minutes. Take the pie out of the oven and allow it to cool to room temperature before serving.

Feel like playing?

Feel free to substitute any seafood or fish you have available to you for this pie. If you have been cooking whole fish, use the leftover bones and head to make fish stock and use that in place of the clam juice here.

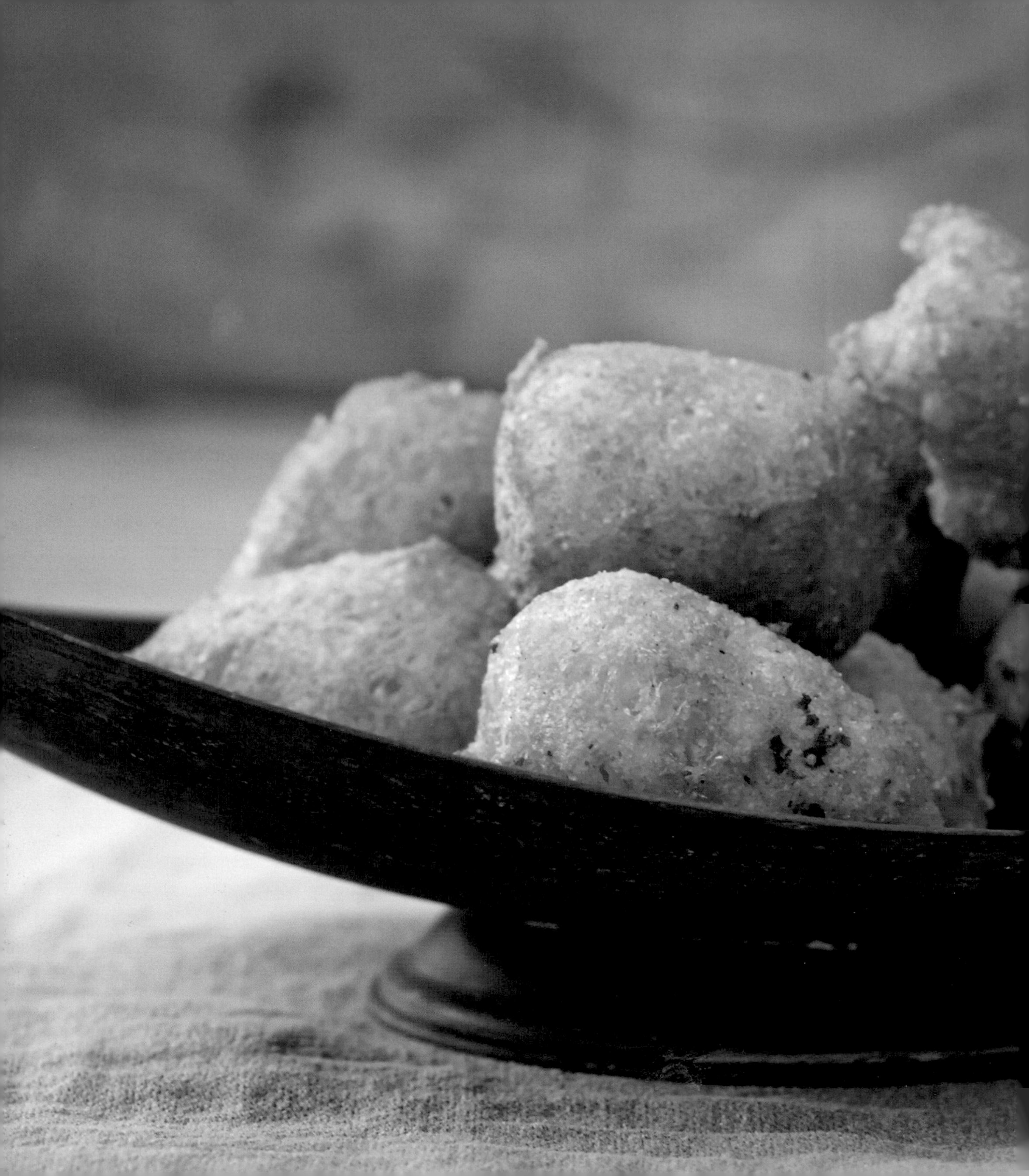

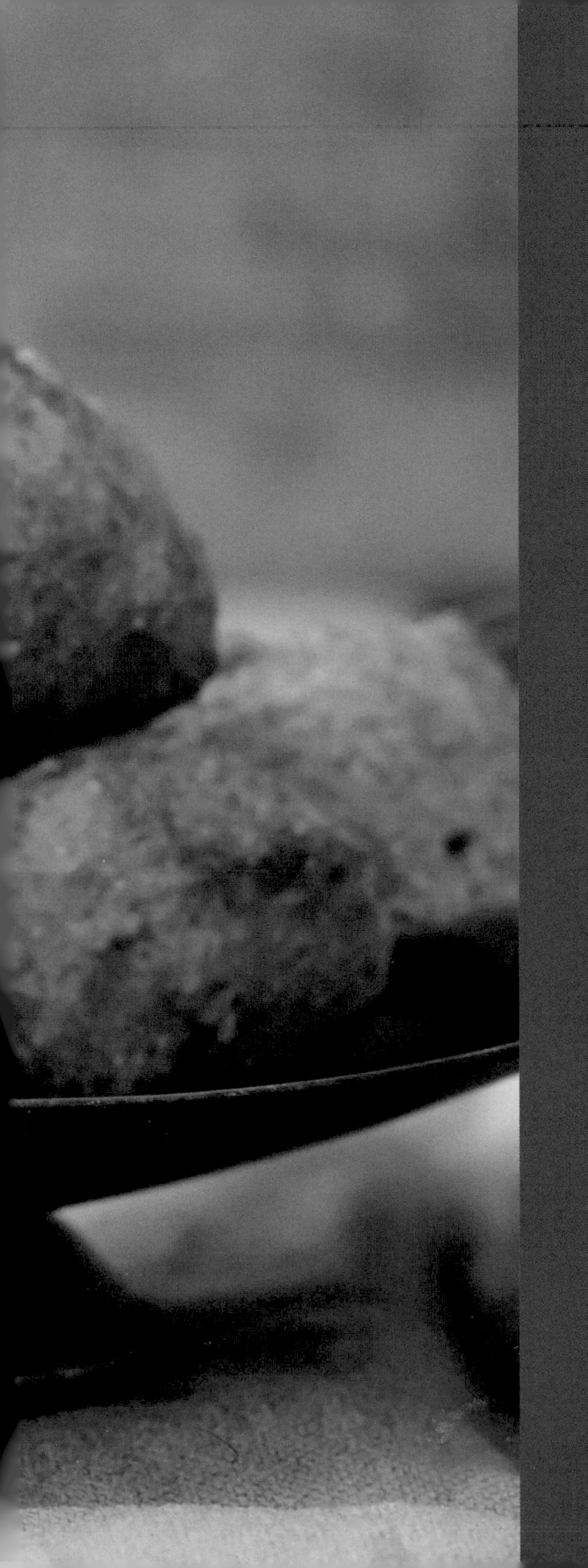

FRIED FOODS

EDNA LEWIS'S FRIED CHICKEN

Feeds 4

There's fast-food fried chicken (ick), there's buttermilk-fried chicken (yum), and then there's Edna Lewis's fried chicken (holy heck, yes!). This is fried chicken for those of you who are not faint of heart. Edna Lewis was one of the preeminent chefs of the American South, her life an incredible story. She was the granddaughter of a man who had been emancipated from slavery and founded the town of Freetown, Virginia, where all citizens were free. She grew up surrounded by fresh food, harvesting and preserving the produce around her, as so many Americans did in the early twentieth century. She moved to New York City as a young woman, making dresses for rich women and young starlets and writing for The Daily Worker. *In the late 1940s, she began cooking at a restaurant called Café Nicholson, which quickly became the favorite restaurant of Southerners away from home, such as William Faulkner and Truman Capote. By the 1970s, Lewis had turned to writing. Her cookbook and memoir,* The Taste of Country Cooking, *is still considered a classic of Southern cuisine. (It's also one of our favorite cookbooks of all time.) She lived to be nearly ninety years old, until the end still cooking and creating community. And this is her fried chicken recipe, transcribed by her cooking partner and friend, Scott Peacock, and we made it gluten-free. Some of you might faint at the amount of fat it takes to fry this chicken. But heck—fried chicken isn't diet food. And if it worked for Edna Lewis, it works for us.*

FOR THE BRINE

½ cup kosher salt

2 quarts cold water

2 chicken breasts, skin on

2 chicken thighs

2 chicken legs

2 chicken wings

FOR THE FRIED CHICKEN

4 cups low-fat buttermilk

2 cups (1 pound) lard

8 tablespoons (115 grams) unsalted butter

½ cup thick-sliced ham cut into long strips (if you can find country ham from the South, even better)

140 grams All-Purpose Gluten-Free Flour Blend (page 17)

2 tablespoons arrowroot flour

1 teaspoon kosher salt

½ teaspoon freshly ground black pepper

Brine the chicken. The day before you intend to fry the chicken, set a Dutch oven over high heat. Add the salt and water. Bring the water to a boil and stir until the salt is dissolved. Take the pot off the heat and allow the brine to cool completely.

Put the chicken into the brine and let it sit overnight in the refrigerator.

CONTINUED

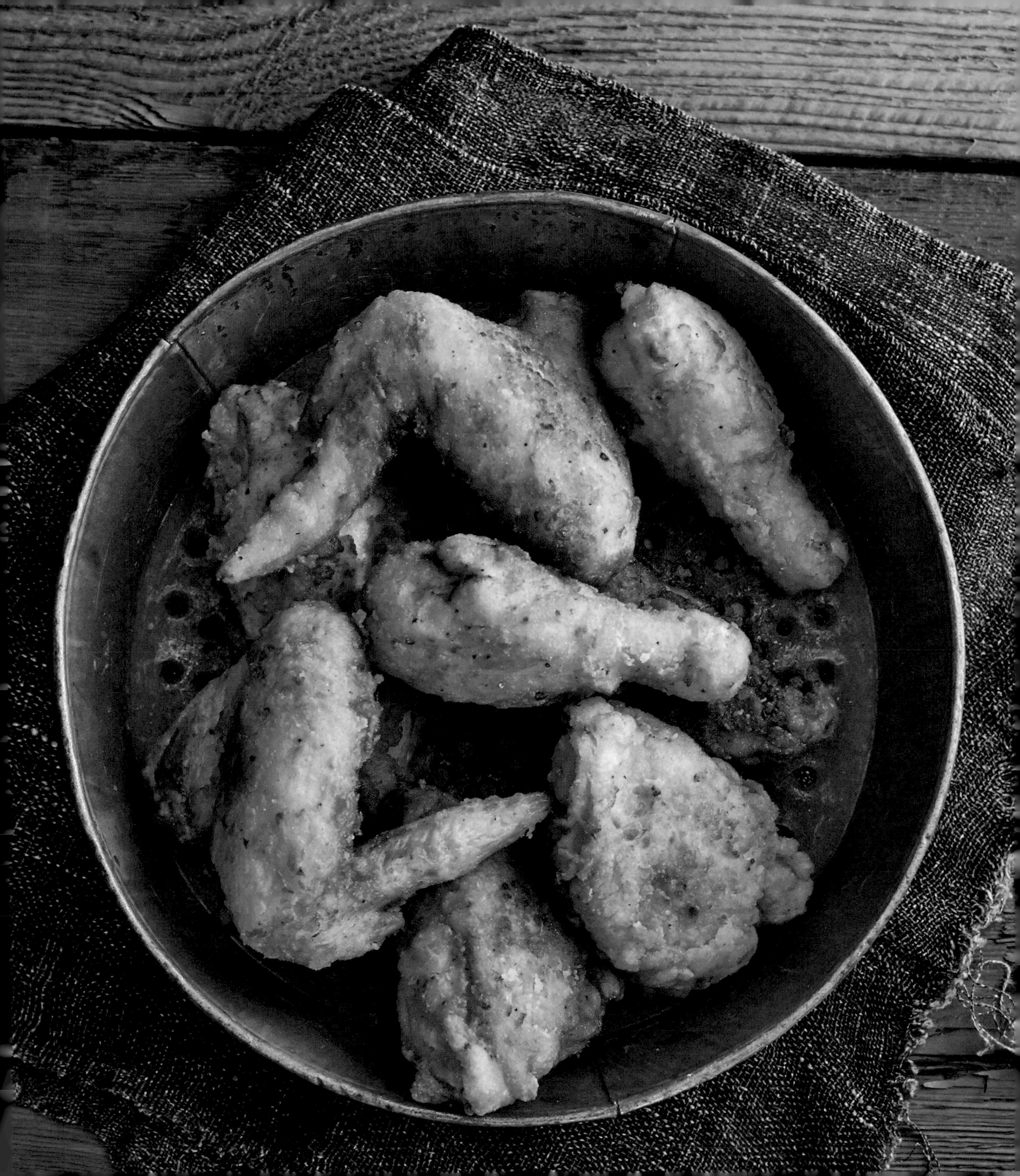

Soak the chicken. The next morning, take the chicken out of the brine and put it in a large bowl. Pour the buttermilk over it. Cover and refrigerate for at least 8 hours.

Drain the chicken. Just before you are ready to cook, take the chicken out of the buttermilk. Put the chicken pieces on a wire rack set over a parchment-lined baking sheet, allowing the chicken to dry a bit.

Get the fat hot. Set a large cast-iron skillet over low heat. Put the lard, butter, and ham pieces into the skillet and heat the fats. The butter will foam up. Skim off the foam and nudge the ham around a bit in the fat. When the ham is completely browned and the fats are hot, after 30 to 45 minutes, remove the ham. (You can discard it or eat it.)

Dredge the chicken. Turn the heat up to medium-high and heat the fat until it's 335°F on an instant-read thermometer. As the fat is coming to heat, whisk together the flour blend, arrowroot, salt, and pepper in a wide bowl. Dredge the chicken pieces in the flour, making sure each piece is thoroughly coated. Lift up each chicken piece, tap it over the bowl to remove any excess flour, then set it on a plate. When the plate is filled with dredged chicken and the fat is hot, it's time to fry.

Fry the chicken. Put 3 or 4 pieces of the dredged chicken into the fat, gently. (We suggest using tongs or a Chinese spider.) Do not overcrowd the skillet, as that will reduce the temperature of the fat and make the chicken taste greasy. Cook until the bottom of the chicken is golden brown, 8 to 10 minutes. The fat should be bubbling the entire time, so it if cools down, turn up the heat. Flip the chicken and continue cooking until the internal temperature is 155°F for the breasts and wings, and 185°F for the thighs and legs, another 8 to 10 minutes. Drain the fried chicken on a paper towel–lined plate and eat as soon as it's not volcanically hot.

Feel like playing?

If you don't have access to arrowroot flour, use cornstarch or potato starch instead. There's no need to use every part of the chicken; that's best suited for when you buy an entire chicken and cut it up. Danny and I like fried chicken legs best, so you could make this recipe for 8 drumsticks instead.

If this recipe terrifies you, you can make an easy oven-baked chicken. Use the recipe for oven-baked pork chops on page 177 and substitute chicken thighs or drumsticks in place of the pork chops.

WISCONSIN FISH FRY

Feeds 4

When my friend Sharon and I drove across the country, we made sure to stop in Madison, Wisconsin, in honor of my dear friend Tita. Raised in Madison and on a farm just outside the city, Tita has more common sense about food than anyone I have ever met. She eats lots of vegetables without knowing what antioxidants are in them. She loves butter, full-fat dairy, and ice cream. (She's from Wisconsin!) She plans her meals for the week to make balanced meals that don't cost much, and she eats pie whenever it feels right. In other words, she's really healthy, both physically and psychologically. So when Tita told me I couldn't drive across the United States without experiencing a Friday night Wisconsin fish fry, I listened. Sharon and I ate some of the best beer-battered fish I've ever eaten. This recipe is in honor of that night in a bar in Madison and Tita.

350 grams All-Purpose Gluten-Free Flour Blend (page 17)

1½ teaspoons kosher salt

1 teaspoon baking powder

1¾ cups gluten-free beer (the darker the better)

3 cups fat or oil of your choice for frying (we use rice bran oil)

Four 6-ounce portions cod (or another fish like haddock or halibut)

Make the batter. In a bowl, whisk together 210 grams of the flour blend, the salt, and baking powder. Slowly, while whisking, pour in the beer. When the batter is smooth, with only a few lumps, put it in the refrigerator for 15 minutes.

Put the remaining 140 grams of flour blend in a wide bowl.

Heat the oil. Set a large wok over medium-high heat. Pour in the oil. Heat until the oil is 350°F.

Fry the fish. Take the beer batter out of the refrigerator. Dredge the fish in the flour, then dunk it in the beer batter. Hold up the piece of fish and let the excess batter drip off. Gently, put the fish in the oil, putting the edge closest to you down first and laying it down away from you to avoid oil splattering on you. Dredge and batter another piece of fish and fry it too. Fry the fish for 4 minutes, then turn them over and fry the other side for another 4 minutes. Continue flipping the fish and frying until they are golden brown and crisp, another 2 to 5 minutes, depending on the thickness of the fish. Put the fried fish on a paper towel–lined plate, draining the oil. Fry the rest of the fish in the same manner. Serve immediately.

Feel like playing?

If you'd like to dip your fish in tartar sauce, combine 1 cup of mayonnaise, 2 tablespoons of capers, 1 tablespoon of finely chopped fresh Italian parsley, 2 teaspoons of lemon juice, and salt and black pepper to taste.

FRIED CLAMS

Feeds 4 to 6

On our New England potluck tour, we had the joy of spending a day in Rockport, Massachusetts, with our friend Stephanie. This might be the sweetest small town we've ever seen, right on the sea. Steph showed us every street she walked as a child. We walked to a great little seafood shack where we pointed to fresh lobsters in a tank and fifteen minutes later someone brought them to us cooked, with a bowl of warm butter, as we sat by the ocean. We never wanted to leave. Danny had the chance to eat the fried clams at Top Dog, a hot dog and fried clam shack. Steph told us, with the confidence of a hometown girl, that these were the best fried clams on the New England coast. I'm sure others would disagree, but Danny is on her side. Watching him eat those little golden brown furls of fried clams made me jealous. So we came home and made these, based on his eating experience.

1 cup cornmeal (make sure it's gluten-free)

105 grams All-Purpose Gluten-Free Flour Blend (page 17)

35 grams milk powder (preferably whole milk powder, if you can find it)

1 teaspoon baking powder

1 teaspoon kosher salt

1 cup low-fat buttermilk

1½ pounds whole-belly clams, shucked (Ipswich or razor clams)

About 6 cups fat or oil of your choice for frying (we use rice bran oil)

Prepare to fry. Grind the cornmeal in a blender until it's very finely ground. In a wide bowl, whisk together the ground cornmeal, flour blend, milk powder, baking powder, and salt. Pour the buttermilk into another wide bowl and set it by the side of the dry ingredients.

Dredge the clams. Dredge each clam in flour, then dip it in the buttermilk (pause to let the excess buttermilk drip back into the bowl), and then in the flour again. Set all the dredged clams on a wire rack set over a baking sheet.

Heat the oil. Set a large wok or Dutch oven over medium-high heat. Pour in the oil. Bring it to 375°F, as registered on an instant-read thermometer. Gently, lower 3 or 4 clams into the hot oil, which should bubble up a bit. Fry the clams for 30 seconds without touching them, then gently nudge them apart and cook until they are golden brown, about 1½ minutes. The clams should move around a bit in the oil, meaning you don't have to flip them, but nudge them a bit once in a while to ensure even cooking. Using a Chinese spider or slotted spoon, move the fried clams to a paper towel–lined baking sheet to drain. Allow the oil to come back to 375°F and continue frying the rest of the clams the same way.

Eat immediately. In fact, you might want to feed the first batch of clams to friends and family while you are frying the remaining batches. You want to eat these as hot as possible.

Feel like playing?

Of course, many of you reading won't have access to whole clams from New England or razor clams from Washington, which have a very short season. But there's really no way to make this with canned clams, which are minced into small pieces. There are places online to buy whole frozen clams. Or it might be worth taking a vacation to New England. (We have to go back soon.) Or, you could steam mussels, open them, and dip them into this batter before frying. Shrimp would work well with this recipe too. By the way, if you can't eat dairy, you could substitute coconut milk or clam juice for the buttermilk. You'll notice there aren't any seasonings in here besides salt. According to Jasper White, one of the great chefs of New England, you don't want any added flavors mucking up the taste of the clams. However, if you want to add some onion powder or fresh parsley, feel free.

FRIED PICKLES

Feeds 4 to 6

I must admit that when I heard about fried pickles, a much-loved Southern side dish, I immediately thought of them as an abomination, like deep-fried Twinkies. Oh, but I was wrong. Take a great dill pickle, slice it up, dip it into a simple batter made of flour, egg, and milk, and fry up those slices in hot peanut oil. Oh my. This sometimes treat deserves its adulation. Nothing wrong with this at all.

1 cup All-Purpose Gluten-Free Flour Blend (page 17)

½ teaspoon baking powder

Kosher salt and freshly ground black pepper

1 large egg

½ cup full-fat milk

3 cups fat or oil of your choice for frying (we use peanut oil)

4 whole dill pickles, cut into ½-inch slices

Make the batter. In a large bowl, whisk the flour blend, baking powder, and salt and pepper. Make a well in the center of the ingredients and add the egg and milk. Stir together all the ingredients with a rubber spatula.

Heat the oil. Set a large wok over high heat. Pour in the oil. Heat the oil to 375°F.

Fry the pickles. Using a pair of tongs, dip a pickle slice into the batter and put it directly into the hot oil. Put in no more than 10 pickle slices at a time, to avoid overcrowding. Fry for 1 minute or so, then flip the pickles and fry until golden brown, about 2 more minutes. Move the fried pickles to a paper towel–lined plate. Bring the oil back up to 375°F and fry the remaining pickles the same way.

Serve immediately. (Most people seem to like ranch dressing for dipping.)

Feel like playing?

If you can't do dairy, you could try coconut milk or another nondairy milk here. You can also use this batter for onion rings, fried okra, fried mushrooms, fried zucchini, or any fried vegetable you want to eat.

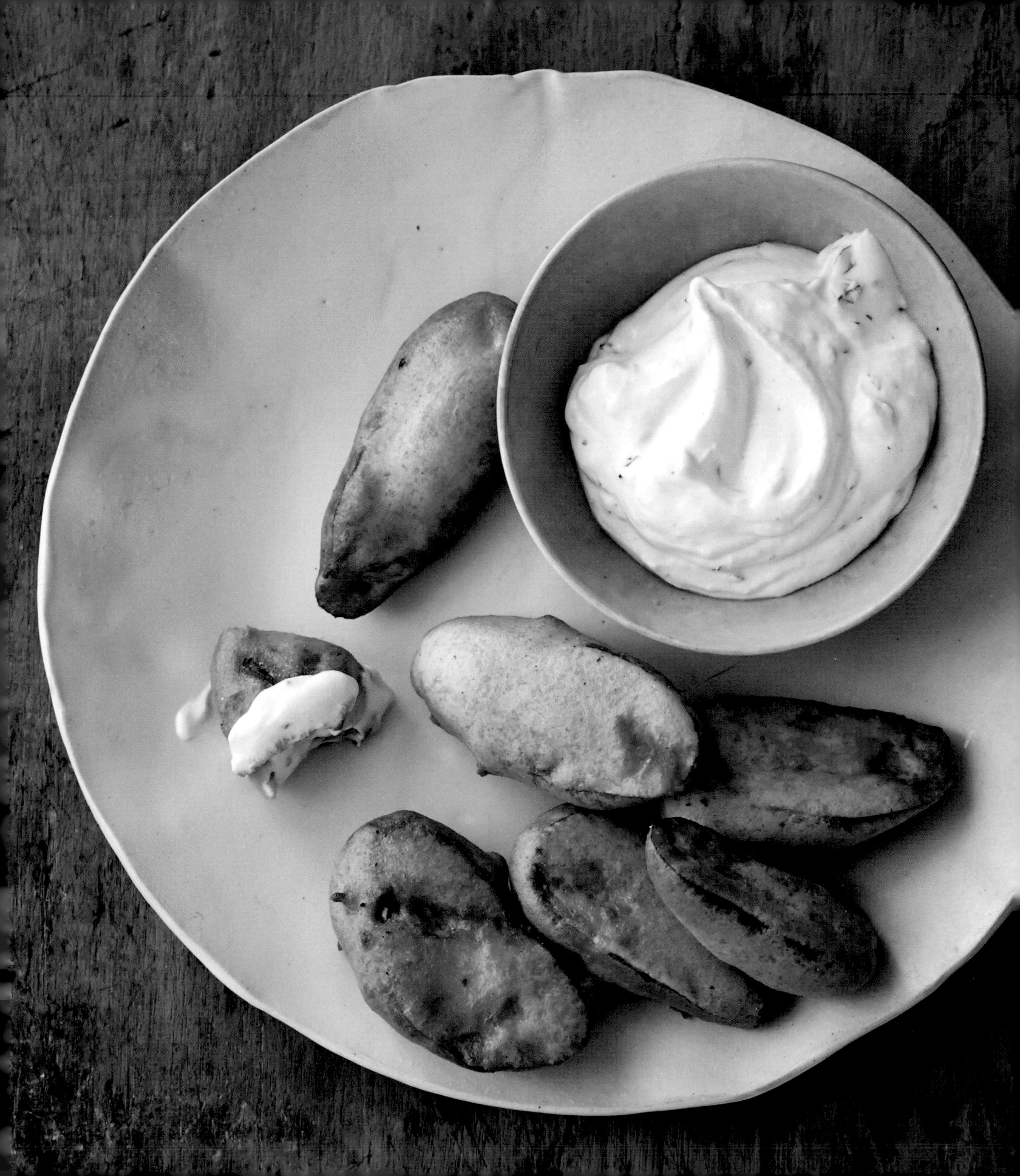

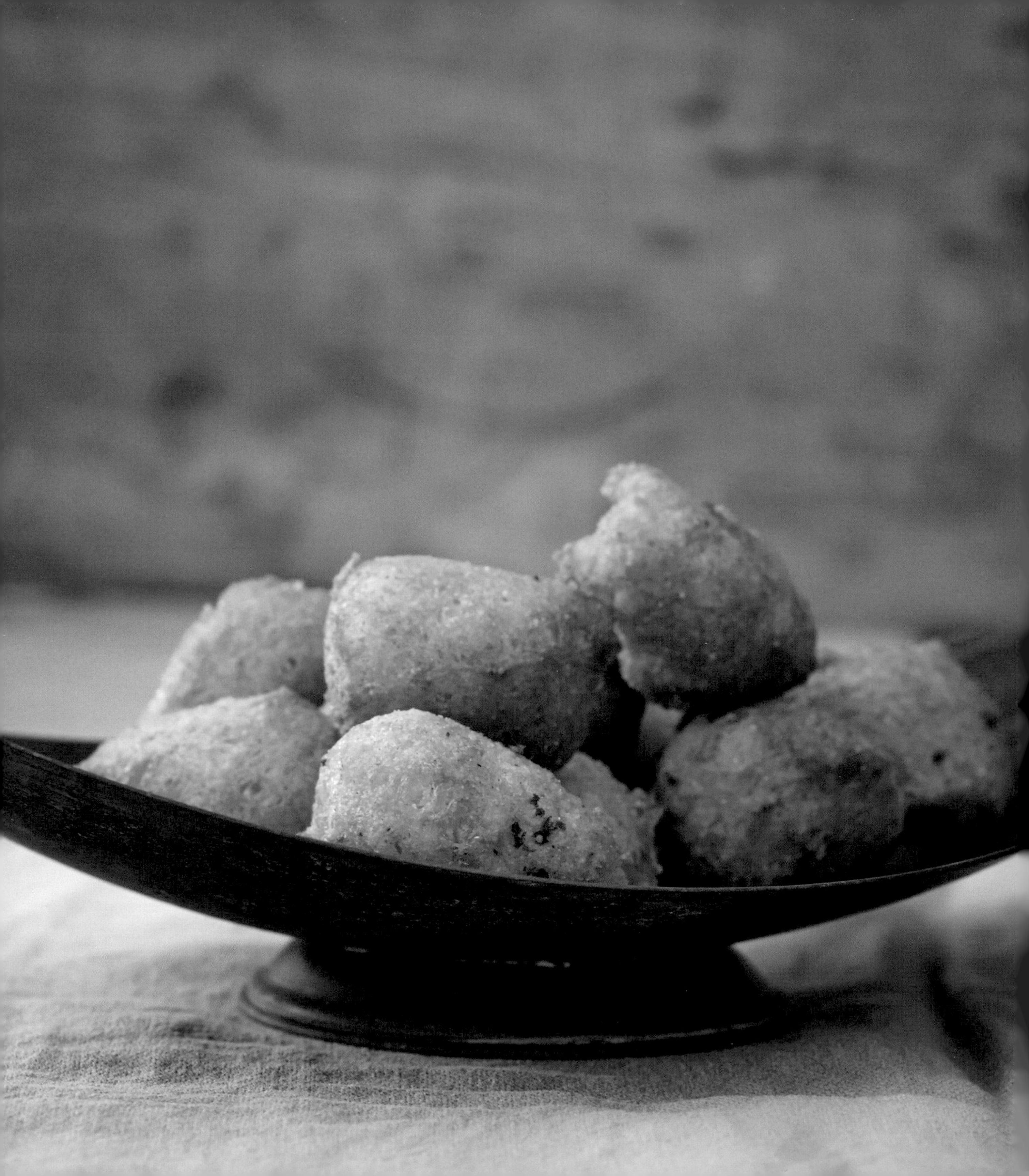

HUSH PUPPIES

Feeds 6 to 8, depending on how hungry your guests are

This classic Southern dish owes its ingredients to the Native Americans who lived in the southeastern part of what became the United States. Those native tribes were cultivating corn long before anyone else arrived. Corn is one of the staple ingredients of what is thought as Southern cuisine, thanks to the natives who shared their growing secrets. It may be legend, but many believe that this dish came from cooks who fried up bits of a cornmeal batter they intended for fish, in order to keep their dogs from howling with hunger. Hush, puppies!

¾ cup cornmeal (make sure it's gluten-free)

70 grams All-Purpose Gluten-Free Flour Blend (page 17)

1 teaspoon baking soda

½ teaspoon kosher salt

¼ teaspoon freshly ground black pepper

2 tablespoons bacon grease

2 tablespoons unsalted butter, softened

1 cup low-fat buttermilk

6 cups fat or oil of your choice for frying (we suggest peanut oil)

Make the hush puppy batter. In a bowl, whisk together the cornmeal, flour blend, baking soda, and salt and pepper. Add the bacon grease and butter and work the fats into the flour with your fingers. Make a well in the center of the flour and pour in the buttermilk. Using a rubber spatula, combine all the ingredients until the batter is smooth.

Heat the oil. Set a Dutch oven over medium-high heat. Pour in the oil. Heat the oil to 350°F on an instant-read thermometer.

Fry the hush puppies. When the oil is hot, drop 1 teaspoonful of batter into the hot oil. Fry up about 8 hush puppies at a time, taking care to not overcrowd the pot. Fry until the hush puppies are golden brown, about 3 minutes. Allow the oil to come to full heat again and fry the remaining hush puppies. Serve immediately.

Feel like playing?

Hush puppies are always, traditionally, corn. But there's no reason you can't play with buckwheat or quinoa flakes ground into a meal here, if you cannot tolerate corn.

BAJA FISH TACOS

Feeds 4

Fish tacos are really a gift from the gods. Actually, they're a gift from the hard-working cooks in Baja California, who have been making tacos of homemade tortillas, lightly fried fish, finely shredded cabbage slaw, and Mexican crema with lime for decades. I've seen a lot of fish tacos on a lot of menus across the country, and most of them get it wrong. We don't need pineapple salsa, blackened fish, smoke flavor, or anything with chipotle. This dish is a lesson in textures: hot fried fish with crisp cabbage and soft avocados with the unctuous ooze of cold crema. Oh dear, now I need another one.

FOR THE LIME CREMA

2 cups sour cream (if you can get Mexican crema, use that instead)

½ cup crumbled queso fresco

Freshly grated zest and freshly squeezed juice of 1 lime

3 tablespoons finely chopped fresh cilantro

Kosher salt and freshly ground black pepper

FOR THE CABBAGE SLAW

½ head green cabbage, thinly slivered (if you have a mandoline, use it)

2 tablespoons apple cider vinegar

FOR THE FRIED FISH

140 grams All-Purpose Gluten-Free Flour Blend (page 17)

¾ teaspoon kosher salt

½ teaspoon baking powder

¾ cup gluten-free beer (the darker the better)

3 cups fat or oil of your choice for frying (we like rice bran oil)

1 pound cod (or another firm white fish), cut into 8 strips

8 store-bought or homemade gluten-free tortillas (see page 109)

1 ripe avocado, pitted, peeled, and thinly sliced

½ cup finely chopped fresh cilantro

Make the crema. In a bowl, combine the sour cream, queso fresco, lime zest and juice, and cilantro. Season with salt and pepper. Refrigerate.

Make the slaw. Combine the cabbage, most of the lime crema (reserve ½ cup for the final dish), and the vinegar in a large bowl. Let sit in the refrigerator to grow cold.

CONTINUED

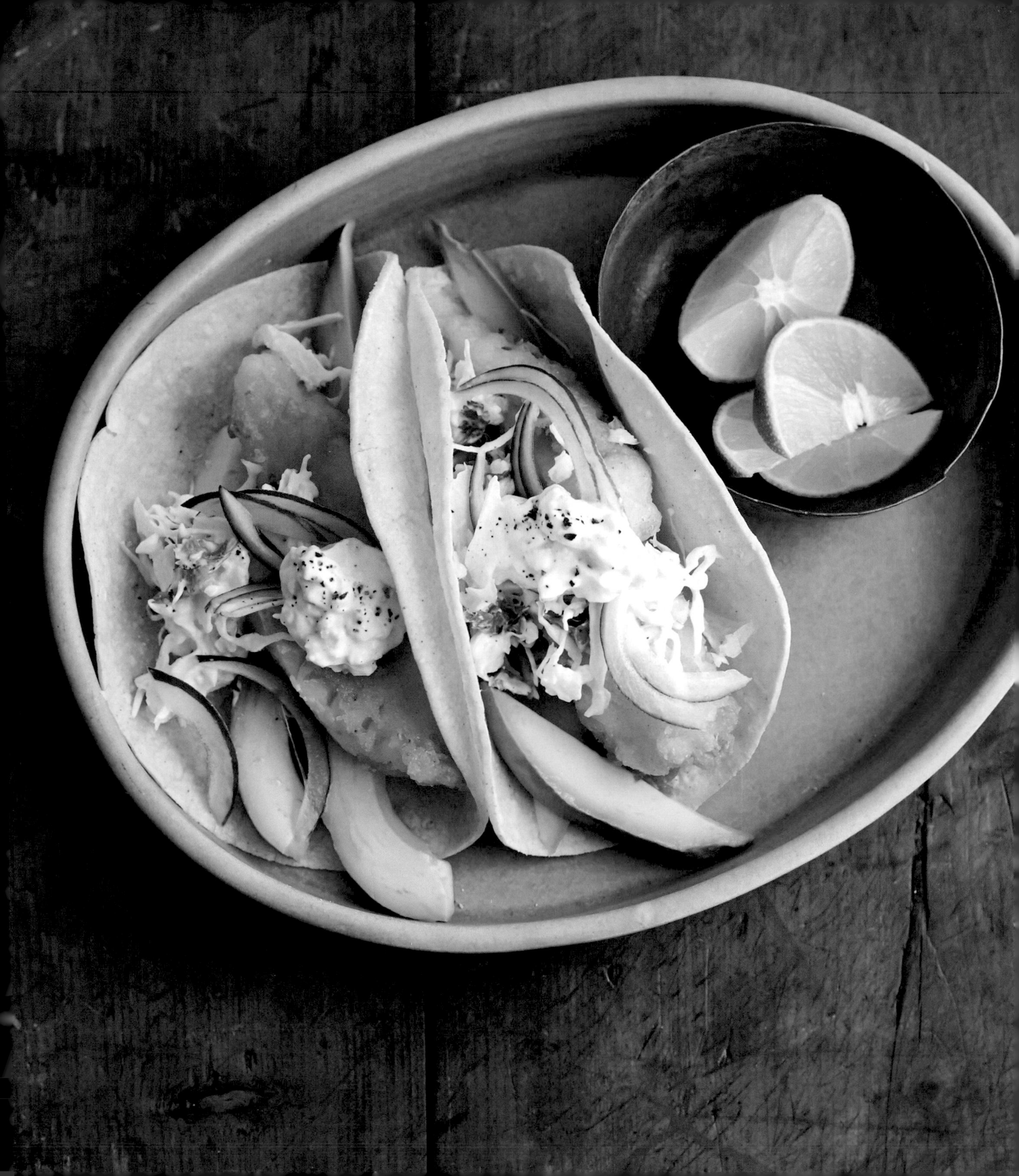

Make the batter. In a bowl, whisk together the flour blend, salt, baking powder, and beer. It should feel like pancake batter. Let the batter sit for 15 minutes.

Heat the oil. Set a large wok over medium-high heat. Add the oil and bring it to 350°F.

Fry the fish. Dip a piece of fish in the batter, letting it drip back into the batter for a moment. Gently, put the fish into the oil, taking care to not splatter yourself with oil. Batter another piece of fish and fry that too. Fry for 1 minute, then flip the pieces of fish and fry until golden brown and crisp, 1 to 2 minutes. Drain the fish on paper towel–lined plates and season with salt. Fry the rest of the fish in the same fashion.

Assemble the tacos. On each tortilla, place a slice of avocado, a piece of hot fish, a bit of the cabbage slaw, and a dollop of the reserved lime crema. Top with cilantro and serve.

Feel like playing?

There's not much to improve here. If you cannot do beer, use an equal volume of club soda for the batter. If you are one of those folks who tastes cilantro as soapy, I'm so sorry. Feel free to skip it here and use something like parsley instead.

FRIED GREEN TOMATOES

Feeds 4 to 6

These Southern specialties are a seasonal delicacy. Can't wait for the tomatoes to ripen? Pick some of them green and fry them up in cornmeal and buttermilk. There's nothing about this recipe that requires the elastic protein of gluten, so there's nothing lost by using the all-purpose flour blend we created for this book. And when you eat, if you're anything like me, you might find you have a hankering to watch the movie Fried Green Tomatoes *again with a plate of these in front of you and your friends. Towanda!*

½ cup cornmeal (make sure it's gluten-free)

70 grams All-Purpose Gluten-Free Flour Blend (page 17)

Kosher salt and freshly ground black pepper

1 cup low-fat buttermilk

1 large egg

3 firm green tomatoes, cut into ½-inch slices

1 cup fat or oil of your choice for frying (we use peanut oil)

3 tablespoons bacon grease

Set up the dredging station. In a wide bowl, whisk together the cornmeal, half the flour blend, and salt and pepper. In another wide bowl, beat together the buttermilk and egg. Put the cornmeal mixture and beaten egg mixture side by side. Put the remaining flour blend in a third bowl.

Dredge the tomatoes. Dredge each tomato in the flour blend, then the buttermilk, then the cornmeal mixture. Put each tomato on a wire rack and repeat with the rest of the tomatoes.

Heat the oil. Set a large cast-iron skillet over medium-high heat. Pour in the oil and bacon grease and give them a good stir. When the oil has come to 375°F on an instant-read thermometer, put several of the dredged tomatoes into the oil. Cook until the bottom is golden brown, about 2 minutes, then flip the tomatoes and cook until the other side is golden brown, another 2 minutes. Move the tomatoes to a paper towel–lined plate and immediately season with salt. Continue frying the remaining tomatoes in the same way.

Feel like playing?

The traditional ingredient for the crust is cornmeal, but if you can't eat cornmeal, try ground buckwheat flakes or quinoa flakes here. If you can't do dairy, then make buttermilk out of your favorite nondairy milk by adding a good squeeze of lemon juice to 1 cup of milk and letting it sit for 20 minutes before using it.

NAVAJO FRY BREAD

Feeds 6

So many folks requested Indian fry bread, a favorite fair snack, as a recipe for this book that we immediately put it on the list of recipes. I'm not sure everyone who requested the recipe knows the sad story behind it. I didn't before I started researching for this book. The Navajo tribe lived in the southwestern part of what became the United States, including Arizona, Colorado, and Utah. In the mid 1800s, American forces starved out the Navajo and herded the survivors into overcrowded camps. The U.S. government provided only meager supplies of food to those Navajo left during those four years of captivity after the Long Walks: flour, lard, powdered milk, baking powder, and salt. Navajo fry bread may have become fair food, but its origins are in starvation and resilience. When you eat this fry bread—as a base for tacos or with cinnamon sugar—raise a piece to the sky in thanks.

350 grams All-Purpose Gluten-Free Flour Blend (page 17)

½ cup powdered milk

1 tablespoon baking powder

1½ teaspoons psyllium husks

1 teaspoon kosher salt

4 cups fat or oil of your choice for frying (we use peanut oil but if you have enough lard, it's even better)

Make the dough. In a large bowl, whisk together the flour blend, powdered milk, baking powder, psyllium husks, and salt. Add enough water to combine the ingredients and make a just-combined soft dough, usually about ½ cup. Form the dough into a ball.

Let the dough rest. Brush some oil over the top of the dough and let it rest for at least 30 minutes and up to 2 hours, covered by a damp cloth.

Fry the dough. Set a large wok over medium-high heat. Pour in the oil. Heat the oil to 375°F.

Quickly, pull off pieces of dough about the size of an egg and roll each one out to the size of a small plate. (Rolling it out between two pieces of lightly greased parchment paper helps make this easier.) Make the dough a bit thicker at the edges than in the middle. Dock the dough with a fork all over the dough. Using your hands and patting it out is fine here. Gently, put the dough into the hot oil and cook for about 2 minutes. Turn the dough with tongs and cook until golden brown, about 2 minutes more. Remove the dough and lay it on a paper towel–lined plate. Continue with the rest of the dough balls.

Feel like playing?

If you have ever eaten elephant ears at the fair and want to experience them gluten-free, simply drizzle honey all over the fry bread, then sprinkle cinnamon sugar on top. If you can't use the milk powder, you can replace it with the same weight of more flour blend. The fry breads will lose a bit of softness, but they will still be good.

APPLE CIDER DOUGHNUTS

Feeds 6 to 8

The first time I visited Vermont, one of my favorite states in the union, my friend Sharon and I were barely over the border before we spotted a quaint shop selling apple cider, country crafts, and apple cider doughnuts. We ran in. (We didn't know we'd see about 50 of these quaint shops in the next three days.) The women running the shop had finished making the doughnut holes mere moments before we walked in. We ordered a dozen. We didn't even pretend to peruse the shop. Instead, we ran out to the car to eat our warm apple cider doughnut holes in silence together. Upon the first bite of that warm doughnut, our lips sprinkled with sugar, Sharon moaned and said, "Oh my god, we have to go in and order another dozen, right now." Somehow, I persuaded her to slow down, to savor the ones in front of us, and remember that there would be more apple cider doughnuts. And even now, without gluten, there are apple cider doughnuts.

1 cup apple cider (the better the quality, the better the doughnuts)

385 grams All-Purpose Gluten-Free Flour Blend (page 17)

1 tablespoon baking powder

1 teaspoon fine sea salt

¼ teaspoon freshly grated nutmeg

⅔ cup plus ½ cup organic cane sugar

2 tablespoons vegetable shortening or lard

1 large egg, at room temperature

1 large egg yolk

⅓ cup low-fat buttermilk

4 cups fat or oil of your choice for frying (we use rice bran oil)

1 tablespoon ground cinnamon

Reduce the apple cider. Set a small pot over medium heat. Pour in the apple cider. Simmer the apple cider until it has reduced to ⅓ cup. Turn off the heat.

Combine the dry ingredients. In a small bowl, whisk together the flour blend, baking powder, salt, and nutmeg.

Cream the sugar and shortening. In the bowl of a stand mixer with the paddle attachment, mix ⅔ cup of the sugar and the shortening until fluffy, about 5 minutes. Scrape down the sides of the bowl with a rubber spatula. Add the egg. When it is fully incorporated into the sugar, add the egg yolk. Scrape down the sides of the bowl with a rubber spatula.

Finish the dough. Combine the reduced cider and buttermilk in the pot the cider was in. With the stand mixer running, add one-third of the flour mixture, followed by the cider and milk, then the rest of the flour mixture. When all the ingredients are well combined and one color, scrape down the sides of the bowl with a rubber spatula. Push the batter into a ball. Cover the bowl with plastic wrap and refrigerate for 1 hour.

Heat the oil. Set a Dutch oven over medium-high heat. Pour in the oil. Bring the oil to 350°F.

CONTINUED

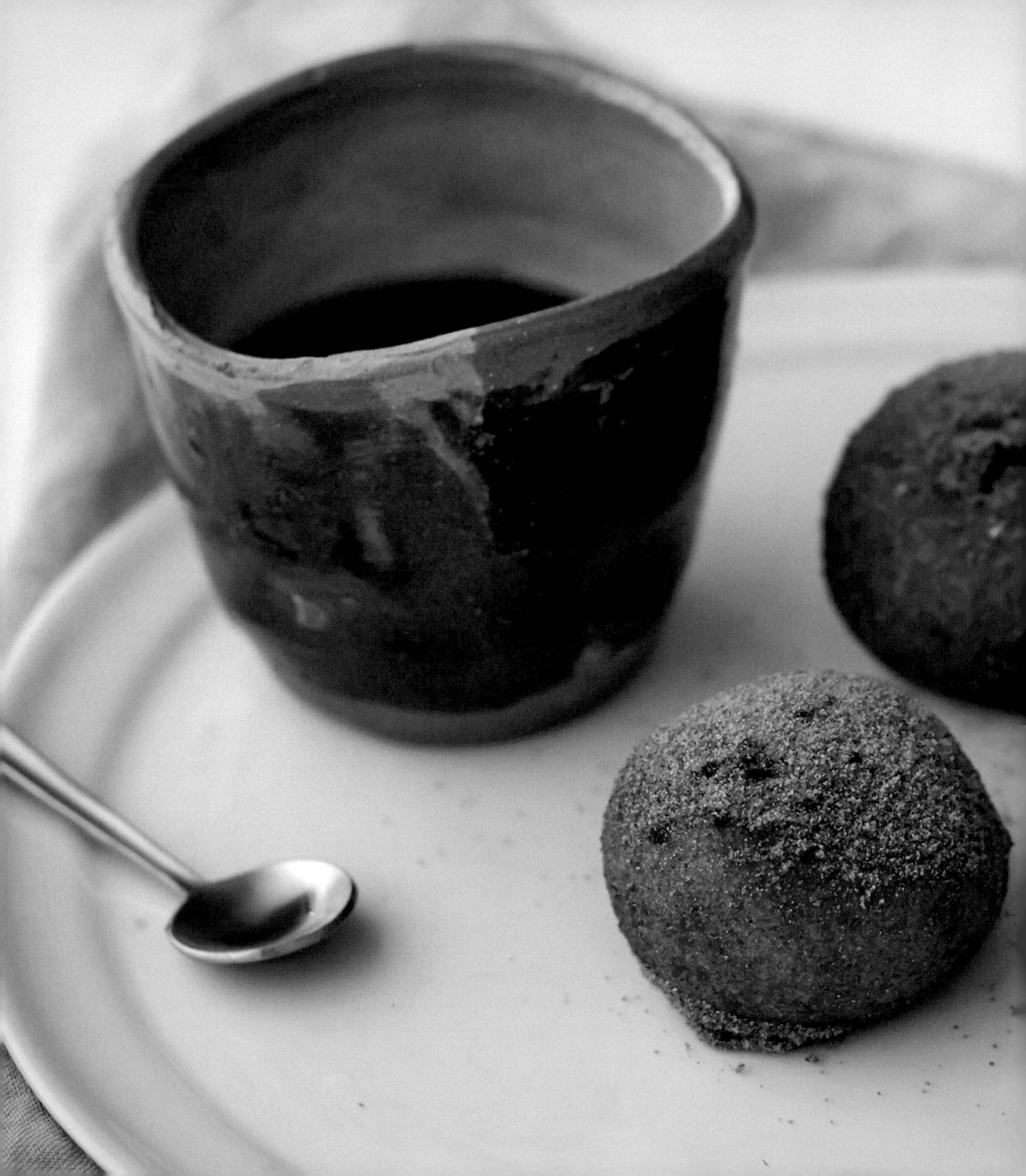

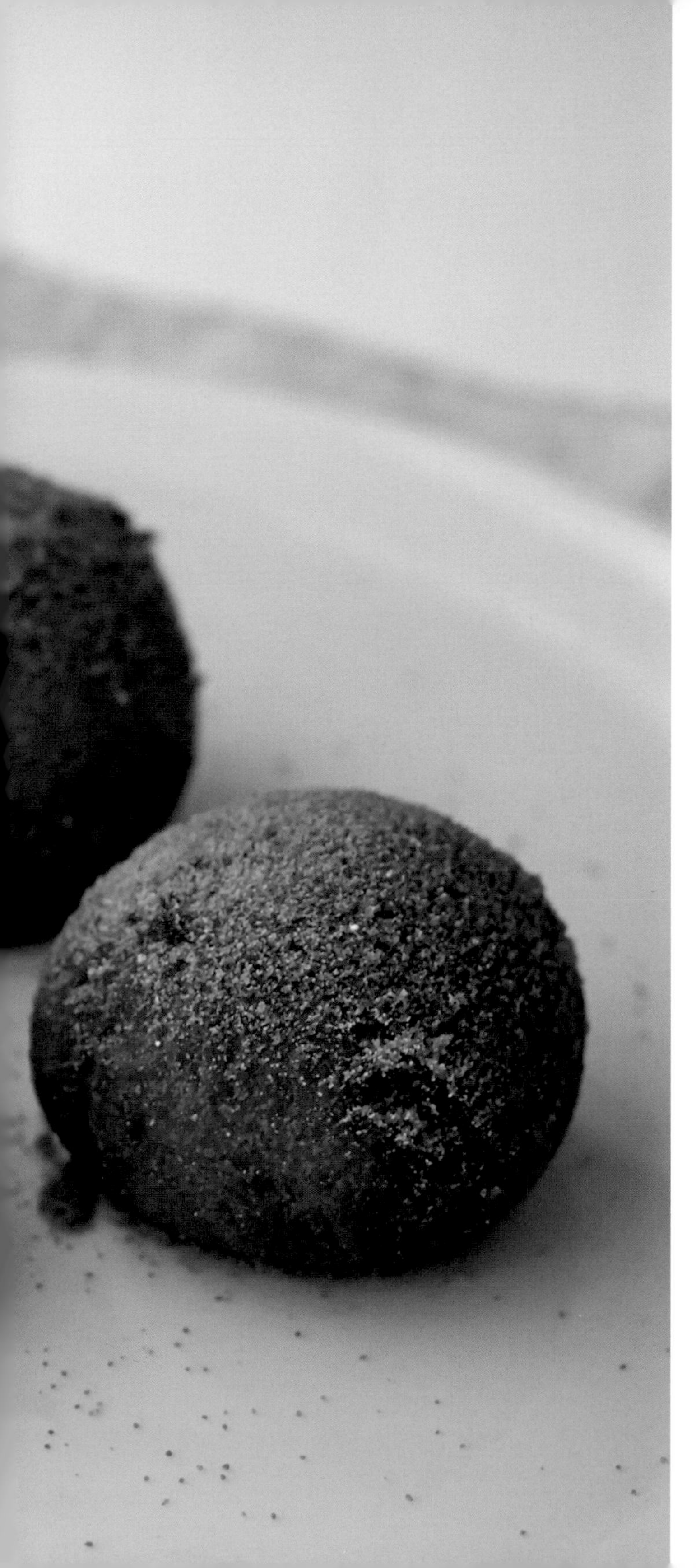

Make the doughnut holes. In a bowl, mix the remaining ½ cup of sugar and the cinnamon. Scoop 2 teaspoons of dough (about 20 grams) and roll it into a ball. Put it on a plate. Quickly, make the rest of the dough into balls.

Fry the doughnut holes. Gently, drop about 10 of the doughnut holes into the oil. Let them sit for a moment, then nudge them around with a Chinese spider or slotted spoon to separate them. Fry the doughnut holes until they are golden brown, 4 or 5 minutes. Take them out of the fryer and drain on paper towels. When they have cooled enough to touch them, roll them in the cinnamon sugar. Repeat with the remaining dough. Serve immediately.

Feel like playing?

If you'd like to make these into doughnuts instead of doughnut holes, let the dough rest much longer—even overnight—then roll the dough out to a 1-inch thickness. Cut out the doughnuts with a biscuit cutter, then make a hole in the middle with your thumb. Fry them in the oil on one side for 3 minutes or so, and then on the other side for another 3 minutes, or until they are golden brown and crispy. Don't forget the cinnamon sugar!

BEIGNETS

Makes about a dozen beignets

I have to admit that I've never eaten a proper beignet. My first and only experience of these glorious fried square doughnuts dusted with powdered sugar was while sitting at a café in New Orleans Square in Disneyland when I was a kid. They may not have been authentic, but oh I craved them after the first time I tried them. Our daughter became obsessed with the idea of beignets after seeing a Disney princess movie set in New Orleans, which made her pretend to make them for us for months. Neither one of us can eat gluten, so neither one of us will ever be able to eat a traditional beignet at Café du Monde in New Orleans, but these are mighty fine.

1 cup warm water (no more than 110°F)

1½ teaspoons active dry yeast

1 teaspoon honey

600 grams All-Purpose Gluten-Free Flour Blend (page 17)

¾ cup whole milk

¼ cup organic cane sugar

1 large egg, at room temperature

1 tablespoon psyllium husks

3 tablespoons lard or vegetable shortening

4 cups fat or oil of your choice for frying (we use rice bran oil)

Powdered sugar for dusting

Proof the yeast. In the bowl of a stand mixer with a paddle attachment, whisk together the warm water, yeast, and honey. Let the mixture sit until the top is foamy, about 15 minutes.

Finish the dough. Add 300 grams of the flour blend, the milk, sugar, egg, and psyllium husks to the yeast mixture. Mix until the dough is smooth, about 4 minutes. With the mixer running, add the lard in little bits, then the remaining 300 grams of the flour blend. Mix until the dough is well combined and fluffy. Scrape down the sides of the bowl with a rubber spatula. Form the dough into a ball. Cover with plastic wrap and chill in the refrigerator overnight.

Shape the dough. The next day, pull the dough out of the refrigerator and let it sit on the counter for 30 minutes before working with it. Grab an egg-size piece of dough, put it between two pieces of lightly greased parchment paper, and roll it out into a 3-inch square.

Heat the oil. Set a large wok over medium-high heat. Pour in the oil. Heat the oil to 365°F on an instant-read thermometer.

Fry the beignets. When the oil has come to heat, add the square of dough to the oil. Fry until the bottom is golden brown, about 2 minutes, then flip the beignet and fry the other side for another 2 minutes. Transfer the beignet to a paper towel–lined plate and immediately dust with an enormous shower of powdered sugar.

While the first beignet is frying on the first side, roll out the next square of dough. Continue with this process until you have made all the beignets. Serve immediately.

Feel like playing?

These will still work with the Grain-Free Flour Mix (page 19) as well, and the taste is pretty great.

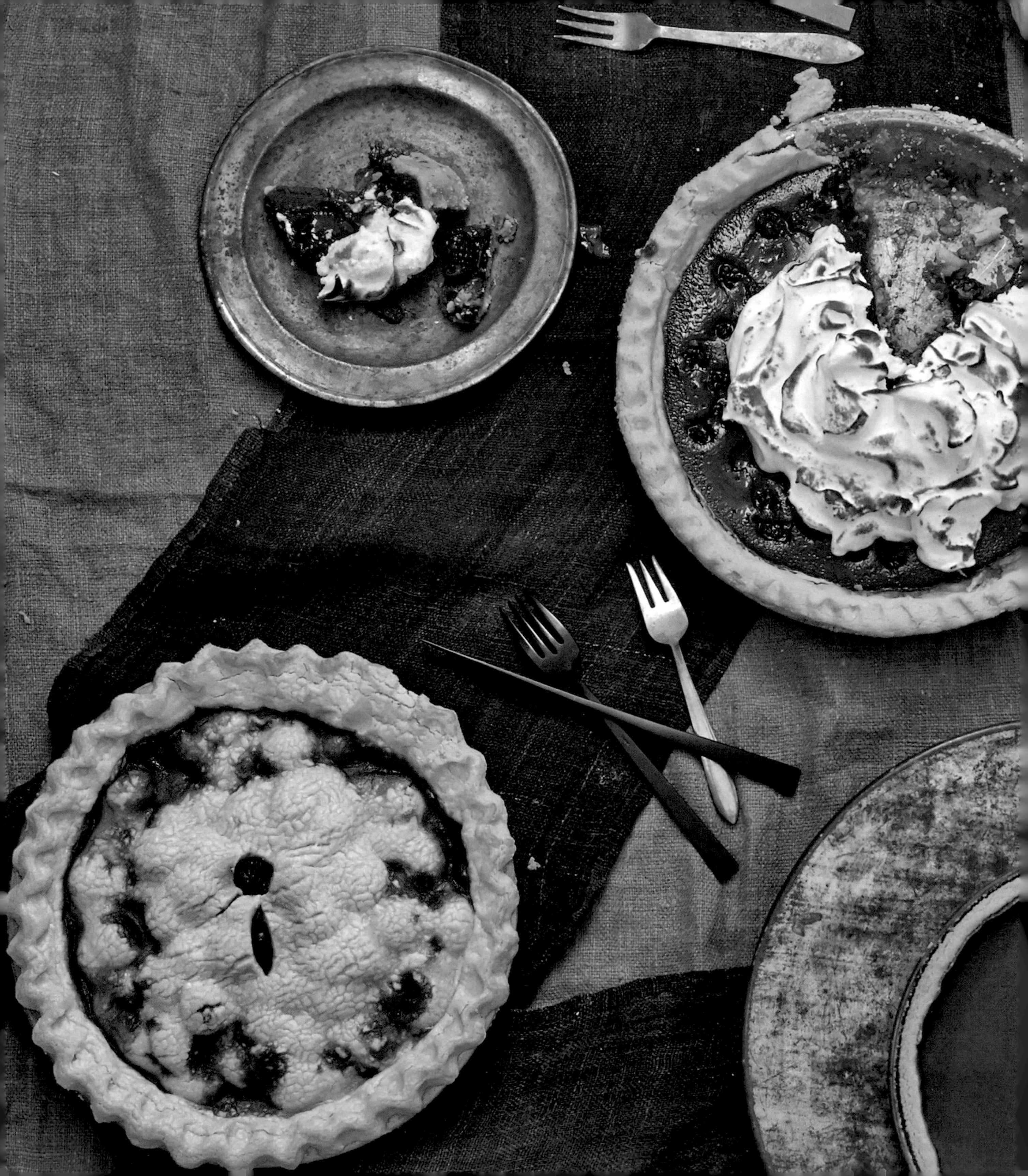

PIES

PIE DOUGH

Makes 2 disks of pie dough

Once you feel comfortable making pie dough by hand, the world opens up to you. Any of the pies in this chapter are yours. What you need: cold butter, a touch of shortening, gluten-free flour, quick hands, and a calm heart. And a lot of practice. Oh darn, you're going to need to make a lot of pies.

14 tablespoons (200 grams) unsalted butter

6 tablespoons (50 grams) lard or vegetable shortening

350 grams All-Purpose Gluten-Free Flour Blend (page 17)

½ teaspoon kosher salt

1 tablespoon cold full-fat sour cream (optional)

4 to 10 tablespoons ice-cold water

Chill the butter. Cut the butter into 1-inch cubes. Put the butter and lard in the freezer, on a saucer, for 15 minutes.

Pulse the flour and butter. Add the flour blend and salt to a large food processor. Pulse them together until the flour is fluffy and aerated. Add the chilled butter cubes and lard to the food processor and pulse 10 times. The flour and fat should look like a sandy mixture, with some chunks about the size of lima beans still visible.

Finish the dough. Mix the sour cream (if using) with 4 tablespoons of the ice-cold water. Pour the water into the food processor and pulse 5 times. The finished dough should not yet be gathered into a solid ball. Instead, it should look like curds of dry cottage cheese. You should also be able to pinch some of it between your fingers and have it stick together. If the dough is dry, add more cold water 1 tablespoon at a time. It's better to have a dough be a little too wet than a little too dry.

Form the dough into disks. Dump the dough onto a clean, cool surface, such as a marble board or a piece of parchment paper. Press the palm of your hand onto one end of the shaggy mess of dough and gently press down and away from your body. This technique, known as fraissage, will create long, buttery flakes throughout the flour, which makes for a flakier crust. Repeat this action with the rest of the dough. When it is all evenly smeared, gently gather the dough together in your hands. (A bench scraper is an enormous help here.) Working quickly, make half the dough into a ball and flatten it into a plump disk, about 2 inches tall. Wrap it in plastic wrap. Repeat with the remaining dough. Transfer the dough disks to the refrigerator to rest for at least 30 minutes. (You can also make the dough the night before you want to make the pie.)

Get ready to make a pie. When you are ready to bake, take the dough disks out of the refrigerator. Let them sit on the counter for at least 10 minutes to allow the dough to come to room temperature before you attempt to work with it.

Roll out the dough. Put two pieces of wax paper on the kitchen counter. (You can also use parchment paper, a floured marble pastry board, or a floured countertop, if you wish.) To prevent sticking, lightly oil the sides of the wax paper that will be touching the dough. Put one of the disks of dough between the pieces of wax paper. Pat down the disk a bit and lay the rolling pin on it. Imagine the dough is the face of a clock. Roll out once at 12 o'clock. Then, lift the rolling pin and roll out the dough at 12:10. Moving in "10-minute" increments, roll out the pie dough to be slightly larger than the pie pan. Don't rush. Think of this as pie meditation. Roll out the dough evenly.

Lift the top piece of wax paper. Put a 9-inch glass pie pan upside down on top of the dough. Flip the pan and dough over together. Carefully, strip away the remaining piece of wax paper. Pat the dough down into the pan, gently. If some of the pie dough sticks to the wax paper, no worries. Peel off that dough and pat it into the rest of the pie dough. There's no gluten, so the crust won't get tough.

Crimp the edges. Flour your fingers. Crimp the edges of the dough by pressing from the inside of the pie pan with the thumb and first finger on your left hand while pressing between those from the outside with the first finger of your right hand. Go slowly and enjoy it.

Now, you are ready to fill your pie.

Feel like playing?

Ready for this? There are SO many ways to play here.

If you have access to good lard (meaning not-grocery-store lard but leaf lard rendered by a good butcher or farmer) and you're not a vegetarian, use lard in this pie dough. Lard makes piecrusts even more flaky and tender than an all-butter crust or a butter and vegetable shortening crust. We use 200 grams of butter and 50 grams of lard, giving the pie dough a buttery taste but the flake of lard. You really can't beat that piecrust.

CONTINUED

You can easily skip the food processor and make the dough by hand, and you probably will once you feel confident. Simply spread the flour out in a rectangle on a clean, cool surface. Lay the pats of butter all over the flour. Use a bench scraper to swoop and cut, swoop and cut, moving the butter into the flour. Beat the egg and pour it over the dough and move it into the dough with the bench scraper. Flick the water over the surface of the flour. And then, fraissage that dough.

You can easily substitute the sour cream with anything that adds a little fat and protein to the dough, such as 3 tablespoons of thick yogurt or coconut milk, or 1 egg yolk. You can also use more water. The dough will be a little leaner, making it a bit tougher to work with for beginners. But you'll get the hang of it.

If you can't eat butter, you can substitute nondairy buttery sticks instead and use them the same way here. Of course, some people swear by vegetable shortening for pie dough in general. Or you could make an all-lard crust.

If you are a beginner and you don't want to go through the process of making a pie dough this way, use 10 tablespoons of coconut oil instead. Coconut oil will melt quickly in your hands, so you won't achieve the same level of flakiness as you might with a butter pie. Simply rub the oil and flour together until you have a sandy mix that looks like little pebbles. Gather the dough together and refrigerate it the same way you do the butter dough. Work quickly when you roll out the dough. When that dough grows warm, it seeps.

Play. Make a pie every week and see what works best in your kitchen.

PEACH PIE

Makes 1 (9-inch) pie

I thought we grew good peaches in eastern Washington. The peaches from California come as a lovely treat in the early summer. But the most memorable peach I have ever eaten was grown on the western slopes of Colorado. These Palisade peaches are firm and plump and their juice runs down your arm in a sweet little trickle you find as a surprise after you are done eating. Peach pie made with these beauties is about the best pie you'll ever eat.

8 large ripe peaches (about 4 pounds)

½ cup (105 grams) organic cane sugar

35 grams All-Purpose Gluten-Free Flour Blend (page 17)

1 tablespoon freshly squeezed lemon juice

½ teaspoon ground cinnamon

¼ teaspoon freshly grated nutmeg

¼ teaspoon fine sea salt

2 disks chilled Pie Dough (page 226)

1 large egg, beaten

Make the filling. Peel the peaches. Cut them in half and remove the pits and jagged edges around the pits. Cut the peaches into ½-inch pieces. (Don't measure them with a ruler! Just try to make the pieces a uniform size.) In a large bowl, combine the peaches, sugar, flour blend, lemon juice, cinnamon, nutmeg, and salt. Make sure all the peaches are evenly coated. Set aside and let the filling sit for at least 30 minutes before filling the pie.

Preheat the oven to 425°F. Roll out one of the dough disks, put it in a 9-inch pie pan, and crimp the edges.

Fill the pie. Fill the pie dough with the peach mixture. It should mound pretty high.

Put on the top crust. Roll out the remaining dough disk. Lay the top dough onto the pie gently, as though you were putting a blanket on a sleeping child. Tuck the edges into the crimped crust. Make two or three small slits in the top crust to allow the steam out. Brush the top of the dough with the beaten egg.

Bake the pie. Put the pie on a parchment-lined baking sheet and put it in the oven. Bake for 15 minutes. Turn down the temperature to 375°F and bake the pie until the top crust is golden brown, the juices are sizzling on the edges of the crust, and the bottom crust is browned when you look at it from the bottom of the pan, 45 minutes to 1 hour.

Wait! Allow the pie to cool for at least 2 hours before you cut into it. I know. It's hard but it's worth the wait.

Feel like playing?

I love the addition of fresh herbs in a peach pie. Try a handful of chopped fresh basil in the peach filling, or fresh thyme or tarragon. They're all good.

SOUR CHERRY PIE

Makes 1 (9-inch) pie

Sour cherries, also known as Montmorency cherries, are the perfect cherries for pie. Where we live in western Washington, we buy beautifully sweet Bing cherries from the farmers' market. We eat them until our chins are stained with cherry juice. But for pie, I want sour cherries. A specialty of northern Michigan and Oregon, these cherries are small and tart, a jewel of a cherry that looks more like a red currant. If you can't go to the Michigan's upper peninsula to visit a cherry grower, try to find sour cherries in season near you and freeze enough to make pies all winter. You won't be sorry for the trouble you took to find them.

6 cups sour cherries, pitted

1¼ cups (260 grams) organic cane sugar

35 grams All-Purpose Gluten-Free Flour Blend (page 17)

Freshly grated zest and freshly squeezed juice of 1 lime

¼ teaspoon ground cinnamon

¼ teaspoon almond extract

Pinch salt

2 disks chilled Pie Dough (page 226)

1 large egg, beaten

Feel like playing?

If you can't find fresh or frozen sour cherries near you, you can use canned cherries. Make sure to use 72 ounces of cherries to make up the bulk of the pie. Add more acid to cut the sweetness—try 2 or 3 limes here instead, with a little more flour to soak up the extra liquid—and cut the sugar in half.

Make the filling. In a large bowl, combine the cherries, sugar, flour blend, lime zest and juice, cinnamon, almond extract, and salt. Make sure all the cherries are evenly coated. Set aside and let the filling sit for at least 30 minutes before filling the pie.

Preheat the oven to 425°F. Roll out one of the dough disks, press it into a 9-inch pie pan, and crimp the edges.

Fill the pie. Fill the pie dough with the cherry mixture. It should mound pretty high.

Put on the top crust. Roll out the remaining dough disk. Lay the top dough onto the pie gently, as though you were putting a blanket on a sleeping child. Tuck the edges into the crimped crust. Make two or three small slits in the top crust to allow the steam out. Brush the top of the dough with the beaten egg.

Bake the pie. Slide the pie into the oven. Bake for 15 minutes. Turn down the temperature to 375°F and bake the pie until the top crust is golden brown, the juices are sizzling on the edges of the crust, and the bottom crust is browned when you look at it from the bottom of the pan, 45 minutes to 1 hour.

Wait! Allow the pie to cool for at least 2 hours before you cut into it. I know. It's hard but it's worth the wait.

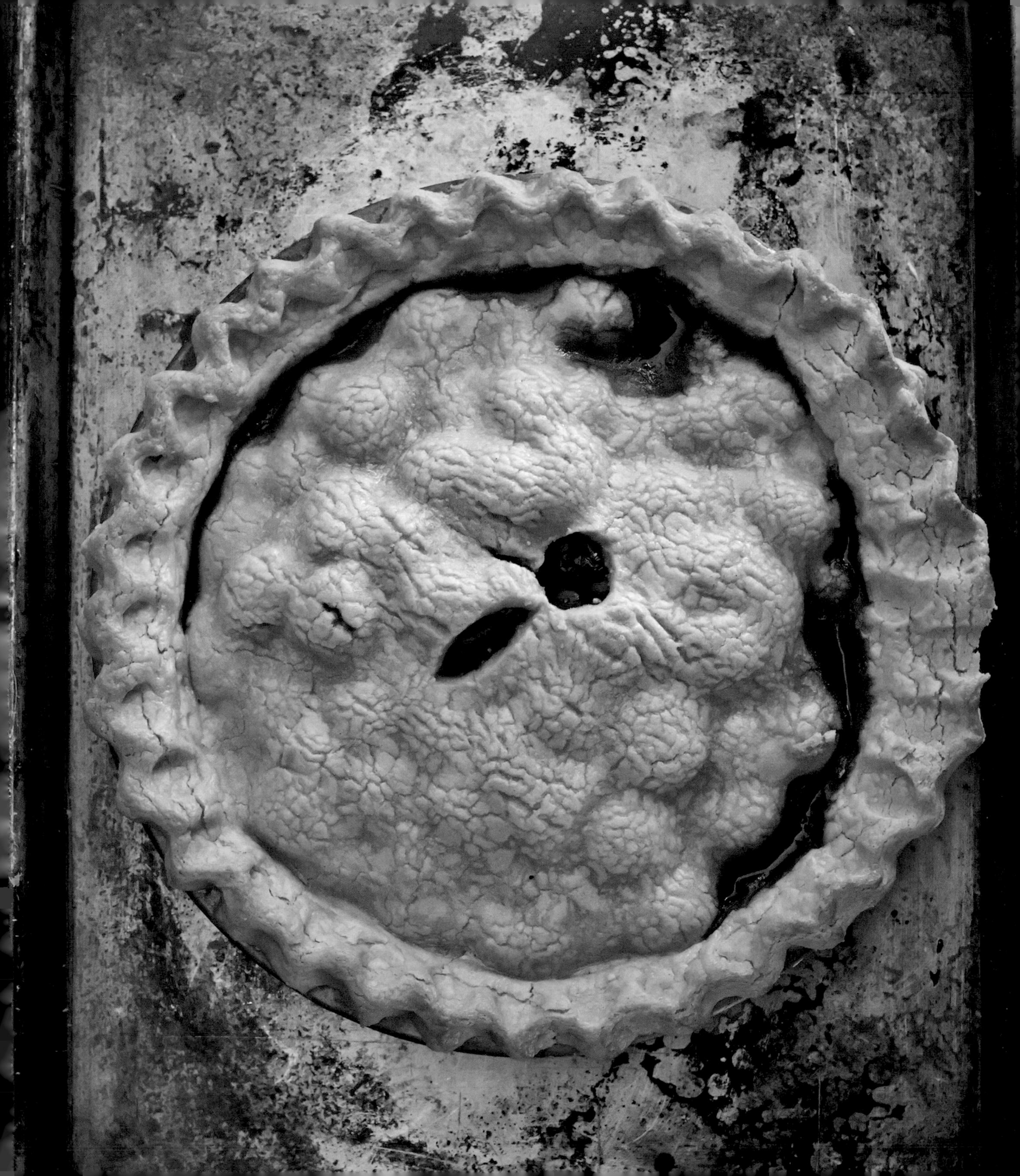

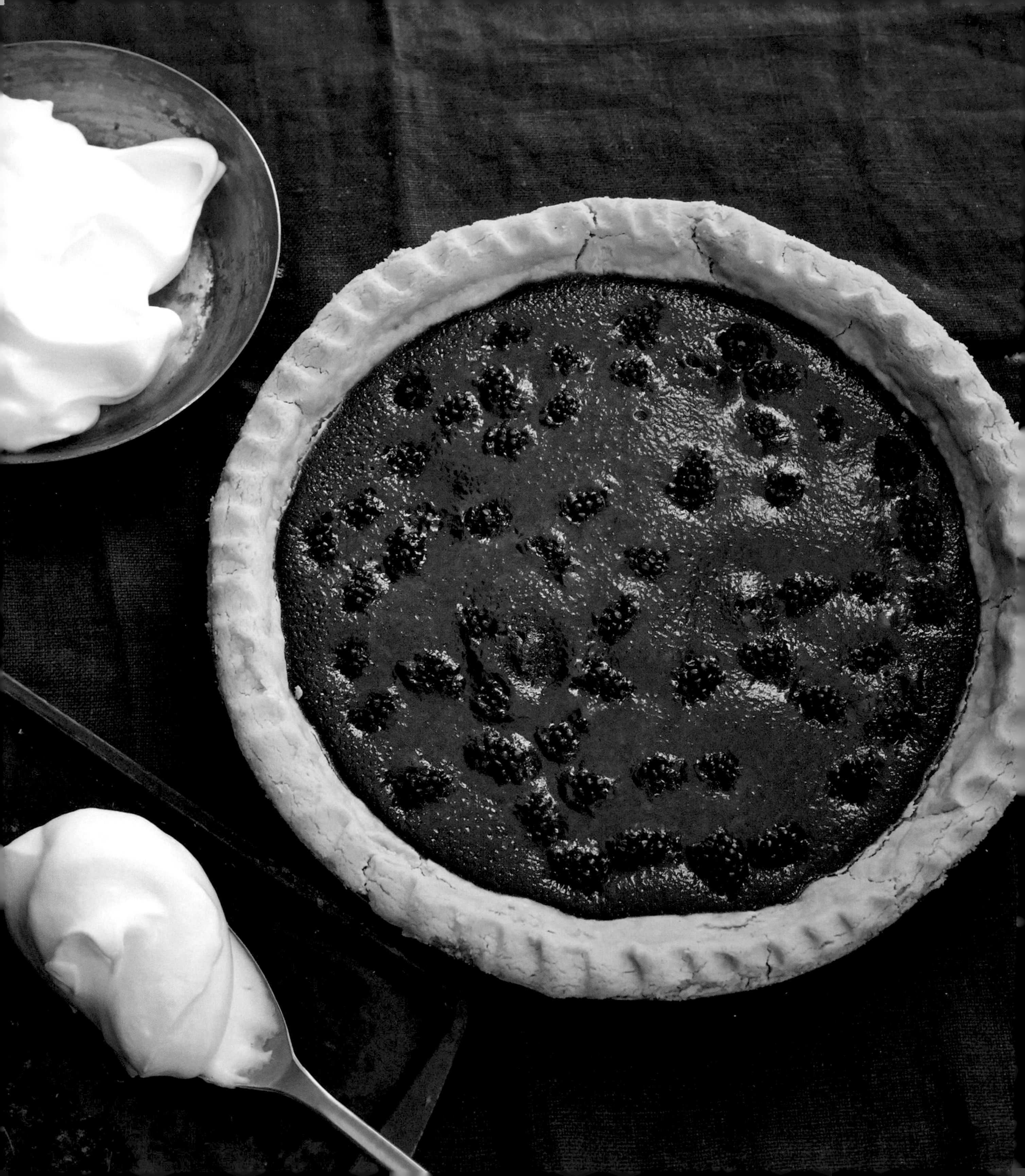

BLACKBERRY MERINGUE PIE

Makes 1 (9-inch) pie

If you live in the Pacific Northwest, you have a relationship with blackberries. Blackberry vines grow wild along the roadside and sprawl along every property here. Some people work hard to hack away at these weeds (some people rent herds of goats to chomp up the vines, believe it or not). We have an entire row of blackberry bushes on the property line of our yard. We wouldn't think of having them removed. Come late August, we walk outside every morning for fresh blackberries for breakfast, pick blackberries for smoothies and yogurt popsicles, and brave the thorns to fill buckets of blackberries to freeze for the winter. But really, we look forward to blackberry season for the pies. This riff on lemon meringue pie requires plump blackberries pureed into dark purple juice for blackberry curd. I like my relationship with blackberries.

1 disk chilled Pie Dough (page 226)

5 cups fresh blackberries (frozen would be fine too)

1⅓ cups (280 grams) organic cane sugar

6 tablespoons (86 grams) unsalted butter, softened

Freshly grated zest and freshly squeezed juice of 1 lemon

6 large eggs

6 large egg yolks

½ teaspoon fine sea salt

3 large egg whites

1 tablespoon arrowroot flour

Bake the piecrust. Preheat the oven to 425°F. Roll out the pie dough, put it in a 9-inch pie pan, and crimp the edges. Grease a piece of aluminum foil and lay it down on the top of the pie dough. Fill the aluminum foil with dried beans. Bake until the edges of the pie dough have set, about 15 minutes. Take the aluminum foil off the pie dough and bake until the crust is golden, another 5 to 10 minutes. Remove from the oven. Cool the crust completely.

Make the juice. Set a large pot over medium heat. Add 4 cups of the blackberries and ½ cup water. Simmer the blackberries, stirring occasionally, until they have softened, about 5 minutes. Put the blackberries into a blender and puree them. Push the puree through a fine-mesh sieve with a rubber spatula to remove the seeds and pulp. This should yield about 1 cup of blackberry juice.

Cream the butter and sugar. Put 1 cup of the sugar and 4 tablespoons of the butter into the bowl of a stand mixer with the paddle attachment. On low speed, cream the sugar and butter together until they are light and fluffy, about 5 minutes.

Make the curd. With the mixer running on low, add the lemon zest and juice. Then add the eggs, one at a time, making sure each egg is fully incorporated into the butter and sugar. After all the eggs have been added, add the egg yolks. Pour in the blackberry juice. Finish with the salt. The final liquid should be thick.

CONTINUED

Cook the curd. Pour the curd into a large pot set over medium heat. Cook, stirring frequently, until the liquid thickens. At first, you might think it will never happen. Keep stirring, constantly at this point, to prevent the curd from burning. After 10 minutes or so, the curd will suddenly thicken, pull away from the edges of the pot a bit, and bubble vigorously. (If you have an instant-read thermometer, you can also use it here to make sure the curd has reached 170°F.) Stick a spoon into the curd. When you drag your finger down the back of the spoon, does it leave a clean trail? You're done. Pull the pot off the heat. Add the remaining 2 tablespoons of butter to the curd and stir until the mixture is smooth. Allow the curd to cool to room temperature.

Prepare to bake. Preheat the oven to 450°F, if the oven isn't already on. Pour the curd into the prepared piecrust, spreading it out evenly. Strew the remaining 1 cup of fresh blackberries over the top of the curd.

Make the meringue. In the bowl of a stand mixer with the whisk attachment, add the egg whites, the remaining ⅓ cup of sugar, and the arrowroot until the egg whites are stiff. Spread the stiff egg whites onto the top of the pie, allowing the edges of the crust to peek through. Bake until the meringue is brown at the tips, 5 to 7 minutes. Serve immediately.

Feel like playing?

If you want to make a great lemon meringue pie, simply use 2 cups of lemon juice instead of making the blackberry juice. Omit the fresh berries on top. Voilà! Lemon meringue pie. You probably don't need me to tell you that blackberry curd is a gorgeous concoction. It's wonderful mixed into thick yogurt or spooned on top of pavlovas or tucked into a tart shell for an easy dessert. But really, you probably just want to eat it out of the jar with a spoon.

KEY LIME PIE

Makes 1 (9-inch) pie

Talk about American pies and you have to include Key lime pie in the conversation. This tart little thing is easy to make and utterly delicious. Originating from Key West, perhaps brought to Florida by settlers from the Bahamas, this pie takes nothing more than waiting for it to chill. (That's hard, however.) There's no real consensus on the right way to make this pie—baked or not baked, with eggs or without, topped with sour cream or meringue. We like this version, which uses a coconut-date crust in place of the typical graham cracker crust. Sweetened with honey, this pie is delightfully tart and subtly sweet. In the heat of the summer, there's nothing better.

1½ cups (240 grams) pitted dried dates

2 cups (180 grams) shredded unsweetened coconut

4 large egg yolks

One 14-ounce can sweetened condensed milk

½ cup lime juice (use Key limes if you can get them)

¼ teaspoon salt

Coconut whipped cream, whipped cream, or sour cream for serving (optional)

Prepare to bake. Preheat the oven to 350°F.

Make the crust. Soak the dates in warm water to cover for 20 minutes. Drain the dates, squeezing them as dry as you can. Put the dates and coconut into the bowl of a food processor. Mix them together until they are finely chopped together and form a large ball around the blade. Press the mixture into a 9-inch pie pan, making sure to distribute it evenly on the bottom and up the sides of the pan. Put the pie pan in the refrigerator.

Make the filling. In a bowl, whisk together the egg yolks and condensed milk. Stir in the lime juice and salt. Stir until the mixture is thick and smooth.

Bake the pie. Pour the filling into the prepared pie pan. Put the pie on a parchment-lined baking sheet and put it in the oven. Bake until the top is just starting to set, about 15 minutes. Put the pie on a wire rack and cool completely, at least 2 hours. Set the pie in the refrigerator and let it chill overnight.

Top with coconut whipped cream, whipped cream, or sour cream, as desired.

Feel like playing?

If you can't find Key limes—they're only briefly available in Seattle—you could buy a jar of the juice. (We like the Manhattan brand, which is a pretty funny name for juice from Key West.)

SWEET POTATO PIE

Makes 1 (9-inch) pie

Our friend Tita always serves preacher sweet potatoes for Thanksgiving dinner. She cooks sweet potatoes with lots of grated fresh ginger and other spices, and sweetened condensed milk, and dots them with marshmallows. She learned this recipe from a Junior League recipe from Valdosta, Georgia. We took all the flavors of her much-loved recipe, switched in coconut milk, and made this sweet potato pie. This one has been on our Thanksgiving table ever since.

1 disk chilled Pie Dough (page 226)

2 cups sweet potato puree (see Note)

½ cup (105 grams) organic cane sugar

½ cup (100 grams) coconut sugar

1 teaspoon peeled and grated fresh ginger

1 teaspoon ground cinnamon

1 teaspoon fine sea salt

½ teaspoon freshly grated nutmeg

¼ teaspoon ground cloves

3 large eggs, at room temperature

One 14-ounce can full-fat coconut milk

Prepare to bake. Preheat the oven to 425°F.

Roll out the dough, press it into a 9-inch pie pan, and crimp the edges, if desired. Put it in the freezer while you make the filling.

Make the filling. In the bowl of a stand mixer with the paddle attachment, mix the sweet potato puree, sugar, coconut sugar, ginger, cinnamon, salt, nutmeg, and cloves. Add the eggs, one at a time, making sure each egg is fully incorporated before adding the next. With the mixer running on low, slowly pour in the coconut milk. Pour the filling into the prepared pie pan.

Bake the pie. Put the pie on a parchment-lined baking sheet and put it in the oven. Bake for 15 minutes. Turn the heat down to 375°F. Bake until the crust is golden brown and the filling feels firm when you touch it gently, about 45 minutes.

Cool the pie. Allow the pie to cool to room temperature on the counter. For best taste, refrigerate it overnight before serving.

Note: To make sweet potato puree, bake 3 large sweet potatoes in a 400°F oven until they are tender to the touch. Peel the skins and put the soft flesh in a food processor. Pulse until they are pureed.

Feel like playing?

You could easily use pumpkin puree or butternut squash puree in place of the sweet potatoes. But really, we think sweet potatoes are best.

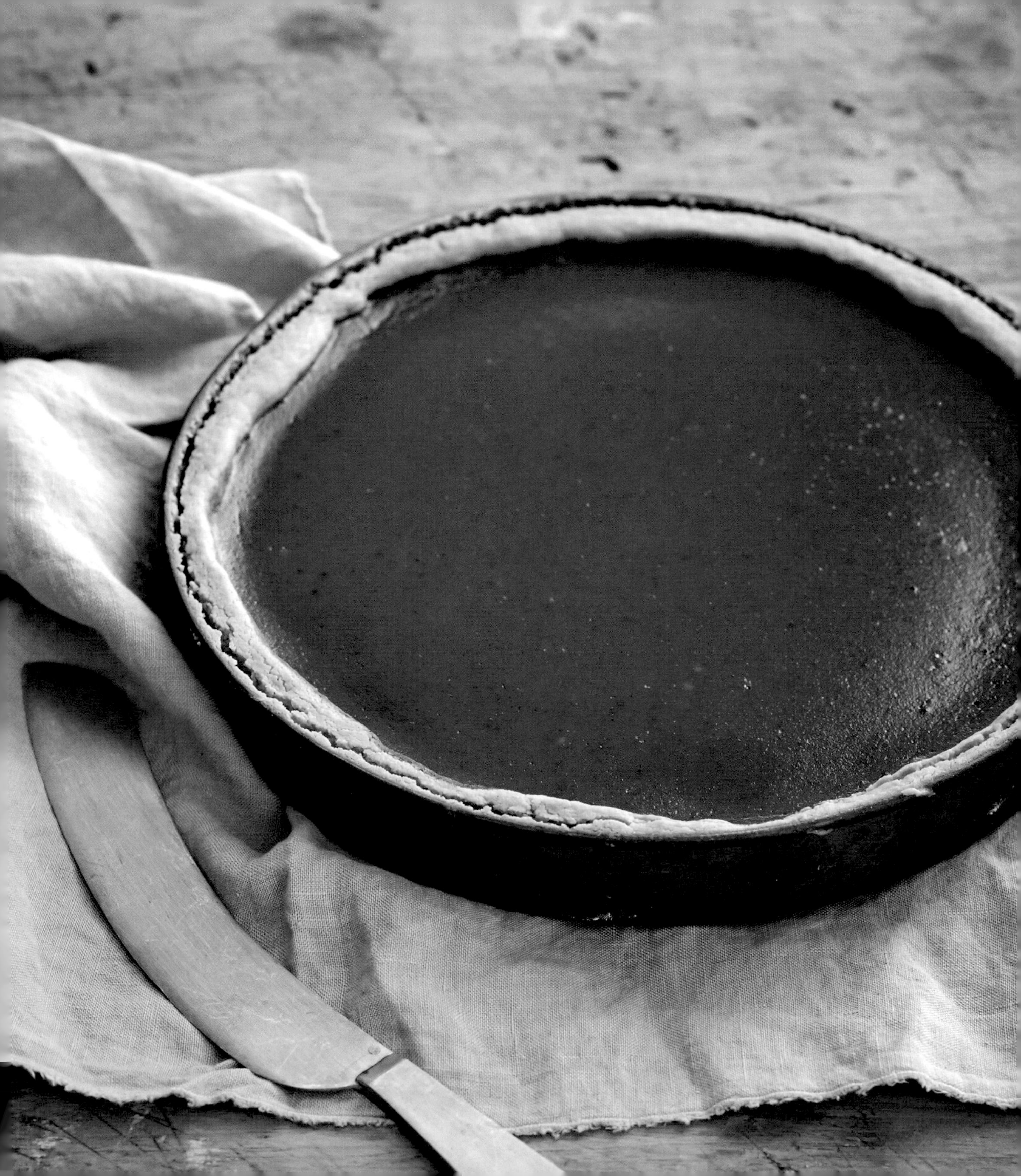

PECAN PIE

Makes 1 (9-inch) pie

Southern pie makers, you have made our lives much sweeter. Sure, there are pies made all over the country, but some of the most classic American pies originated in the South, including pecan pie. No one is quite sure of the origin, but it might be that French bakers who settled in New Orleans invented this pie after tasting pecans. Whoever it was who first made this sweet custard cut with pecan halves? We salute you. After a corn syrup company in the 1930s started promoting the use of its product to make this pie, pecan pie seemed naked without sticky corn syrup. But we prefer the sweetness of pure cane syrup here. You can play and make it yours, of course.

1 disk chilled Pie Dough (page 226)

1 cup (370 grams) pure cane syrup (see Note)

3 large eggs, beaten

½ cup (100 grams) organic cane sugar

2 tablespoons (29 grams) unsalted butter, melted

1 teaspoon vanilla extract

½ teaspoon fine sea salt

½ teaspoon ground cinnamon

2 cups (225 grams) pecan halves

Prepare to bake. Preheat the oven to 350°F.

Roll out the dough, press it into a 9-inch pie pan, and crimp the edges. Put the pie pan in the freezer as you make the filling.

Warm the cane syrup. Set a small pot over medium heat. Fill it halfway with water. Fill a tall coffee cup with the cane syrup and set the coffee cup in the simmering water until the syrup is thinned enough to pour.

Make the filling. Pour the warm cane syrup into a large bowl. Add the eggs, sugar, butter, vanilla, salt, and cinnamon. Stir with a rubber spatula until everything is well combined. Add the pecans and stir.

Bake the pie. Pour the filling into the prepared pie pan and move the pecans around until they are spread evenly throughout. Put the pie on a parchment-lined baking sheet and put it in the oven. Bake until the crust is golden brown and the filling feels firm when you touch it gently, about 50 minutes.

Cool the pie. Allow the pie to cool on the counter to room temperature, then put it in the refrigerator overnight.

Note: Pure cane syrup is concentrated juice from sugarcane, traditionally made by cooking it slowly in large, open kettles. It's liquid sweetness, far better than corn syrup in a pecan pie. We're pretty crazy about Steen's cane syrup, which has been made in Abbeville, Louisiana, since 1910, and it's available online.

Feel like playing?

If you want, you can use corn syrup in place of the cane syrup. Also, if you want this pie sweeter—some people like their pecan pie very sweet—use 1 cup of sugar instead of ½ cup. The cinnamon isn't traditional, but we feel it adds a little warmth to the taste of the pie.

SHOOFLY PIE

Makes 1 (9-inch) pie

"Shoo fly, don't bother me." It's almost impossible to hear the phrase shoofly pie *and not sing this song in your head. This Pennsylvania Dutch pie, which also became traditional in the South, is a basic pantry pie. Rather than using luscious seasonal fruit, this pie makes do with what's left when the cupboard is nearly bare and you want something sweet to eat. The dark taste of molasses and the tumble of flour and sugar on top of the filling are so appealing that the flies are said to draw too near. Shoo away, fly. This pie is mine.*

- 1 disk chilled Pie Dough (page 226)
- 140 grams All-Purpose Gluten-Free Flour Blend (page 17)
- ⅔ cup (140 grams) coconut sugar
- 1 tablespoon (13 grams) coconut oil, melted
- 1 cup molasses
- 1 large egg
- 1 teaspoon baking soda
- ¾ cup boiling water

Prepare to bake. Preheat the oven to 425°F.

Roll out the dough, press it into a 9-inch pie pan, and crimp the edges. Put the pie pan in the freezer as you make the filling.

Make the filling. In a bowl, whisk together the flour blend and sugar. Add the coconut oil and mix until the oil is fully integrated into the flour. Set aside ½ cup of the mixture.

Add the molasses, egg, and baking soda to the flour and sugar mixture and stir with a rubber spatula until well combined. Pour in the boiling water and stir until everything is thoroughly mixed.

Bake the pie. Pour the filling into the prepared pie pan. Scatter the reserved flour mixture evenly over the top of the filling. Put the pie on a parchment-lined baking sheet and put it in the oven. Bake the pie for 15 minutes. Lower the temperature to 375°F and bake until the crust is golden brown and the center of the pie is mostly set but still a tiny bit jiggly, 18 to 20 minutes.

Allow the pie to cool on the counter until it comes to room temperature. Serve.

Feel like playing?

Traditionally, the filling uses vegetable shortening rather than coconut oil. We like the unctuous nature of coconut oil here, but butter would be good too.

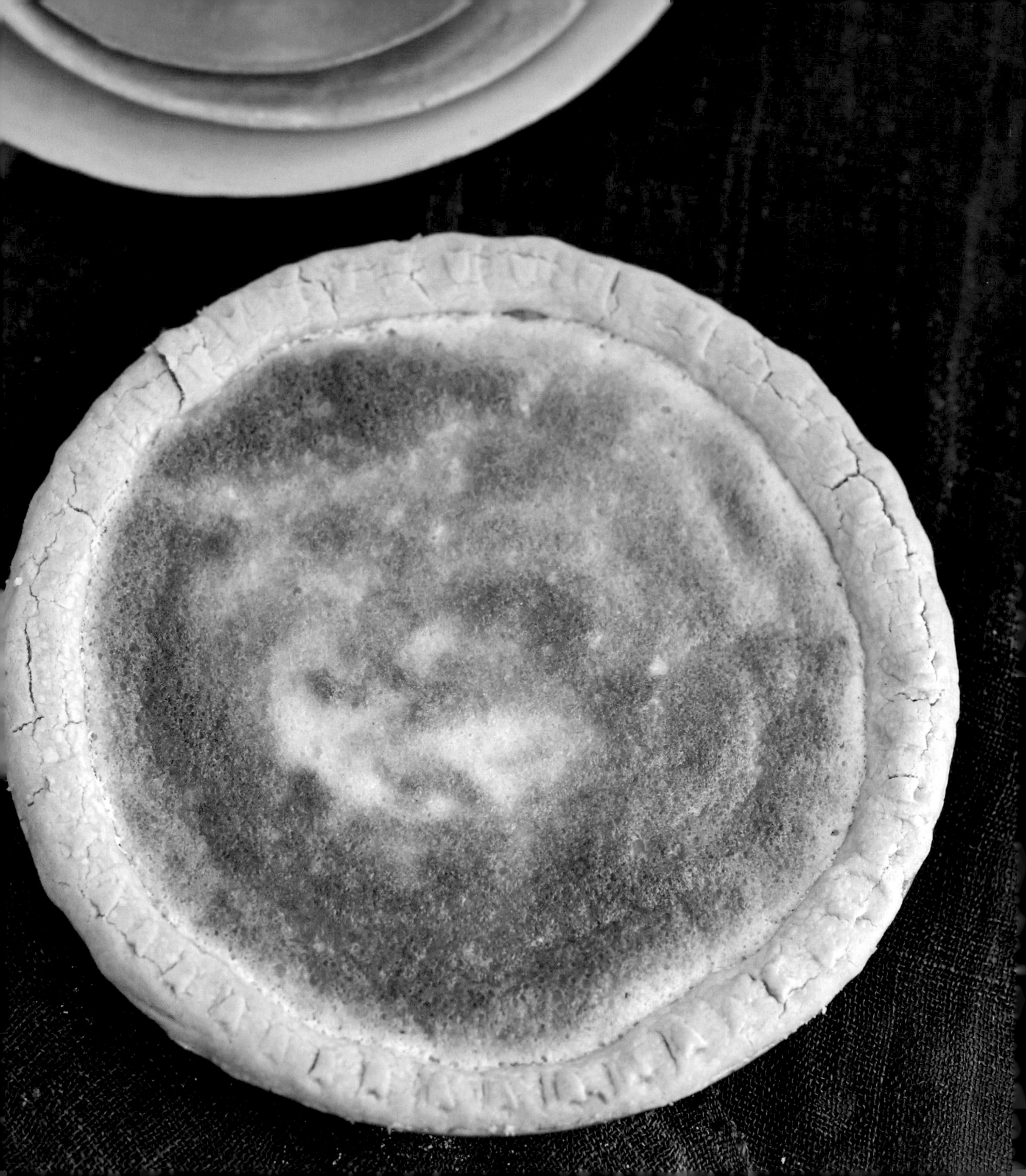

BUTTERMILK CHESS PIE

Makes 1 (9-inch) pie

The recipe for this traditional Southern pie is adapted from one sent by a reader of our site, Liz Meier. As she wrote, "This recipe is from my great-aunt's housekeeper, Quintella. They lived on a tobacco farm in a small town in southern Kentucky. It was the late '50s, early '60s. My great-aunt and -uncle were affluent and had domestic help in the house. (If you're having visions of the movie The Help, *you're about dead-on.) Quintella worked for the family for a long time. She helped care for my brother and me in the late '60s. To this day, older members of the family still talk about what a great cook she was, and this pie was a real favorite. I seem to remember this being more of an everyday pie than a special holiday pie." I'd be happy to eat this pie every day. It's pretty humble looking and more delicious for it. Thank you for sharing this with us, Liz.*

1 disk chilled Pie Dough (page 226)

1 cup (210 grams) organic cane sugar

2 large eggs, at room temperature and separated

¼ cup low-fat buttermilk

4 tablespoons (65 grams) unsalted butter, softened

Freshly grated zest and freshly squeezed juice of 1 lemon

Prepare to bake. Preheat the oven to 350°F.

Roll out the dough, press it into a 9-inch pie pan, and crimp the edges, if desired. Put the pie pan in the freezer as you make the filling.

Make the filling. In the bowl of a stand mixer with the whisk attachment, beat the sugar and egg yolks until they are fluffy. With the mixer running, pour in the buttermilk, Add the butter in little pieces, then the lemon zest and juice. Pour the filling into a large bowl.

Beat the egg whites. Clean the bowl of the stand mixer and the whisk attachment thoroughly and wipe them entirely dry. Add the egg whites to the bowl and beat them until they form stiff peaks.

Finish the filling. Fold the stiff egg whites into the pie filling. Pour it into the prepared pie pan.

Bake the pie. Put the pie on a parchment-lined baking sheet and put it in the oven. Bake until the crust is golden brown and the pie filling is set, about 45 minutes.

Cool the pie. Cool the pie on the counter until it is room temperature. Serve.

Feel like playing?

For a more traditional chess pie, you can use ¼ cup of milk instead of buttermilk, take out the lemon juice and zest, add 1 tablespoon of apple cider vinegar, and increase the sugar to 2 cups. (Some folks like their pies mighty sweet.)

CHOCOLATE MERINGUE PIE

Makes 1 (9-inch) pie

It's not clear who first made a chocolate meringue pie. Is it a pie of the Deep South or big Texas? I don't think it matters much. What does matter is that you experience the flaky crust topped with chocolate custard and not-too-sweet meringue, fluffed as high as you can go. The traditional pie gets its chocolate taste from the custard made with cocoa powder, which we blend with coconut milk for a more lush taste. Somehow, however, that just didn't deliver enough of the chocolate promise for us, so we added a layer of melted bittersweet chocolate, sandwiched between the slight saltiness of the piecrust and the smooth chocolate of the custard.

1 disk chilled Pie Dough (page 226)

3 ounces (85 grams) bittersweet chocolate, chopped

1 cup (210 grams) organic cane sugar

¼ cup unsweetened cocoa powder

27 grams All-Purpose Gluten-Free Flour Blend (page 17)

1 tablespoon arrowroot flour

½ teaspoon fine sea salt

One 12-ounce can full-fat coconut milk

3 large eggs, separated

3 tablespoons (39 grams) coconut oil, melted

1 teaspoon vanilla extract

½ teaspoon cream of tartar

Bake the crust. Preheat the oven to 425°F. Roll out the pie dough, put it in a 9-inch pie pan, and crimp the edges. Grease a piece of aluminum foil and lay it down on the top of the pie dough. Fill the aluminum foil with dried beans. Bake until the edges of the pie dough have set, about 15 minutes. Take the aluminum foil off the pie dough and bake until the crust is golden, another 5 to 10 minutes. Remove from the oven. Cool the crust completely.

Melt the chocolate. Set a pot of water over medium-high heat. When the water comes to a boil, turn the heat down to low and put a metal bowl on top of the pot. Add the chopped chocolate to the bowl. Using a rubber spatula, stir the chocolate until it is completely melted and smooth. Take the bowl off the heat and scrape the melted chocolate onto the cooled crust. Spread it evenly and allow the melted chocolate to cool completely.

Make the chocolate filling. Whisk together ⅔ cup of the sugar, the cocoa powder, flour blend, arrowroot, and salt in a bowl. Put them in a large pot. Slowly, whisk in the coconut milk until everything is one color. Whisk in the egg yolks.

Set the pot over medium heat. Cook the chocolate filling, whisking continuously, until it starts to boil, about 5 minutes. Turn the heat down to low and whisk vigorously for 1 minute.

Pour the hot chocolate filling into a fine-mesh sieve set over a large bowl. Using a rubber spatula, push the chocolate filling through the sieve. Whisk in the coconut oil and vanilla until they are fully incorporated.

Chill the pie. Pour the warm filling into the baked crust, on top of the layer of chocolate. Set the pie in the refrigerator and chill for at least 2 hours, preferably overnight.

Prepare to bake. After the pie has chilled, preheat the oven to 450°F.

Make the meringue. In the bowl of a stand mixer with the whisk attachment, beat the egg whites, the remaining ⅓ cup of sugar, and the cream of tartar until the egg whites are stiff. Spread the stiff egg whites onto the top of the pie, allowing the edges of the crust to peek through. Bake until the meringue is brown at the tips, 5 to 7 minutes. Serve immediately.

Feel like playing?

Arrowroot flour, in our estimation, makes the best thickener for recipes like this. It thickens without adding any muddy taste. However, if you don't use arrowroot regularly for gluten-free baking, it is expensive to buy it in the supermarket. Feel free to use cornstarch or tapioca flour instead.

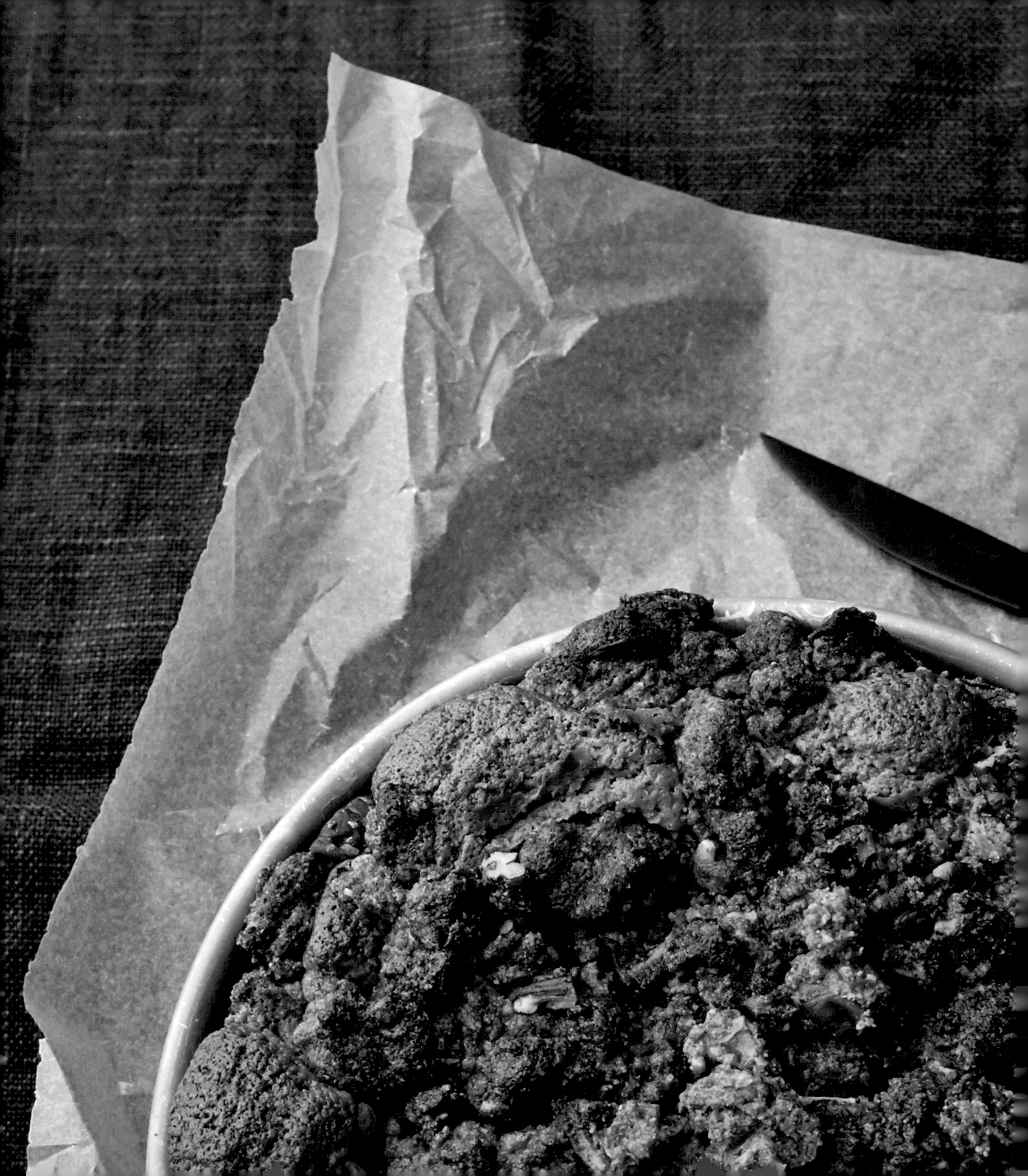

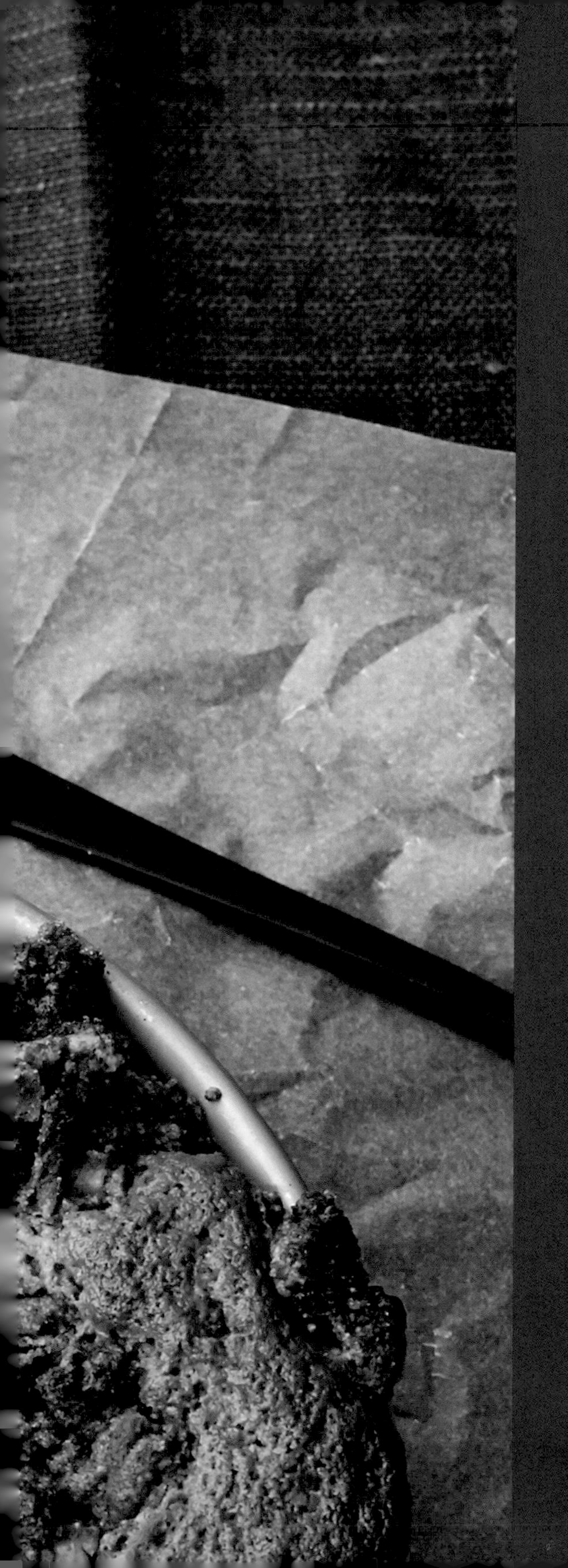

CAKES

YELLOW CAKE

Makes 1 (8-inch) cake

We played with a lot of cakes for this cookbook: the festooned-with-raisins-and-pecans Lane cake, the banana- and pineapple-flavored hummingbird cake, the eight-layered Smith Island cake. They are all much beloved and all rather elaborate. But in the end, we knew the cake most of us would make, most often, is this basic yellow layer cake.

This recipe is the template recipe for most of the cakes in this chapter. Once you feel confident making this cake, you can make spice cake, coconut cake, pineapple upside-down cake, and any coffee cake you want. But make two of these yellow cakes, slather them with chocolate buttercream frosting, and stack them on top of each other on a cake plate—you're going to make any birthday kid happy.

P.S. once you know how to make this cake, you could also figure out how to adapt the Lane cake, hummingbird cake, and Smith Island cake to make them gluten-free too. You can do it.

Fat for greasing the pan

280 grams All-Purpose Gluten-Free Flour Blend (page 17)

1 teaspoon baking powder

½ teaspoon baking soda

½ teaspoon kosher salt

2 large eggs, at room temperature

1¼ cups (260 grams) organic cane sugar

½ cup (100 grams) coconut oil, melted

1 cup (210 grams) full-fat sour cream

2 to 5 tablespoons water

Prepare to bake. Preheat the oven to 350°F. Grease an 8-inch cake pan. Lay a greased round of parchment paper into the pan.

Combine the dry ingredients. In a large bowl, whisk together the flour blend, baking powder, baking soda, and salt. Set aside.

Cream the eggs and sugar. Add the eggs to the bowl of a stand mixer with the paddle attachment. Add the sugar and cream them together on medium speed until they are light and fluffy. With the mixer running on low, pour in the melted coconut oil. Stop the mixer and scrape down the bowl with a rubber spatula.

Finish the batter. With the mixer running, add approximately one-third of the flour mixture to the cake batter. When the flour has disappeared into the batter, add half the sour cream. When the sour cream has blended in with the batter, stop the mixer and scrape down the sides of the bowl with a rubber spatula. Repeat, varying between the flour and sour cream, ending with the flour. The batter should be light and fluffy, sliding easily off the paddle. If the batter is too thick, add water, 1 tablespoon at a time with the mixer running on low, until the batter is pourable.

CONTINUED

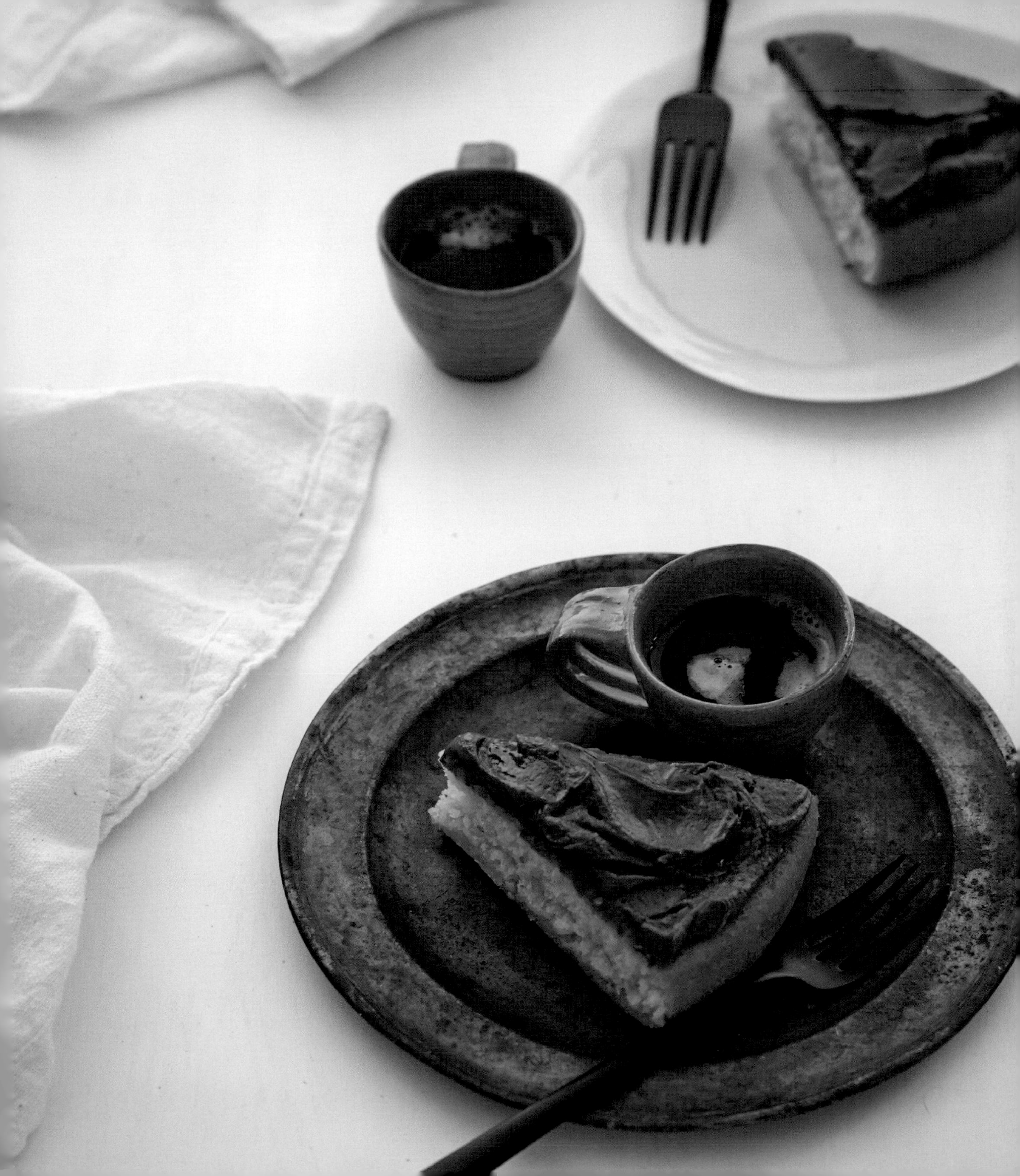

Bake the cake. Pour the batter into the prepared cake pan. Give it a little thump on the counter to settle the batter evenly. Put it on the middle rack in the oven. Bake until the cake has started to pull away from the edges of the pan and the center has a little athletic jiggle when you touch it, and a toothpick inserted into the center comes out clean, 18 to 25 minutes.

Cool the cake. Let the cake pan rest on the counter for 10 minutes. Gently, run a table knife around the edges of the cake. Invert the cake pan onto a plate, then invert the plate onto a wire rack. Allow the cake to cool completely before frosting it.

Feel like playing?

If you add ⅓ cup of cocoa powder to the dry ingredients, you'll have a moist chocolate cake. Add cinnamon, cloves, ginger, and nutmeg and you'll have a wonderful spice cake. Add lemon juice and zest for a lemon cake. Once you know how to make this cake, you'll be playing with cake recipes for a while.

COCONUT CREAM CAKE

Makes 1 (8-inch) cake

This classic Southern cake is inspired by the work of Nancie McDermott, a wonderful food writer and cooking instructor from North Carolina. Our friend Pableaux from New Orleans introduced me to her by saying, "I would drag my head through broken glass to eat one of her pies." I hear her cakes are mighty fine too. Nancie's book, Southern Cakes, *is a treasure trove of jelly rolls, Lane cakes, caramel cakes, and all the much-loved traditional cakes from the South. This coconut cake, made gluten-free and even more coconutty with the addition of coconut milk and oil, will be staying in our repertoire for decades.*

Fat for greasing the pan

280 grams All-Purpose Gluten-Free Flour Blend (page 17)

1 teaspoon baking powder

½ teaspoon baking soda

½ teaspoon fine sea salt

2 large eggs, at room temperature

1¼ cups (260 grams) organic cane sugar

½ cup (100 grams) coconut oil, melted

½ cup (100 grams) coconut milk

⅓ cup (100 grams) sour cream

½ cup (50 grams) finely shredded unsweetened coconut

About 5 tablespoons water

1 batch Coconut Frosting (page 269)

Prepare to bake. Preheat the oven to 350°F. Grease an 8-inch cake pan. Lay a greased round of parchment paper into the pan.

Combine the dry ingredients. In a large bowl, whisk together the flour blend, baking powder, baking soda, and salt. Set aside.

Cream the eggs and sugar. Add the eggs to the bowl of a stand mixer with the paddle attachment. Add the sugar and cream them together until they are light and fluffy. With the mixer running on low, pour in the melted coconut oil. Stop the mixer and scrape down the bowl with a rubber spatula.

Mix the wet ingredients. In a small bowl, whisk together the coconut milk and sour cream.

Finish the batter. With the mixer running, add approximately one-third of the flour mixture to the cake batter. When the flour has disappeared into the batter, add half the sour cream mixture. When the sour cream has blended in with the batter, stop the mixer and scrape down the sides of the bowl with a rubber spatula. Repeat, varying between the flour and sour cream, ending with the flour. Add the shredded coconut and mix.

The batter should be light and fluffy, sliding easily off the paddle. If the batter is too thick, add water, 1 tablespoon at a time with the mixer running, until the batter feels like cake batter to you. (This cake will probably require about 5 tablespoons.)

Bake the cake. Pour the batter into the prepared cake pan. Give it a little thump on the counter to settle the batter evenly. Put it on the middle rack in the oven. Bake until the cake has started to pull away from the edges of the pan and the center has a little athletic jiggle when you touch it, and a toothpick inserted into the center comes out clean, 18 to 25 minutes.

Cool the cake. Let the cake pan rest on the counter for 10 minutes. Gently, run a table knife around the edges of the cake. Invert the cake pan onto a plate, then invert the plate onto a wire rack. Allow the cake to cool completely before frosting it with the coconut frosting.

Feel like playing?

If you want to make a dramatic-looking cake, make two of these cakes. Once they have fully cooled, cut across each cake horizontally to make four layers. Slather the coconut frosting between each layer and across the top and watch people go gaga.

PINEAPPLE UPSIDE-DOWN CAKE

Makes 1 (8-inch) cake

When my mom made a pineapple upside-down cake in a blue Pyrex pan, I thought we were eating the most exotic dessert, straight from Hawaii. I'm still pretty excited by it now.

About ¼ cup (50 grams) coconut oil

⅔ cup (140 grams) coconut sugar

One 14-ounce can pineapple slices

280 grams All-Purpose Gluten-Free Flour Blend (page 17)

1 teaspoon baking powder

½ teaspoon baking soda

½ teaspoon kosher salt

2 large eggs

1¼ cup (260 grams) organic cane sugar

½ cup (100 grams) coconut oil, melted

⅔ cup plus 1 tablespoon (210 grams) full-fat sour cream

2 to 5 tablespoons water

Prepare to bake. Preheat the oven to 350°F.

Caramelize the pineapple. Set a 10-inch cast-iron skillet over medium heat. Add the coconut oil. When it has melted, add the coconut sugar and simmer, stirring, until the mixture turns a dark caramel color, about 4 minutes. Remove the skillet from the heat. Lay the pineapple slices on top of the caramel in concentric circles. Imperfect is best here.

(If you don't have a cast-iron skillet, pour the caramel into a greased 8-inch cake pan and lay the pineapple slices over that.)

Combine the dry ingredients. In a large bowl, whisk together the flour blend, baking powder, baking soda, and salt. Set aside.

Cream the eggs and sugar. Add the eggs to the bowl of a stand mixer with the paddle attachment. Add the sugar and cream them together until they are light and fluffy. With the mixer running on low, pour in the melted coconut oil. Stop the mixer and scrape down the bowl with a rubber spatula.

Finish the batter. With the mixer running, add approximately one-third of the flour mixture to the cake batter. When the flour has disappeared into the batter, add half the sour cream. When the sour cream has blended in with the batter, stop the mixer and scrape down the sides of the bowl with a rubber spatula. Repeat, varying between the flour and sour cream, ending with the flour. The batter should be light and fluffy, sliding easily off the paddle. If the batter is too thick, add water, 1 tablespoon at a time with the mixer running on low, until the batter is pourable.

Bake the cake. Pour the batter evenly onto the pineapple in the skillet. Give it a little thump on the counter to settle the batter evenly. Put it on the middle rack in the oven. Bake until the cake has started to pull away from the edges of the pan and the center has a little athletic jiggle when you touch it, and a toothpick inserted into the center comes out clean, 20 to 30 minutes.

Cool the cake. Let the cake pan rest on the counter for 10 minutes. Gently, run a table knife around the edges of the cake. Put a plate over the skillet and turn the skillet upside down onto the plate. (Be sure to keep them firmly pressed together.) If there are any pineapple bits left in the skillet, put them onto the cake. Serve the cake warm.

Feel like playing?

Using the same technique as above, you could caramelize any fruit for this cake. We like a peach-thyme cake, a cherry-basil cake, and a plum-tarragon cake made using this method.

SEATTLE COFFEE CAKE

Makes 1 (8-inch) cake

We can't write an American cookbook without including something with coffee from Seattle. It really is true, folks. We like our coffee here. Most of us drink it all day long. And when it's time for dessert, we're happy to serve a moist, delicious layer cake made with espresso, brushed with coffee syrup, and topped with a coffee buttercream frosting (page 271).

You might want to go with decaf for the cake, however.

Fat for greasing the pan

280 grams All-Purpose Gluten-Free Flour Blend (page 17)

1 teaspoon baking powder

½ teaspoon baking soda

½ teaspoon kosher salt

2 large eggs, at room temperature

1¼ cups (260 grams) organic cane sugar

½ cup (100 grams) coconut oil, melted

1 cup (210 grams) full-fat sour cream

3 to 5 tablespoons cooled brewed espresso

⅓ cup warm coffee syrup (page 309)

Prepare to bake. Preheat the oven to 350°F. Grease an 8-inch cake pan. Lay a greased round of parchment paper into the pan.

Combine the dry ingredients. In a large bowl, whisk together the flour blend, baking powder, baking soda, and salt. Set aside.

Cream the eggs and sugar. Add the eggs to the bowl of a stand mixer with the paddle attachment. Add the sugar and cream them together on medium speed until they are light and fluffy. With the mixer running on low, pour in the melted coconut oil. Stop the mixer and scrape down the bowl with a rubber spatula.

Finish the batter. With the mixer running, add approximately one-third of the flour mixture to the cake batter. When the flour has disappeared into the batter, add half the sour cream. When the sour cream has blended in with the batter, stop the mixer and scrape down the sides of the bowl with a rubber spatula. Repeat, varying between the flour and sour cream, ending with the flour. Add the cooled espresso, 1 tablespoon at a time, with the mixer running on low. The batter should be light and fluffy, sliding easily off the paddle.

Bake the cake. Pour the batter into the prepared cake pan. Give it a little thump on the counter to settle the batter evenly. Put it on the middle rack in the oven. Bake until the cake has started to pull away from the edges of the pan and the center has a little athletic jiggle when you touch it, and a toothpick inserted into the center comes out clean, 18 to 25 minutes.

Cool the cake and slather it in coffee syrup. Let the cake pan rest on the counter for 10 minutes. Gently, run a table knife around the edges of the cake. Invert the cake pan onto a plate, then invert the plate onto a wire rack. Use a sharp skewer to poke holes gently all over the top of the cake. Brush the warm coffee syrup over the top of the cake, slowly, allowing the coffee syrup to drip into the cake evenly. Allow the cake to cool completely before frosting it.

Feel like playing?

If you don't have any coffee syrup on hand, you can make a quick simple coffee syrup with ⅓ cup coarsely ground coffee, ⅓ cup sugar, and ⅓ cup water. Bring to a boil, then simmer for 10 minutes. Let it sit off the heat for 30 minutes for the flavors to infuse. Strain the syrup really well, then brush that over the top of the cake.

RED VELVET CAKE

Makes 2 (8-inch) cakes

This was, by far, the most requested recipe for this cookbook. People, you love your red velvet cake! The red velvet cake has become a thing. Not only are red velvet cupcakes the most popular cupcake flavor in America, but also, some manufacturer has begun producing red velvet cupcake roll-on perfume. Now that's America.

For years, I thought the original cake was made with beets and that modern convenience switched the beets to red food coloring. However, thanks to the baking research done by our pastry chef friend Stella Parks, whose food site Brave Tart is brilliant, red velvet *meant something different in the nineteenth century than it does today.* Red *meant made with red sugar, which we call brown sugar today. And* velvet *referred to the tight, fine crumb on a really well-made cake. A food dye company in the 1950s concocted a recipe for a cake they called red velvet cake, which called for a full ounce of their food coloring. Somehow, it spread and became a thing. But we didn't want to use a bottle of red food coloring in our cake. Just a little more work yields a truly delicious cake. The earthy sweetness of pureed beets, coupled with cocoa powder, mixes with the sweetness of organic cane sugar and the tang of buttermilk and champagne vinegar. Now this cake? This cake makes me understand why people lose their minds for red velvet.*

Fat for greasing the pan

1 medium beet

280 grams All-Purpose Gluten-Free Flour Blend (page 17)

4 tablespoons (15 grams) unsweetened cocoa powder

2 teaspoons baking powder

1 teaspoon kosher salt

1½ cups (300 grams) organic cane sugar

¾ cup (150 grams) coconut oil, melted

2 large eggs, at room temperature

1 teaspoon vanilla extract

¾ cup (180 grams) low-fat buttermilk

1 tablespoon champagne vinegar

2 to 5 tablespoons water

Prepare to bake. Preheat the oven to 350°F. Grease two 8-inch cake pans. Lay a greased round of parchment paper into each pan.

Boil the beets. Set a medium pot filled with water over high heat. Put the beet in the water. Bring the water to a boil and let it continue to boil until a knife inserted into the beet slides right through, about 20 minutes. Remove the beet from the pot, reserving the water, and let the beet cool completely. Slide the skin off the beet. Chop the beet into pieces. Put the beet in a blender, along with about ¼ cup

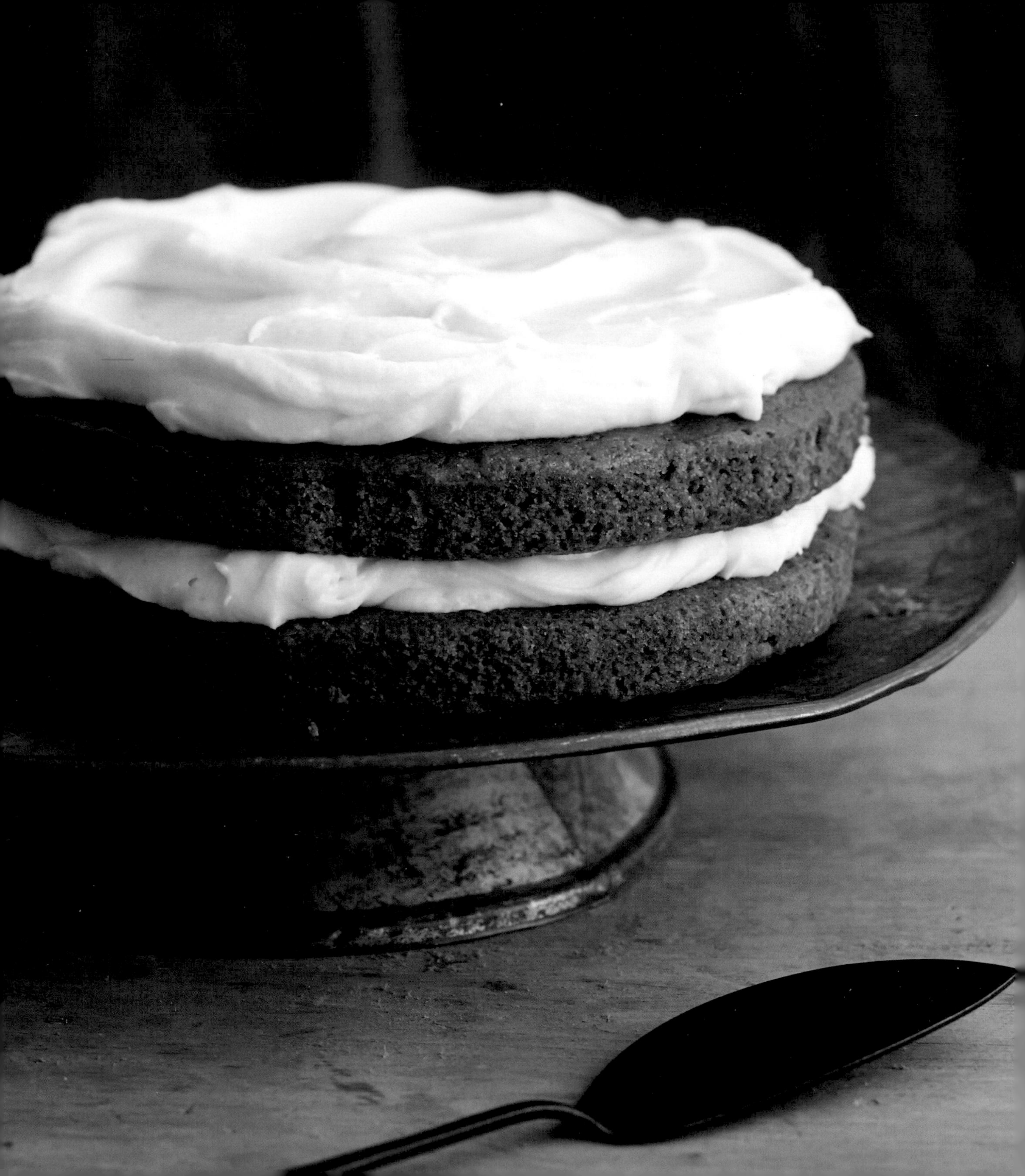

of the reserved cooking water. Blend until the beet puree is smooth. It should be the consistency of waffle batter. If it is too thick, add more water.

Reduce the beet puree. Set a medium pot over low heat. Spoon in the beet puree. Simmer the puree, stirring frequently, until it is thickened and reduced to about 1⁄4 cup. Take the pot off the heat. Spread the puree out evenly on a plate. Put the plate in the refrigerator. Cool the beet puree completely.

Combine the dry ingredients. In a bowl, whisk together the flour blend, cocoa powder, baking powder, and salt.

Cream the oil and sugar. In the bowl of a stand mixer with the paddle attachment, place the sugar and coconut oil. Cream them together on medium speed until they are light and fluffy. Add the eggs, one at a time, making sure each egg is fully incorporated before moving on. Pour in the vanilla. Add the cooled beet puree to the bowl and mix until the batter is evenly pink.

Make the buttermilk mixture. In a bowl, combine the buttermilk and vinegar.

Finish the batter. With the mixer running on medium, add one-third of the flour mixture to the cake batter. When the flour has disappeared into the batter, pour in half of the buttermilk and vinegar. Scrape down the sides of the bowl with a rubber spatula. Repeat this process, adding flour and then buttermilk, ending with the last third of the flour mixture. Scrape down the sides of the bowl with a rubber spatula. The batter should be light and fluffy, sliding easily off the paddle. If the batter is too thick, add water, 1 tablespoon at a time with the mixer running on low, until the batter has the right consistency.

Bake the cake. Pour the batter evenly into the prepared cake pans. Give each pan a little thump to settle the batter evenly. Put the pans on the middle rack in the oven. Bake until the cakes have started to pull away from the edges of the pans and the centers have a little athletic jiggle when you touch them, and a toothpick inserted into the center comes out clean, 25 to 35 minutes.

Cool the cake. Let the cake pans rest on the counter for 10 minutes. Gently, run a table knife around the edges of each cake. Invert each cake pan onto a plate, then invert the plate onto a wire rack. Allow the cakes to cool completely before frosting.

Feel like playing?

You can make your own buttermilk, with whatever kind of milk you drink, by squeezing 1 tablespoon of lemon juice into 1 cup of milk. Let it sit for 15 minutes and voilà! Buttermilk.

APPLE-WALNUT CRUMB CAKE

Makes 1 (8-inch) cake

When we traveled around New England together, Danny bought a slice of apple crumb cake from small cafés or bakeries several times. He knew I couldn't share, since that cake was made with gluten flour, but he just called it research for this book. This cake is quintessential New England in the fall: tart apples, cinnamon, and a caramel sweetness from coconut sugar. This cake gets its apple flavor from homemade roasted applesauce. But any good chunky applesauce will do here. Even after eating apple cake around New England, Danny likes this apple crumb cake the best.

Fat for greasing the pan

FOR THE WALNUT TOPPING

2¼ cups (170 grams) chopped walnuts

85 grams Grain-Free Flour Mix (page 19)

½ cup (85 grams) packed coconut sugar

5 tablespoons (55 grams) coconut oil, melted

1 teaspoon ground cinnamon

FOR THE CAKE

280 grams All-Purpose Gluten-Free Flour Blend (page 17)

1 teaspoon ground cinnamon

1 teaspoon baking powder

½ teaspoon baking soda

½ teaspoon fine sea salt

2 large eggs, at room temperature

1¼ cups (260 grams) organic cane sugar

½ cup (100 grams) coconut oil, melted

¾ cup roasted applesauce (see box)

1 cup (210 grams) sour cream

2 to 5 tablespoons water

Prepare to bake. Preheat the oven to 350°F. Grease an 8-inch cake pan. Lay a greased round of parchment paper into the pan.

Make the walnut topping. In a large bowl, mix the walnuts, flour mix, sugar, oil, and cinnamon together until they are all evenly coated with the oil. Set aside.

Combine the dry ingredients. In a large bowl, whisk together the flour blend, cinnamon, baking powder, baking soda, and salt. Set aside.

Cream the eggs and sugar. Add the eggs to the bowl of a stand mixer with the paddle attachment. Add the sugar and cream them together on medium speed until they are light and fluffy. With the mixer running on low, pour in the melted coconut oil. Mix in the applesauce. Stop the mixer and scrape down the bowl with a rubber spatula.

Finish the batter. With the mixer running, add approximately one-third of the flour mixture to the cake batter. When the flour has disappeared into the batter, add half the sour cream. When the sour cream has blended in with the batter, stop the mixer and scrape down the sides of the bowl with a rubber spatula. Repeat, varying between the flour and sour cream, ending with the flour. The batter should be light and fluffy, sliding easily off the paddle. If the batter is too thick, add water, 1 tablespoon at a time with the mixer running on low, until the batter is pourable.

Bake the cake. Pour the batter into the prepared cake pan. Put it on the middle rack in the oven. Bake the cake for 15 minutes. Carefully, open the oven and slide the rack with the cake pan out toward you. Gently, pat the walnut topping onto the top of the cake. Close the oven and bake the cake until a knife inserted into the center comes out clean, about 30 more minutes. If you find the top of the cake is starting to brown too much, make a tent of aluminum foil over the top of the cake and continue baking until the cake is fully baked.

Cool the cake. Let the cake pan rest on the counter for 10 minutes. Cut slices right from the pan. Serve warm.

Feel like playing?

Try roasting apples to make applesauce, like Judy Rodgers's The Zuni Café Cookbook *recommends. Peel, core, and quarter 3 to 4 pounds of apples. Toss them with a pinch of salt and a couple of teaspoons of sugar. Put them in a 9 x 13-inch baking pan, with dots of butter on top. Cover with aluminum foil and roast in a 375°F oven until the apples have begun to soften, about 30 minutes. Take the foil off and roast at 500°F until the tips of the apples have browned, about 10 minutes. Take the apples out of the oven and mash them, adding a bit more sugar or a spoonful of apple cider vinegar, if you wish.*

DATE SHAKE COFFEE CAKE

Makes 1 (8-inch) cake

According to legend, a date farmer in the Coachella Valley in southern California came up with this simple, intoxicating taste: chopped Medjool dates, vanilla ice cream, and whole milk, blended into a shake. Sweet and creamy, this rich treat is a cool splurge in intense heat.

We wanted to take the flavors of this shake and make it into a coffee cake, a classic American baked good. Make this cake for a Sunday morning, throw on a big pot of coffee, and invite friends over for brunch—you have a new tradition.

Fat for greasing the pan

FOR THE DATE TOPPING

85 grams Grain-Free Flour Mix (page 19)

5 large (85 grams) pitted dates, chopped

1 cup (85 grams) chopped pecans

½ cup (85 grams) packed coconut sugar

5 tablespoons (55 grams) coconut oil, melted

1 teaspoon ground cinnamon

FOR THE CAKE

275 grams Grain-Free Flour Mix (page 19)

1 teaspoon baking powder

½ teaspoon baking soda

½ teaspoon freshly grated nutmeg

½ teaspoon kosher salt

2 large eggs, at room temperature

1¼ cups (260 grams) organic cane sugar

½ cup (100 grams) coconut oil, melted

1 cup (210 grams) full-fat sour cream

1 cup (150 grams) dates, pitted and chopped

5 to 8 tablespoons water

Prepare to bake. Preheat the oven to 350°F. Grease an 8-inch cake pan. Lay a greased round of parchment paper into the pan.

Make the date topping. In a large bowl, mix all the ingredients together until they are all evenly coated with the oil.

Combine the dry ingredients. In a large bowl, whisk together the flour mix, baking powder, baking soda, nutmeg, and salt. Set aside.

Cream the eggs and sugar. Add the eggs to the bowl of a stand mixer with the paddle attachment. Add the sugar and cream them together until they are light and fluffy. With the mixer running on low, pour in the melted coconut oil. Stop the mixer and scrape down the bowl with a rubber spatula.

CONTINUED

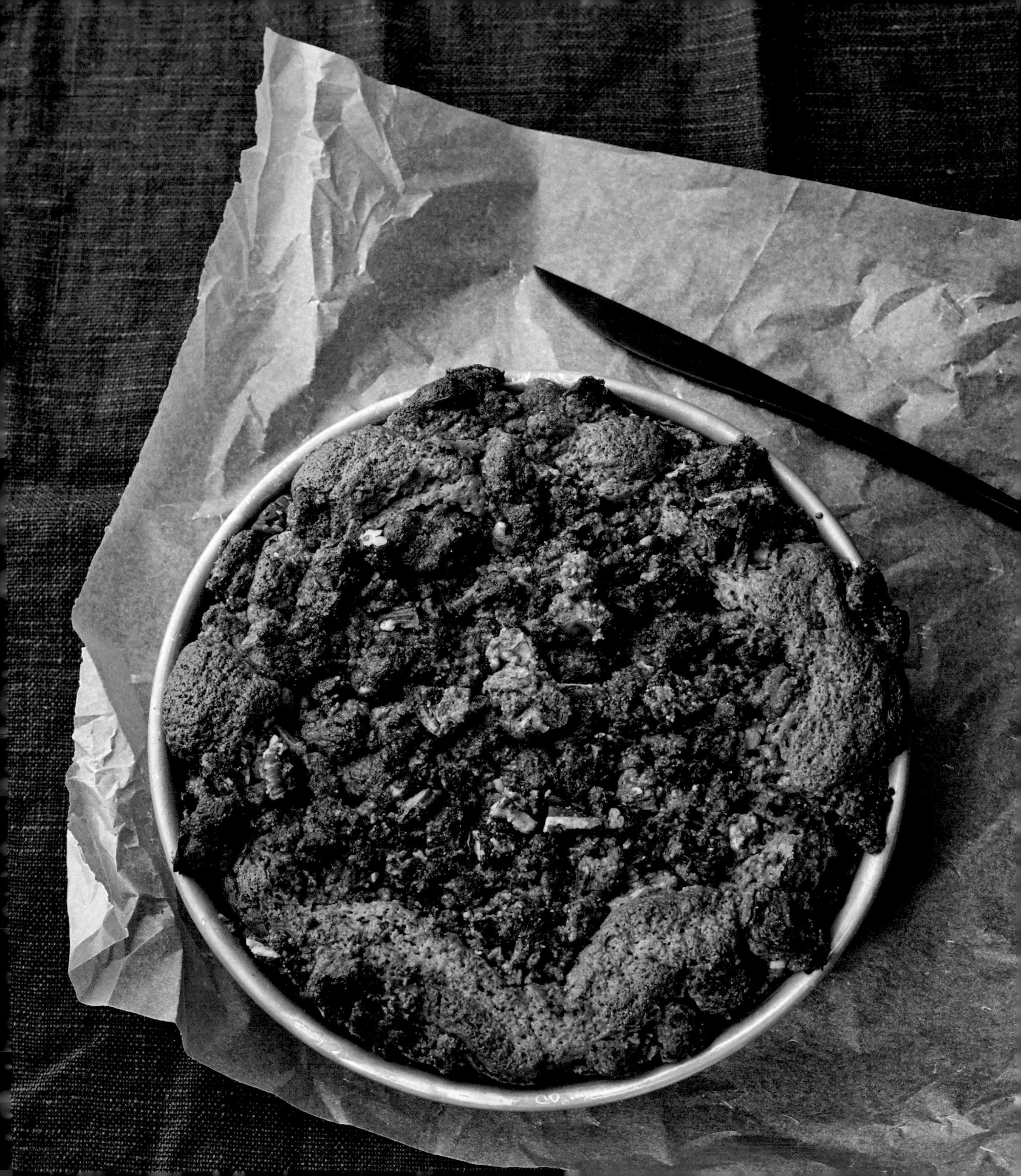

Finish the batter. With the mixer running, add approximately one-third of the flour mixture to the cake batter. When the flour has disappeared into the batter, add half the sour cream. When the sour cream has blended in with the batter, stop the mixer and scrape down the sides of the bowl with a rubber spatula. Repeat, varying between the flour and sour cream, ending with the flour. Add the chopped dates and mix until they are part of the batter. The batter should be light and fluffy, sliding easily off the paddle. If the batter is too thick, add water, 1 tablespoon at a time with the mixer running, until the batter feels like cake batter.

Bake the cake. Pour the batter into the prepared cake pan. Give it a little thump on the counter to settle the batter evenly. Put it on the middle rack in the oven. Bake until the edges of the cake have just started to set and the top of the cake is a little jiggly, about 15 minutes. Strew the date topping over the cake, covering it evenly. Close the oven door and bake until the topping is golden brown and a toothpick inserted into the middle of the cake emerges with only a few crumbs on it, 25 to 35 minutes. (If the top is browning too quickly before the cake is done, make a tent of aluminum foil over the top of the cake.)

Cool the cake. Let the cake pan rest on the counter for 10 minutes. Cut slices of the cake straight from the pan. Serve warm.

Feel like playing?

We learned the hard way that gluten-free cakes need to bake a bit before the streusel can go on top. When we scattered the date topping on top of the batter, then put it in the oven, it all sank into the cake, which ended up with a funny-looking top. But frankly, it was a great cake! Feel free to make the same mistake and feed it to your friends, as we did.

CREAM CHEESE POUND CAKE

Makes 1 (10-inch) pound cake

Pound cake is named for the way women used to make this confection: a pound of butter, a pound of sugar, a pound of eggs, and a pound of flour. Hey, look at that! Long before we grew convinced that measuring ingredients in cups was the only way to bake, American women used the scale to make cakes.

A pound cake is meant to be dense in texture, to satisfy with just one slice, which is why we use butter here instead of coconut oil. Basic pound cake can run a little dry, so the addition of cream cheese gives this cake a soft, moist crumb. Cream cheese also lends a tiny tang to kick through the wall of sweetness. Thank you, Nancie McDermott, for teaching us this.

Fat for greasing the pan

450 grams All-Purpose Gluten-Free Flour Blend (page 17)

1 teaspoon baking powder

½ teaspoon kosher salt

16 tablespoons (230 grams) unsalted butter, softened

One 8-ounce package full-fat cream cheese, softened

3 cups (600 grams) organic cane sugar

6 large eggs, at room temperature

1 teaspoon vanilla extract

1 batch Citrus Syrup (page 271)

Prepare to bake. Preheat the oven to 325°F. Grease a 10-inch Bundt pan. (You could also grease and line two 5 x 9-inch loaf pans with parchment paper.)

Combine the dry ingredients. In a large bowl, whisk together the flour blend, baking powder, and salt. Set aside.

Cream the butter and sugar. In the bowl of a stand mixer with the paddle attachment, mix the butter and cream cheese together until they are fluffy. With the mixer running on low, pour in the sugar. When the sugar is incorporated fully, after about 2 minutes, scrape down the sides of the bowl with a rubber spatula. Add the eggs, one at a time, beating the batter to incorporate after each egg has been added. Pour in the vanilla.

Finish the batter. With the mixer on low, add one-third of the flour mixture, mixing until the flour disappears into the batter. Scrape down the sides of the bowl with a rubber spatula. Continue this until you have added all the flour mixture.

Bake the cake. Pour the cake batter into the Bundt pan. Give it a little thump on the counter to settle the batter evenly. Put it on the middle rack in the oven. Bake until the edges of the cake are starting to pull away from the pan and the top of the cake has a little athletic jiggle when you touch it, and a toothpick inserted into the center comes out clean, about 1 hour and 15 minutes.

(That's about 55 minutes for the loaf pans.) Set the cake pan on a wire rack. Cool the cake completely before sliding a knife around the edges and turning the pan over to remove the cake. Drizzle the citrus syrup over the pound cake and serve.

Feel like playing?

Do you need to avoid dairy? Use coconut oil instead of the butter. If you can eat soy, you could one of the several nondairy cream cheeses on the market now. Or, try this trick. Put several cans of coconut milk in the refrigerator overnight. In the morning, skim the thickest part of the coconut milk off the top. Weigh out 8 ounces of it and use that in place of the cream cheese.

TEXAS SHEET CAKE

Makes 1 sheet cake

This is a big cake, a Texas-size cake. It's not fancy or frilly. It's a crowd-pleaser, easy as pie to make. In fact, it's easier than pie to make. Just make sure you have plenty of friends willing to come over and eat it with you. Otherwise, you're going to eat the whole thing yourself. And you don't want that, do you?

300 grams All-Purpose Gluten-Free Flour Blend (page 17)

2½ cups (400 grams) organic cane sugar

¼ teaspoon fine sea salt

16 tablespoons (230 grams) unsalted butter

¼ cup (15 grams) unsweetened cocoa powder

1 cup boiling water

½ cup low-fat buttermilk

2 large eggs, beaten

1 teaspoon baking soda

1 teaspoon vanilla extract

Powdered sugar for dusting

Prepare to bake. Preheat the oven to 350°F. Line a large rimmed baking sheet with greased parchment paper.

Combine the flour and sugar. In a large bowl, whisk together the flour blend, sugar, and salt.

Boil the butter and cocoa. Set a small pan over medium-high heat. Add the butter. When the butter has melted, add the cocoa powder and the boiling water. Whisk the mixture and bring it to a boil. Boil for 30 seconds, then turn off the heat. Pour the cocoa mixture over the flour mixture and stir it all up.

Mix the liquids. In a small bowl, whisk together the buttermilk, eggs, baking soda, and vanilla. Pour this into the flour and chocolate mixture. Stir together.

Bake the cake. Pour the cake batter onto the prepared baking sheet. Put it on the middle rack in the oven. Bake until the edges of the cake are starting to pull away from the edges of the pan and the center of the cake has an athletic jiggle to the touch, and a toothpick inserted into the center comes out clean, 20 to 25 minutes.

Cool the cake. Allow the cake to cool to room temperature. Cut a piece of parchment paper the same size as the cake. Dust the parchment paper with powdered sugar, then lay it down on the top of the cake. Turn the sheet cake over onto the parchment paper.

Feel like playing?

This cake freezes really well. Cut up the cake and freeze individual pieces in a freezer bag for a little bit of chocolate every night.

ST. LOUIS GOOEY BUTTERY CAKE

Makes 1 (8-inch) cake

This is a most unusual cake. It has a yeasted batter that requires three hours of rising, a topping made of corn syrup, sugar, and flour, and a final dusting of powdered sugar. As I saw it once described, "It's like a big gooey wedge of buttery sugar."

This is a true splurge cake. And for the folks who grew up near St. Louis, this is a much-loved cake, a tradition, and a family ritual. Who knows? You might just make it your family tradition too.

FOR THE CAKE

275 grams All-Purpose Gluten-Free Flour Blend (page 17)

1 teaspoon fine sea salt

5 tablespoons warm milk (about 100°F)

1 envelope (2¼ teaspoons) active dry yeast

6 tablespoons (13 grams) coconut oil, softened

3 tablespoons organic cane sugar

1 large egg, at room temperature

Fat for greasing the baking dish

FOR THE GOOEY TOPPING

¼ cup light corn syrup

2 tablespoons water

2 teaspoons vanilla extract

13 tablespoons (170 grams) coconut oil, softened

1½ cups (310 grams) organic cane sugar

1 large egg, at room temperature

½ teaspoon fine sea salt

140 grams All-Purpose Gluten-Free Flour Blend (page 17)

Powdered sugar for sprinkling

Combine the dry ingredients. In a bowl, whisk together the flour blend and salt. Set aside.

Proof the yeast. In a small bowl, gently whisk together the warm milk and yeast until the yeast is entirely dissolved. When the milk forms a slight foam on top, the yeast is ready to use.

Make the batter. In a stand mixer with the paddle attachment running on medium speed, cream the coconut oil and sugar until they are light and fluffy. Scrape down the sides of the bowl with a rubber spatula. Mix in the egg. With the mixer running on low, add the flour mixture, then the milk mixture, scraping down the sides of the bowl in between each addition. Mix until the dough is soft and pliable and starting to slump off the paddle, about 5 minutes.

Let the batter rise. Grease a 9 x 13-inch baking dish and press the batter evenly into the dish. The dough will be sticky, so use water or oil on your hands to keep the batter from sticking too much. Cover the baking dish with a clean kitchen towel and let it rise in a warm place until it has doubled in size, about 3 hours.

Prepare to bake. Preheat the oven to 350°F.

Make the topping. In a small bowl, whisk together the corn syrup, water, and vanilla. In the bowl of a stand mixer with the paddle attachment, cream together the coconut oil and sugar. When they are light and fluffy, after about 5 minutes, mix in the egg and salt. Scrape down the sides of the bowl with a rubber spatula. Mix in half of the flour blend, then the corn syrup mixture, then the last of the flour.

Bake the cake. Plop dollops of the gooey topping onto the risen batter. Using an offset spatula, spread the topping evenly over the cake. Put the cake pan on the middle rack in the oven. Bake until the top is golden brown and the center is just a tiny bit liquidy, 30 to 45 minutes. (This will give the cake that gooey texture.)

When the cake has cooled, sprinkle it with powdered sugar and serve.

Feel like playing?

There's not much playing going on here. This is a very specific taste and texture. However, the cake itself, without the gooey topping, is great with a bit of coconut whipped cream and fresh fruit. Also, it may seem strange that it's called "buttery" cake and there's no butter in there. The coconut oil produces a fluffier cake, but feel free to substitute butter if you want to have it in your cake.

CREAM CHEESE FROSTING

Makes about 2 cups

One 8-ounce package full-fat cream cheese, softened

3 tablespoons unsalted butter, softened

3 cups powdered sugar, sifted

1 teaspoon vanilla extract

2 to 5 tablespoons whole milk or water

Mix the cream cheese and butter together in the bowl of a stand mixer with the paddle attachment on medium speed. With the mixer running on low, add the powdered sugar and vanilla. Beat until the frosting is smooth and creamy. If it feels too thick, add 1 tablespoon of milk or water at a time.

Feel like playing?

If you would like to make this without the powdered sugar, substitute ½ cup of honey instead. The frosting will have a different texture, but it will still be sweet. You could also substitute coconut oil for the butter. Feel free to add any spices you like for a different flavor: cinnamon, cardamom, or nutmeg come to mind.

COCONUT FROSTING

Makes about 5 cups

- 1 cup organic cane sugar
- ½ cup water
- 2 large egg whites, at room temperature
- 3 cups freshly grated coconut or finely shredded unsweetened coconut

Make the syrup. Set a small pot over medium-high heat. Stir together the sugar and water in the pot. Cook, without stirring, for 3 minutes. Then cook at a rolling boil, stirring often, until a thick syrup has formed, 5 to 10 minutes. When you spoon up the syrup, it should pour back into the pot in a long, thick thread. If the syrup is not that thick, keep cooking. Set aside the syrup to cool.

Beat the egg whites. In an impeccably clean bowl of a stand mixer, beat the egg whites with the whisk attachment. Beat until the egg whites are pillowy and standing up stiff, about 3 minutes. With the stand mixer running on low, slowly pour in the cooled syrup until the mixture blends to make a fully white frosting, 4 to 5 minutes.

Frost the cake. After you've generously covered a cake with this frosting, pat the grated coconut on top, covering the cake completely.

Feel like playing?

The base of this frosting—the sugar syrup and beaten egg whites—is also known as an Italian meringue. It's a classic frosting to top any cake you wish. It's particularly great for dairy-free folks.

CHOCOLATE BUTTERCREAM FROSTING

Makes about 3 cups

16 tablespoons unsalted butter, softened

3½ cups powdered sugar, sifted

⅔ cup unsweetened cocoa powder

2 teaspoons vanilla extract

½ teaspoon fine sea salt

4 to 6 tablespoons full-fat coconut milk

Whip the butter in the bowl of a stand mixer with the paddle attachment on medium speed until it is light and fluffy, about 1 minute. Add the powdered sugar, slowly, with the mixer on low speed. Add the cocoa powder and mix it in, slowly, until the frosting is whipped. (Powdered sugar and cocoa can waft into the air and onto your shirt easily, so you might want to cover the bowl of the stand mixer with a towel while you do this.) Add the vanilla and salt. If the frosting feels too thick, add the coconut milk, 1 tablespoon at a time, until the frosting is whipped and smooth.

Feel like playing?

You could use the same weight of "buttery" nondairy sticks for this frosting, as well as vegetable shortening, if you cannot eat dairy. Add 1 teaspoon of cinnamon and 1 teaspoon of ancho chile powder to the frosting for a Mexican chocolate frosting. A tablespoon of hazelnut spread, such as Nutella, also works well here.

COFFEE BUTTERCREAM FROSTING

Makes about 3 cups

- 16 tablespoons unsalted butter, softened
- 3 cups powdered sugar, sifted
- 2 tablespoons unsweetened cocoa powder
- 3 to 5 tablespoons coffee syrup (see page 309)

Whip the butter in the bowl of a stand mixer with the paddle attachment on medium speed until it is light and fluffy, about 1 minute. Add the powdered sugar, slowly, with the mixer on low speed. Add the cocoa powder and mix it in, slowly, until the frosting is whipped. (Powdered sugar and cocoa can waft into the air and onto your shirt easily, so you might want to cover the bowl of the stand mixer with a towel while you do this.) Add the coffee syrup, 1 tablespoon at a time, until the frosting is whipped and smooth.

Feel like playing?

If you don't have any coffee syrup on hand, you could use strong brewed espresso here instead. It might make the frosting more bittersweet than sweet, which isn't a bad thing at all.

CITRUS SYRUP

Makes about ¼ cup

- Freshly squeezed juice of 2 lemons
- Freshly squeezed juice of 2 tangerines
- 2 tablespoons honey

Set a small pot over medium heat. Add the lemon and tangerine juices and honey. Stir until the honey is dissolved and the liquids are starting to boil on the edges of the pot. Simmer, stirring frequently, until the mixture forms a syrup, about 5 minutes. Allow it to cool before pouring over a cake.

Feel like playing?

You could use any citrus you want here: tangelos, oranges, and limes would be great too. You could also try maple syrup in place of the honey.

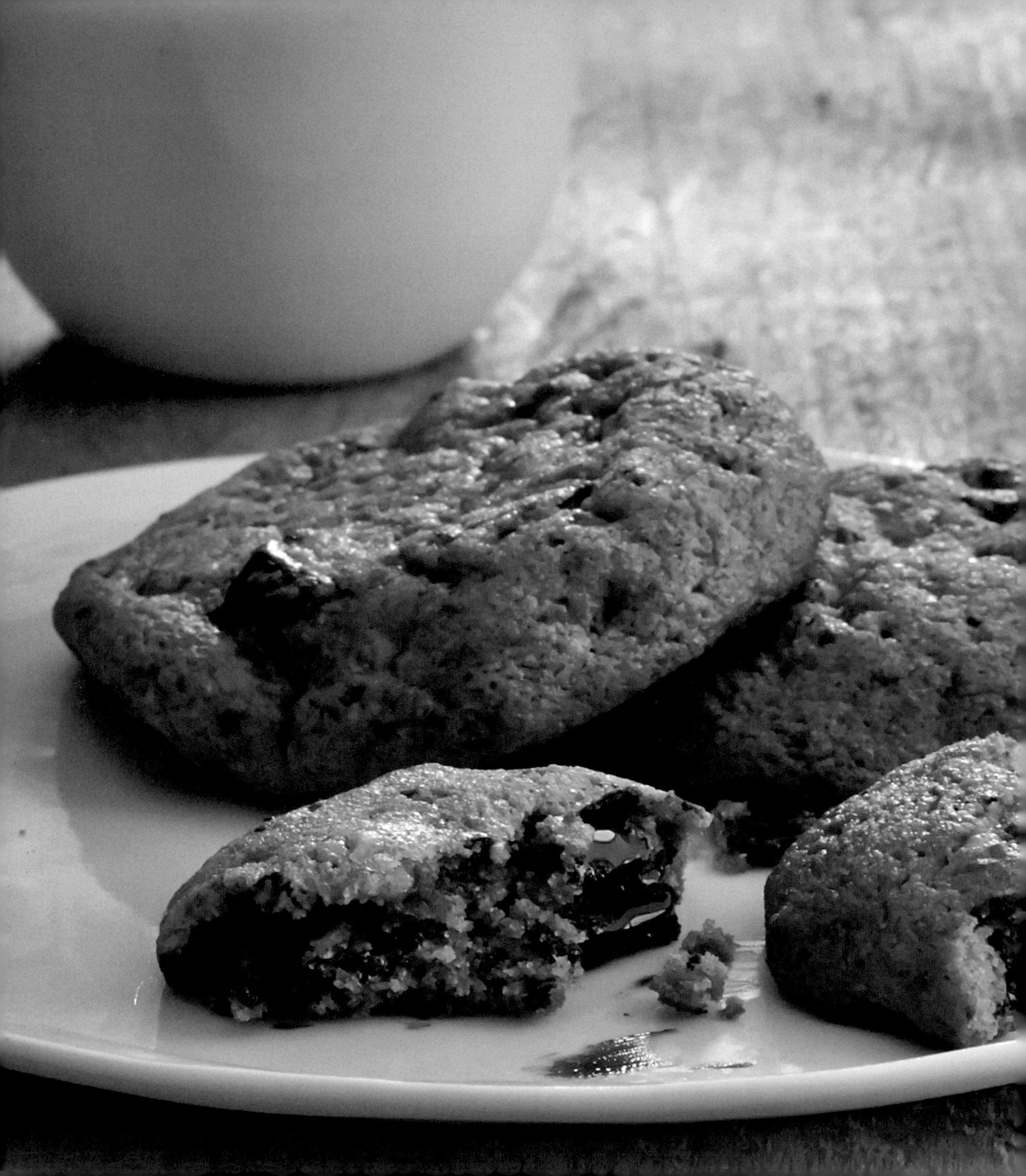

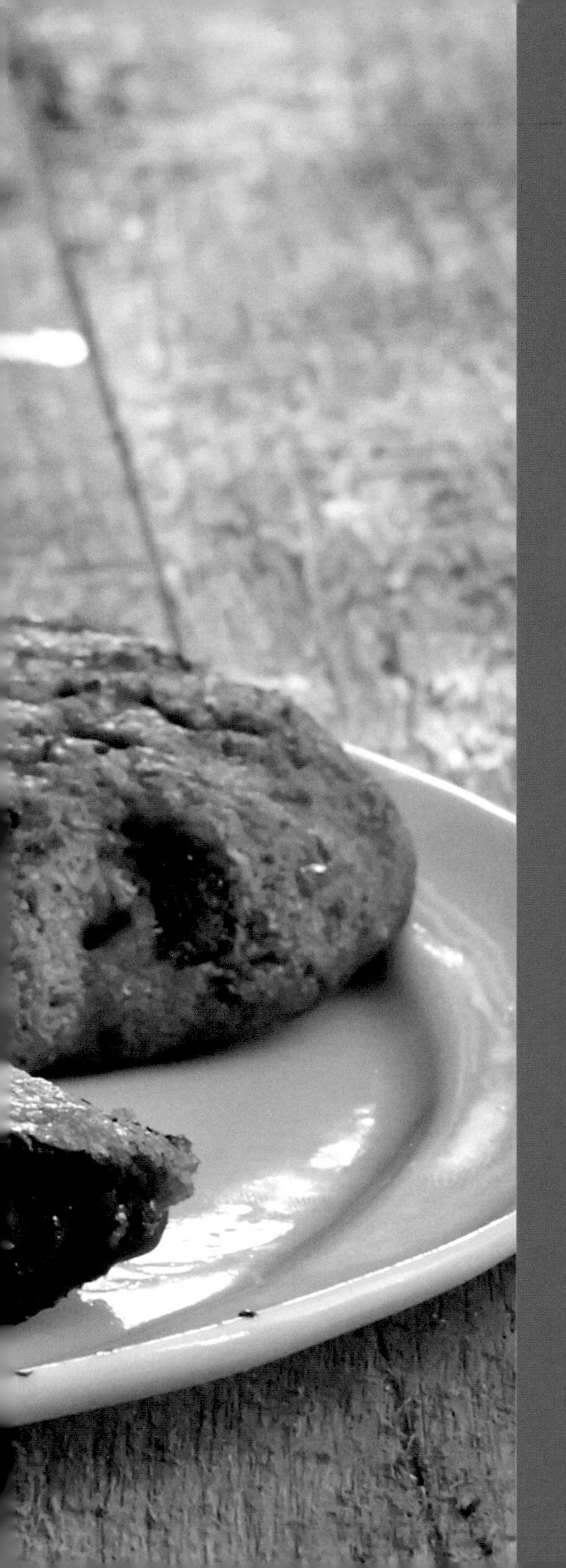

COOKIES

CHOCOLATE CHIP COOKIES

Makes about 20 cookies

Chocolate chip cookies might be the most quintessentially American recipe in this book. (They're adapted from the Nestlé Toll House cookies, the one printed on the back of the package, since that's what most people requested for this book.) One of the secrets is teff flour, a dark whole-grain flour that is filled with iron and good nutrients and also tastes faintly of chocolate. If you are ever baking with chocolate, add some teff. I suppose that makes these cookies not so typically American, but I think that's just fine too.

375 grams All-Purpose Gluten-Free Flour Blend (page 17)

50 grams teff flour

1 teaspoon kosher salt

½ teaspoon baking powder

½ teaspoon baking soda

16 tablespoons (230 grams) unsalted butter, at room temperature, cubed

¾ cup (165 grams) packed light brown sugar

¾ cup (160 grams) organic cane sugar

2 large eggs, at room temperature

1 teaspoon vanilla extract

2 cups (335 grams) bittersweet chocolate, coarsely chopped into ½-inch pieces

½ cup (50 grams) chopped nuts (we prefer hazelnuts)

Flaky sea salt (optional)

Combine the dry ingredients. In a large bowl, whisk together the flour blend, teff flour, salt, baking powder, and baking soda until they have become one color.

Cream the butter and sugar. Put the butter in the bowl of a stand mixer. With the paddle attachment, run the mixer on medium speed until the butter is creamy and softened. Add the brown sugar and cane sugar. Blend them together on medium speed until the mixture is light and fluffy, about 3 minutes. Use a rubber spatula to scrape down the sides of the bowl with a rubber spatula. Add the eggs and mix until all traces of egg disappear into the dough. Mix in the vanilla.

Finish the dough. With the mixer running, add the flour mixture a scoop at a time. When all the flour has been added and all trace of flour has disappeared into the dough, scrape down the sides of the bowl with a rubber spatula. Add the chocolate and nuts. Mix until just combined.

Refrigerate the dough. Wrap the bowl in plastic wrap and put it in the refrigerator. If you have the patience—and oh, it will be worth it—shove the dough to the back of the refrigerator and try to forget it for 3 days. The flours will hydrate fully, the flavors will intensify, and you will be happy. If you can't stand it, please at least refrigerate the dough overnight. (You could also do a science experiment and eat cookies at the same time. Bake one batch after an hour, another after one day, and another after two days or three days. Take notes.)

CONTINUED

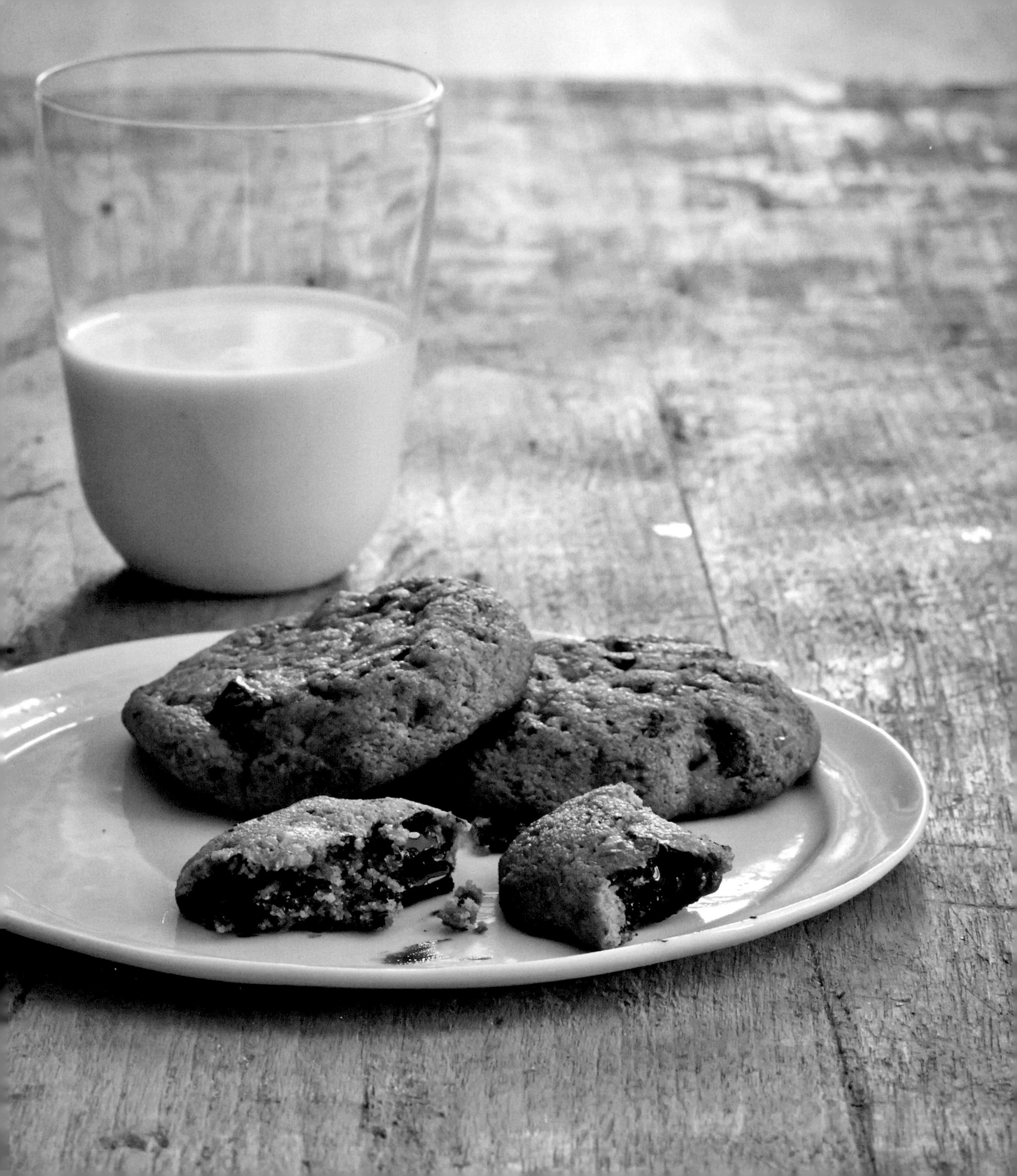

Prepare to bake. Preheat the oven to 375°F. Line a baking sheet with parchment paper.

Bake the cookies. Weigh out 30 grams of cookie dough. Make that into a ball of dough. Put the dough ball on the baking sheet, then gently slightly flatten the dough ball with the palm of your hand. Smooth out the edges of the cookie. Repeat until you end up with 6 cookies on the baking sheet with about 3 inches of space between them. Put the baking sheet in the freezer for 15 minutes.

Bake the cookies until the edges are crisp and the center is still soft to the touch, 8 to 12 minutes, turning the baking sheet 180 degrees in the oven halfway through baking. Take the cookies out of the oven and top each cookie with a pinch of flaky sea salt, if you wish. Allow the cookies to cool on the baking sheet for 10 minutes, then move the cookies to a wire rack. Bake the rest of the cookies in the same fashion.

Feel like playing?

Coconut oil works well here, in place of the butter. If you don't like nuts in your cookies, add more chocolate. Making these with the grain-free flour mix makes the flavor even more incredible, if slightly unfamiliar. These make great log cookies too. Roll the dough into three logs, cover them in plastic wrap, and you have cookie dough waiting to make a couple of cookies an evening, if you prefer.

SUNFLOWER SEED BUTTER COOKIES

Makes about 3 dozen cookies, depending on the size you make them

These days, if you try to take a treat to a preschool in the United States, traditional peanut butter cookies will not work. Someone cannot eat gluten, another kid can't have dairy, and you certainly don't want to bring peanuts into a school with so many kids suffering from potentially fatal peanut allergies. How do you provide a sweet treat for everyone? How about sunflower seed butter cookies made with coconut oil, honey, and a grain-free flour mix? Besides all that, these are great cookies.

1¼ cups (115 grams) coconut oil, softened

¾ cup honey

1 large egg, at room temperature

1 teaspoon vanilla extract

¾ cup (200 grams) salted sunflower seed butter

250 grams Grain-Free Flour Mix (page 19)

½ teaspoon baking soda

¼ teaspoon kosher salt

Combine the wet ingredients. In the bowl of a stand mixer with the paddle attachment, whisk together the coconut oil, honey, egg, and vanilla. When they are well combined, add the sunflower seed butter. Mix until well combined.

Combine the dry ingredients. In a bowl, combine the flour mix, baking soda, and salt. With the stand mixer running, add the flour mixture slowly to the bowl of the stand mixer. Scrape down the sides of the bowl with a rubber spatula and mix again.

Refrigerate the dough. Wrap the bowl in plastic wrap or drape a kitchen towel over it and put the dough into the refrigerator for at least 3 hours, if not overnight.

Prepare to bake. Preheat the oven to 350°F. Line a baking sheet with parchment paper.

Bake the cookies. Form a small ball of dough, no more than 30 grams. Put it on the baking sheet and flatten it slightly. Crisscross the top of the cookie with the tines of a fork. Fill the baking sheet with balls of dough, 2 inches apart from each other. Put the baking sheet in the freezer for 15 minutes.

Bake until the edges of the cookies are just starting to brown and the centers are still a bit soft, 10 to 15 minutes. Let the cookies cool on the baking sheet for 10 minutes, then carefully move them to a wire rack. They will crisp up in the air.

Continue baking the rest of the cookies.

Feel like playing?

If you want to use sugar instead of the honey, try 1 cup of coconut sugar for the best flavor. Use about 10 more grams of coconut oil as well. We like these cookies small, which makes them a great snack size. But you can easily make much bigger cookies.

GINGERSNAPS

Makes 4 dozen cookies

When I was a kid, my favorite cookies were the crisp little gingersnaps that came in a brown and orange box in almost every grocery store in America. Full of ginger flavor, those cookies kept drawing me in. Now that I make my own food, and I have a sense of what might have been in those packaged cookies, I can't imagine eating them. These are the crisp little flavorful cookies I wish I had been eating back then.

600 grams Grain-Free Flour Mix (page 19)

1 tablespoon ground ginger

1¼ teaspoons ground cinnamon

1 teaspoon baking soda

¾ teaspoon kosher salt

½ teaspoon freshly grated nutmeg

¼ teaspoon ground cloves

¼ teaspoon freshly ground black pepper

16 tablespoons (230 grams) unsalted butter, softened

1 cup (200 grams) packed dark brown sugar

⅔ cup molasses

1 large egg, at room temperature

2 teaspoons vanilla extract

1 teaspoon finely grated fresh ginger

¾ teaspoon freshly grated orange zest

Combine the dry ingredients. In a large bowl, whisk together the flour mix, ground ginger, cinnamon, baking soda, salt, nutmeg, cloves, and pepper.

Combine the wet ingredients. In the bowl of a stand mixer with the paddle attachment, mix the butter and brown sugar together until they are fluffy, about 3 minutes. Scrape down the sides of the bowl, then add the molasses, egg, vanilla, fresh ginger, and orange zest. Run the mixer on low until everything is combined thoroughly, about 2 minutes.

Finish the dough. With the stand mixer running on low, add the flour mix, about one-quarter of it at a time, mixing in between until the flour has disappeared entirely into the dough. Scrape down the sides of the bowl with a rubber spatula. Continue this until all the dry ingredients have been added. The dough will be a little sticky to the touch. Don't worry.

Refrigerate the dough. Divide the dough into quarters and shape each piece into a disk. Wrap each disk in plastic wrap and put them in the refrigerator for at least 1 hour.

Prepare to bake. Preheat the oven to 350°F. Line a baking sheet with parchment paper.

Bake the cookies. Form small balls of dough, about 30 grams each. Put the balls onto the baking sheet 2 inches apart. When the baking sheet is filled, bake for 6 minutes, then rotate the baking sheet 180 degrees in the oven. Bake until the edges are starting to crisp and the edges are still soft, about 6 more minutes. If you want crisper cookies, bake for an additional 3 minutes.

Remove the cookies from the oven. Allow the cookies to cool on the baking sheet for 10 minutes, then move them to a wire rack.

Continue baking the rest of the cookies.

Note: We found that the cookies taste even better the next day, so save at least some of them for the day after you bake them. The dough freezes well, so since this makes a lot of cookies, you could easily set yourself up for freshly baked cookies for a while.

Feel like playing?

If you want to add more gingery pizzazz to these, throw a handful of finely chopped candied ginger into the dough. These are wonderful cookies for small ice cream sandwiches. They also make a great gingersnap crust for pies. Finally, if you roll the dough out instead of dropping it, and you frost them after baking, you will have gingerbread men.

SNICKERDOODLES

Makes 4 dozen cookies

Years ago, our friend Irvin made some snickerdoodles with wheat flour on his blog, Eat the Love. Then a reader asked if he could make them gluten-free. He did. And then we adapted them with different flours and no xanthan gum for our website. Somehow, this recipe came from new technology, food friends, and gluten-free flours. That feels like America today.

475 grams All-Purpose Gluten-Free Flour Blend (page 17)

2 teaspoons cream of tartar

1 teaspoon baking soda

½ teaspoon kosher salt

8 tablespoons (115 grams) unsalted butter, softened

½ cup (110 grams) vegetable shortening (please buy the one without trans fats)

1½ cups plus 3 tablespoons (300 grams) organic cane sugar

2 large eggs

1 large egg yolk

2 teaspoons vanilla extract

1 tablespoon ground cinnamon

Combine the dry ingredients. In a large bowl, whisk together the flour blend, cream of tartar, baking soda, and salt.

Cream the butter and sugar. Add the butter to the bowl of a stand mixer with the paddle attachment. Put the shortening in with the butter and blend on medium speed until they are coherent. Scrape down the sides of the bowl with a rubber spatula. With the mixer running, add 1½ cups of the sugar and beat until the mixture is fluffy. Scrape down the sides of the bowl with a rubber spatula. With the mixer running, add the eggs and egg yolk, one at a time, waiting until each egg is fully incorporated into the dough before adding the next. Pour in the vanilla and mix until combined.

Finishing the cookie dough. With the stand mixer running on low, slowly pour in the flour mixture, scraping down the sides of the bowl once in a while. Cover the bowl with plastic wrap and put it in the refrigerator for at least 3 hours and preferably overnight.

Prepare to bake. Preheat the oven to 350°F. Line a baking sheet with parchment paper.

Bake the cookies. Take the dough out of the refrigerator. Form small balls of dough, about 30 grams each. Combine the remaining 3 tablespoons of sugar and the cinnamon in a small bowl. Dunk each ball of dough in the cinnamon sugar and roll it around. Space the cookies 2 inches apart on the baking sheet. Put the baking sheet in the freezer for 15 minutes, then pull it out and immediately place it in the hot oven. Bake until the cookies are flattened, crisp at the edges, and the tops have started to crackle, 10 to 15 minutes. Let the cookies cool on the baking sheet for 10 minutes, then move them to a wire rack and continue baking the rest of the cookie dough the same way.

Feel like playing?

I've made these cookies successfully with all coconut oil. They spread a little more than the butter-shortening version, but they're just as delicious.

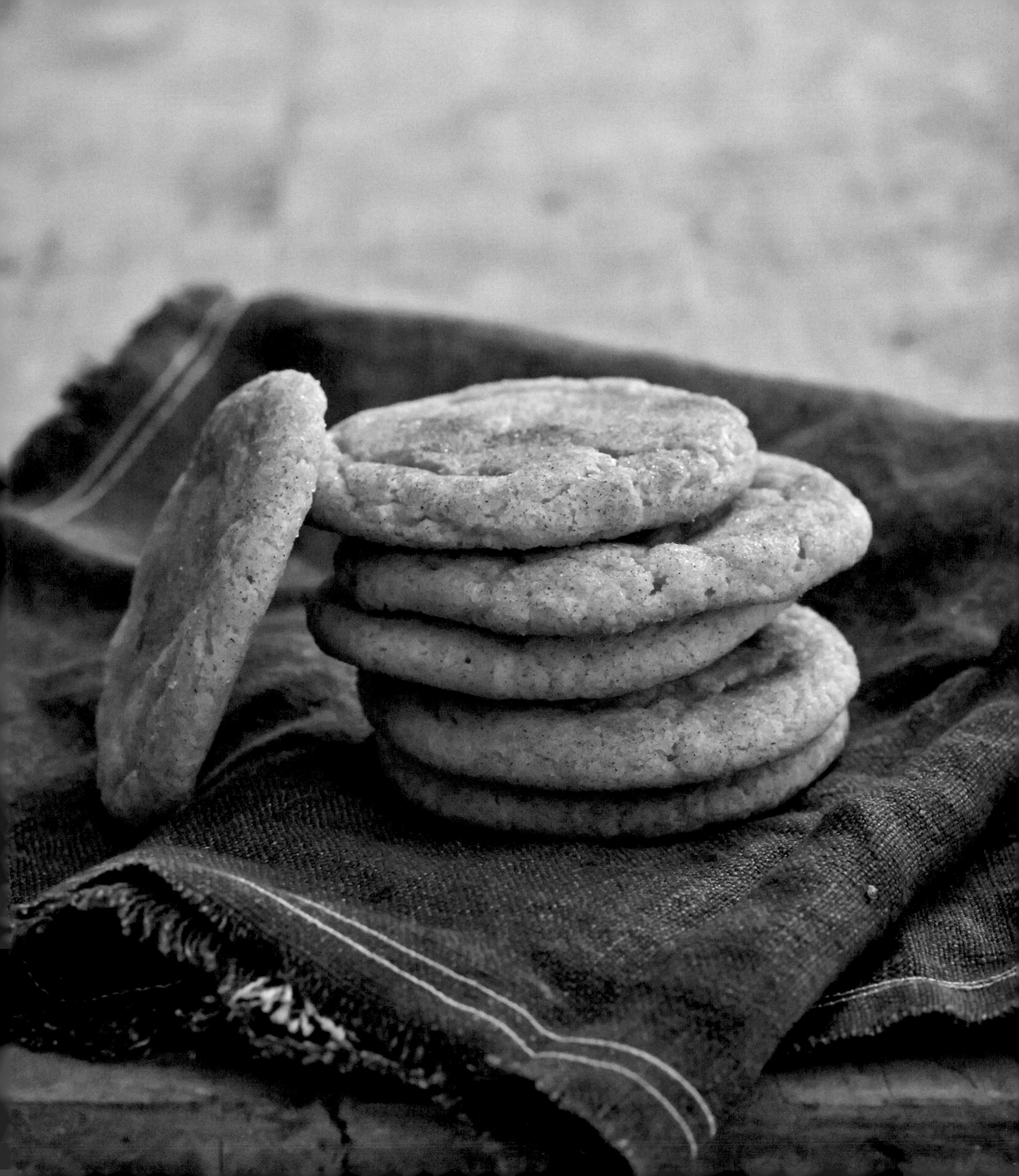

WHOOPIE PIES

Makes about a dozen whoopie pies

When we drove around New England with our daughter, doing potluck events in nearly every state, we saw signs for a treat we don't seem to eat in the Pacific Northwest: whoopie pies! These sweet little cake-like cookies (mostly chocolate, it seemed) sandwiched a creamy filling (marshmallow crème, mostly). Think soft ice cream sandwich, but warm and without ice cream. In Maine, where whoopie pies are the official state treat, every gas station and small store sold them, along with lobster rolls. (Mainers lay claim to the invention of the whoopie pie, but the folks in Pennsylvania beg to disagree. They claim that it's an Amish treat, and when hard-working farmers opened their lunch boxes and found this sweet, they all shouted "Whoopie!") We gluten-free folks can have our whoopie pies easily. I'd venture to say that these are better than the ones you'd buy in a gas station anyway. Instead of marshmallow crème in the middle, we use cream cheese frosting, inspired by the recipe by our talented friend Tara Barker, a gluten-free pastry chef who lives in Maine.

280 grams All-Purpose Gluten-Free Flour Blend (page 17)

½ cup (60 grams) raw cacao powder

1 teaspoon baking powder

½ teaspoon fine sea salt

About 8 tablespoons (115 grams) coconut oil, softened

1 cup (210 grams) organic cane sugar

2 large eggs, at room temperature

2 teaspoons vanilla extract

½ cup coconut milk

2 cups Cream Cheese Frosting (page 268)

Combine the dry ingredients. In a large bowl, whisk together the flour blend, cacao powder, baking powder, and salt.

Mix the wet ingredients. In the bowl of a stand mixer with the paddle attachment, combine the coconut oil and sugar. Mix until they are light and fluffy, about 3 minutes. With the mixer running, add the eggs one at a time, waiting until each egg is fully incorporated before adding the next. Turn off the mixer and scrape down the sides of the bowl with a rubber spatula. Add the vanilla and finish mixing.

Finish the dough. With the mixer running, add half the flour mixture, then the coconut milk, then the remaining flour mix. Scrape down the sides of the bowl with a rubber spatula. The final dough should be like a thick cake batter.

Chill the dough. Cover the bowl with plastic wrap and chill for at least 1 hour.

Prepare to bake. Preheat the oven to 325°F. Line a baking sheet with parchment paper.

Bake the cookies. Gather a heaping tablespoon of dough for each cookie and drop it onto the prepared baking sheet, leaving about 2 inches of space around each cookie. Put the baking sheet in the freezer for 15 minutes.

Bake the cookies until the tops of the cookies spring back slightly when touched, 8 to 10 minutes, rotating the baking sheet halfway through the baking time. Allow the cookies to cool on the baking sheet for 10 minutes, then gently move them to a wire rack. Continue baking the rest of the cookies in this manner.

Fill the whoopie pies. When the cookies are entirely cooled, spread a thick layer of cream cheese frosting on the flat side of one cookie, then top with another cookie. Whoopie! You just made a whoopie pie.

Feel like playing?

You could easily use butter in place of the coconut oil, another nondairy milk or cow's milk in place of the coconut milk, and an alternative sugar such as sucanat or coconut sugar here, if you want.

THIN MINTS (LIKE THE ONES A SCOUT WHO IS A GIRL MIGHT SELL YOU)

Makes 3 to 4 dozen cookies

There are so many great American cookies that the list for this chapter once numbered forty-eight recipes. Oatmeal-raisin cookies! Buckeyes! Animal crackers! Seriously, we could do an entire book of American cookies made gluten-free. But when we were winnowing down that list to the chapter you hold in your hands, Danny had only one request. Thin Mints. You know, like the ones a scout who is also a girl might sell you? We adapted the cookie part of this recipe from the Bouchon Bakery *cookbook, one of the best baking books ever published. These are for you, Chef.*

260 grams All-Purpose Gluten-Free Flour Blend (page 17)

About 1 cup (90 grams) unsweetened Dutch-process cocoa powder

½ teaspoon baking soda

16 tablespoons (227 grams) unsalted butter, softened

2 teaspoons fine sea salt

½ teaspoon peppermint extract

About ¾ cup (160 grams) organic cane sugar

12 ounces (1500 grams) good dark chocolate (at least 72% cacao)

2 tablespoons (26 grams) coconut oil, melted

Combine the dry ingredients. In a large bowl, whisk together the flour blend, cocoa powder, and baking soda.

Cream the butter, salt, and sugar. Put the butter into the bowl of a stand mixer with the paddle attachment. Beat the butter on medium-low speed until it's smooth, about 1 minute. Add the salt and ¼ teaspoon of the peppermint extract and mix for another 30 seconds. Scrape down the sides of the bowl with a rubber spatula. Add the sugar and mix for 2 minutes. Scrape down the sides of the bowl with a rubber spatula.

Finish the dough. With the mixer running, add the flour mixture, a little at a time. When you have finished adding all the flour, scrape down the sides of the bowl with a rubber spatula and mix again. The final dough should be loosely combined.

Dump the dough onto a clean surface. Using a pastry scraper, move the dough around to push it into 2 square blocks.

Chill the dough. Wrap the dough in plastic wrap and chill it for at least 3 hours, and preferably overnight.

Prepare to bake. Preheat the oven to 325°F. Line a baking sheet with parchment paper.

Roll out the dough. Put one block of dough between two pieces of lightly greased parchment paper. Roll out the dough, rotating the block of dough 90 degrees every time you roll, until it is about ⅛ inch thick. Quickly, using a small round cookie cutter, cut out shapes from the dough. Put them on the baking sheet, leaving at least 1 inch between them. When you are done cutting shapes, gather all the leftover dough and roll it into a ball. Put plastic wrap around this and put it back in the refrigerator. Put the baking sheet into the freezer for 15 minutes.

Bake the cookies. Bake the cookies until they are just set on top and small cracks appear on the surface, 9 to 11 minutes. Be sure to rotate the baking sheet halfway through the baking time. (If you made larger cookies than 2 inches across, give the cookies up to 18 minutes to bake.) Let the cookies rest on the baking sheet for 10 minutes, then move them to a wire rack to cool entirely.

Repeat with the remaining dough. Wait to dip the cookies in chocolate until they are all thoroughly cooled.

Melt the chocolate. Set a large pot filled three-quarters full with water over high heat. Bring the water to a boil. Set a large metal pan over the large pot. Add the chocolate, the remaining ¼ teaspoon peppermint extract, and coconut oil to the metal bowl. Grip the bowl with a kitchen towel and stir the chocolate with a rubber spatula until all the ingredients are well combined and the chocolate is lusciously melted. Turn off the heat.

Coat the cookies. Set a wire rack over a parchment-lined baking sheet. Brush the melted chocolate over the bottoms of all the cookies. Set them chocolate side up on the wire rack and let the chocolate solidify. Turn the heat on under the large pot again and re-melt the chocolate. Turn off the heat. Dip the tops of the cookies into the melted chocolate, carefully, then turn them over onto the wire rack and let the excess chocolate drip off. You're probably going to have to lick your fingers. Darn.

Chill the cookies in the refrigerator—they really are better cold—and then feed your friends.

Feel like playing?

You could easily make these into coconut-chocolate cookies by substituting the butter with coconut oil.

BLACK AND WHITE COOKIES

Makes about 2 dozen cookies, depending on the size you make

Do you remember that Seinfeld *episode where they talked about the black and white cookie? Or the scene in* Sex and the City *where Carrie nibbles on a black and white cookie while talking about her Russian lover? Sense a theme? These are New York cookies. If you've never lived in New York, you might not have seen these. You have two options: fly to New York and try to find some or make them yourself. And if you're gluten-free, you couldn't eat the black and white cookies in New York anyway. They're full of gluten.*

The cookie part of the black and white cookie is soft and cakey with a hint of lemon, like a tea cake smooshed down to the size of your hand. And then you make one frosting and add cocoa powder to half of it, and vanilla extract to the other half, and frost the cookie half and half. Oh my.

FOR THE COOKIES

280 grams All-Purpose Gluten-Free Flour Blend (page 17)

1 teaspoon baking powder

¼ teaspoon fine sea salt

⅓ cup whole milk

1 teaspoon vanilla extract

Freshly grated zest of 1 lemon

8 tablespoons (115 grams) unsalted butter, softened

⅔ cup (130 grams) organic cane sugar

2 large eggs, at room temperature

FOR THE FROSTING

2 cups plus 2 tablespoons (250 grams) powdered sugar

4 teaspoons light corn syrup

1 teaspoon vanilla extract

3 tablespoons lukewarm water

3 tablespoons (20 grams) unsweetened Dutch-process cocoa powder

Combine the dry ingredients. In a large bowl, whisk together the flour blend, baking powder, and salt. Set aside.

Combine the wet ingredients. In a small bowl, combine the milk, vanilla, and lemon zest. Set aside.

Cream the butter and sugar. In the bowl of a stand mixer with the paddle attachment, cream together the butter and sugar until they are light and fluffy, about 5 minutes. Scrape down the sides of the bowl with a rubber spatula. With the mixer running, add the eggs, one at a time, until they are all fully incorporated.

Finish the dough. With the mixer running on low, add half the flour mix, then the milk mixture, then the rest of the flour. Scrape down the sides of the bowl with a rubber spatula and finish mixing everything together. Cover the bowl with plastic wrap and put it in the refrigerator for at least 2 hours, if not overnight.

Prepare to bake. Preheat the oven to 375°F. Line a baking sheet with parchment paper.

Bake the cookies. Drop about 50 grams of dough for each cookie onto the baking sheet. Make sure the mounds of batter are 2 inches apart from each other. Put the baking sheet in the freezer for 15 minutes.

Bake the cookies for 7 minutes, then rotate the baking sheet

180 degrees in the oven. Bake until the cookies feel just set in the middle and the edges are just starting to darken, about 8 minutes more. Allow the cookies to cool on the baking sheet for 10 minutes, then move them to a wire rack. Continue baking the rest of the cookies the same way.

Make the frosting. In the bowl of a stand mixer with the paddle attachment, mix 2 cups of the powdered sugar, 2 teaspoons of the corn syrup, the vanilla, and the lukewarm water until the frosting is smooth.

Take half the frosting out of the stand mixer and put it in another bowl. Put the remaining 2 tablespoons of powdered sugar into this other bowl of frosting and mix until it is spreadably thick. This is the "white" frosting.

Add the cocoa powder and the remaining 2 teaspoons of corn syrup to the frosting in the bowl of the stand mixer. This is the "black" frosting. If that frosting feels too thick, add 1 tablespoon of water at a time until the frosting feels right.

Frost the cookies. Turn the cooled cookies over, so the puffy side is down. Using a butter knife or small spatula, frost half of the flat part of each cookie with the white frosting. Spread the black frosting over the other half of each cookie. Let the cookies sit for a moment. Dive in.

Feel like playing?

Making these cookies with coconut oil instead of butter gives them a slightly different texture—they spread a bit more—but they're still delicious.

ALMOND DIM SUM COOKIES

Makes 3 dozen or so cookies

These delicious, crumbly cookies are inspired by the cookies typically served at the end of a dim sum meal at Chinese restaurants in Hawaii. Strangely, most recipes don't call for almonds at all but rather typical bleached all-purpose wheat flour. Our grain-free flour and almond flour take these cookies to a new flavor level, however. The traditional recipes call for lard, which makes for a pretty intoxicating taste. Make sure you're buying good lard from a butcher or farmer, however. The lard off the grocery store shelf is pretty bad stuff. You don't want to feed your kids cookies made with that.

125 grams Grain-Free Flour Mix (page 19)

100 grams almond flour

1 cup (210 grams) organic cane sugar

½ teaspoon baking powder

½ teaspoon fine sea salt

1 cup (225 grams) lard

1 large egg, at room temperature

36 whole raw almonds

Combine the dry ingredients. In a large bowl, whisk together the flour mix, sugar, baking powder, and salt.

Finish the dough. Drop the lard in spoonfuls into the dry ingredients. Work the lard into the flour until the dough is sandy and crumbly. Add the egg and stir to combine. Refrigerate the dough for at least 3 hours and preferably overnight.

Prepare to bake. Preheat the oven to 325°F. Line a baking sheet with parchment paper.

Bake the cookies. Roll the dough into 1-inch balls (for even baking, make each ball 30 grams). Put balls of dough onto the parchment paper, flatten the top, and put an almond in the center. Space the cookies 2 inches apart. Bake the cookies until they are set at the edges and just starting to brown, 15 to 18 minutes. Let the cookies cool on the baking sheet for 10 minutes, then move them to a wire rack. Finish baking the rest of the cookies the same way.

Feel like playing?

Substitute an equal amount of vegetable shortening for the lard if you are vegetarian. Many folks seem to skip the almond topping and use a dot of red food dye instead. We're pretty partial to the almonds, however.

BISCOCHITOS

Makes 4 to 5 dozen cookies, depending on the size of the cookie cutters you use

You might not have encountered a biscochito *cookie if you live far from the Southwest. But there's a reason why this is the state cookie of New Mexico. These cookies, made with lard, sugar, anise seed, cinnamon, and sweet white wine, are a cross between cutout sugar cookies and shortbread. Traditionally in New Mexico, they're served at the holidays as well as weddings and baptisms. Need a reason to celebrate? Bring out the* biscochitos! *This recipe is inspired by one on Gabriela's Kitchen, a food blog begun by a Latina food lover dedicated to honoring the women in her life who taught her to cook.*

420 grams All-Purpose Gluten-Free Flour Blend (page 17)

1½ teaspoons baking powder

½ teaspoon fine sea salt

¾ cup (168 grams) lard (make it the good stuff, to avoid trans fats)

¾ cup (158 grams) organic cane sugar

2 large eggs, at room temperature

1½ teaspoons anise seed

½ teaspoon ground cinnamon

¼ cup sweet white wine, such as Sauternes or a sweet sherry

FOR THE TOPPING

¼ cup (53 grams) organic cane sugar

2 teaspoons ground cinnamon

Combine the dry ingredients. In a large bowl, whisk together the flour blend, baking powder, and salt.

Cream the lard and sugar. In the bowl of a stand mixer with the paddle attachment, combine the lard and sugar. Mix until they are light and fluffy, about 3 minutes.

Add the eggs, one at a time, making sure each one is incorporated fully before adding the next one. Scrape down the sides of the bowl with a rubber spatula. Add the anise seed and cinnamon and mix fully.

Finish the dough. With the stand mixer running on low, add the flour mixture to the dough, stopping to scrape down the sides of the bowl with a rubber spatula a couple of times. Add the wine, a tablespoon at a time, until the dough comes together as a ball.

Chill the dough. Divide the dough in half and form each into a ball. Wrap each in plastic wrap and refrigerate overnight.

Prepare to bake. The next day, preheat the oven to 350°F. Line a baking sheet with parchment paper. Pull the balls of dough out of the refrigerator. Mix the sugar and cinnamon together in a small bowl.

Roll out the cookies. Put one of the balls of dough between two pieces of lightly greased parchment paper. Roll out the dough gently until it's about ⅛ inch thick. Cut the dough into the shapes you are using with cookie cutters. (We like stars here.) Dip one side of the cookie into the cinnamon sugar and put it on the baking sheet, sugar side up. Continue until the baking sheet is filled.

Bake the cookies. Bake the cookies until the bottom of the cookies are browned and the tops are set, 10 to 15 minutes, rotating the baking sheet 180 degrees halfway through the baking time.

Let the cookies cool for 5 minutes on the baking sheet, then dip both sides of the warm cookies in the cinnamon sugar and set them on a wire rack. Be nimble—the cookies can fall apart when warm.

Continue baking the rest of the cookies the same way.

Feel like playing?

I know that you might be tempted to substitute another fat for the lard, but please try the lard first. It gives a really special taste here. Of course, if you're a vegetarian, you can use coconut oil instead. Just know you'll have a different cookie than the traditional biscochito.

RUGELACH

Makes 32 cookies

I first ate rugelach in New York City, and I have never forgotten it. Part flaky pastry, part bite-size cookie, and all delicious, this sweet is often served at Hanukkah. Think super-easy croissant with any filling you wish. This recipe owes its structure to the wonderful Dorie Greenspan, who is one of my favorite baking gurus and such a lovely person. If Dorie thinks you should eat these, you should listen to her. We just made them gluten-free for you.

4 ounces cold cream cheese

8 tablespoons (115 grams) cold unsalted butter

575 grams All-Purpose Gluten-Free Flour Blend (page 17)

½ teaspoon fine sea salt

⅔ cup apricot jam

½ teaspoon ground cinnamon

1 cup (100 grams) chopped walnuts

1 large egg, beaten

Prepare to bake. Set the cream cheese and butter out on the counter 10 minutes before you intend to start working with them. Cut the cream cheese and butter into 4 pieces each.

Combine the dry ingredients. Put the flour blend and salt in the bowl of a food processor. Whirl them up.

Form the dough. Drop the cream cheese and butter pieces into the flour. Pulse the dough 5 to 10 times to break up the pieces of fat, then turn on the processor. At first, the flours will spin round and round and you'll think you need some liquid to make them stick. Be patient. After a few moments, you'll see the forces start to gather. Watch carefully. Stop the processor when the dough looks like giant curds, before it has formed a solid ball.

Chill the dough. Form 2 balls of dough. Cover them in plastic wrap and refrigerate them for at least 2 hours, or overnight.

Make the filling. Set a small pot over low heat. Add the jam and cinnamon and stir together. Heat the jam until it turns to liquid. Set aside.

Roll out the dough. Pull one of the balls of dough out of the refrigerator. Roll out the dough between two pieces of lightly greased parchment paper to an even 10-inch circle.

Peel off the top layer of parchment paper and spread half of the jam and walnuts onto the dough, leaving at least 1 inch of space around the edges. Press the parchment paper lightly onto the filing to press it into the dough, then remove the parchment again.

Make the crescents. Cut the dough into 16 triangles. (A pizza wheel

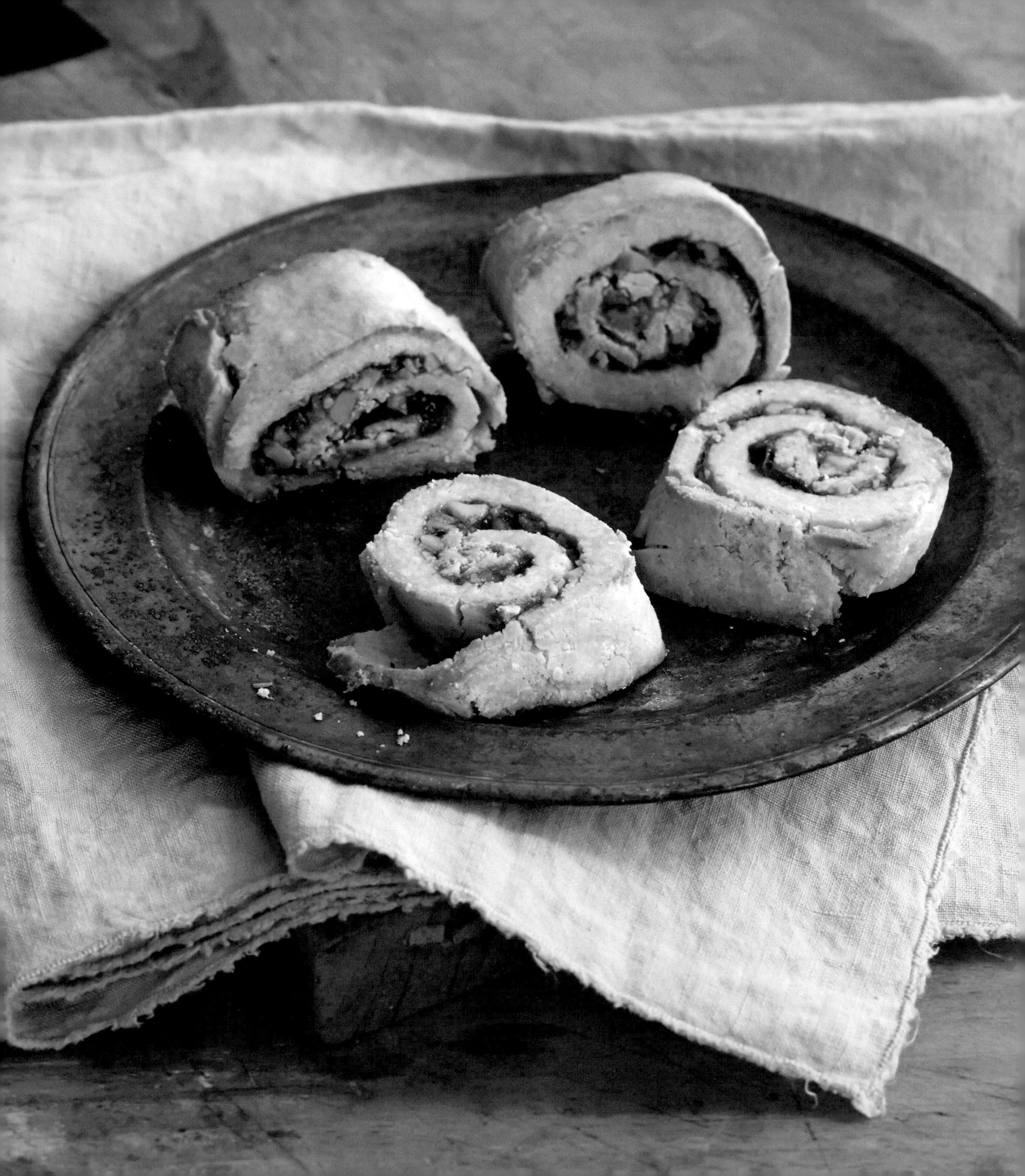

is the best tool for this.) Start with the widest part of each triangle as the base and roll up the triangle into a little crescent roll. Put the rollups onto a baking sheet, tucking the point at the end of the crescent under the roll. When the baking sheet is filled, put it in the freezer for 30 minutes.

Repeat with the remaining dough and another baking sheet.

Preheat the oven to 350°F.

Bake the rugelach. Pull the rugelach out of the freezer. Brush some of the beaten egg gently over the cookies. Bake the cookies for 10 minutes, then rotate the baking sheet 180 degrees. Bake until the rugelach are deeply golden brown and slightly puffed, about 10 minutes more. Cool the rugelach on the baking sheet for 10 minutes, then carefully transfer them to a wire rack.

You may eat the rugelach when they have cooled to room temperature.

Feel like playing?

You can fill these with any filling you wish. The apricot jam and walnut filling is only the traditional. I particularly liked one we made with a stewed prune puree and dark chocolate. You can also make these savory. Think tiny pizza rolls for the kids!

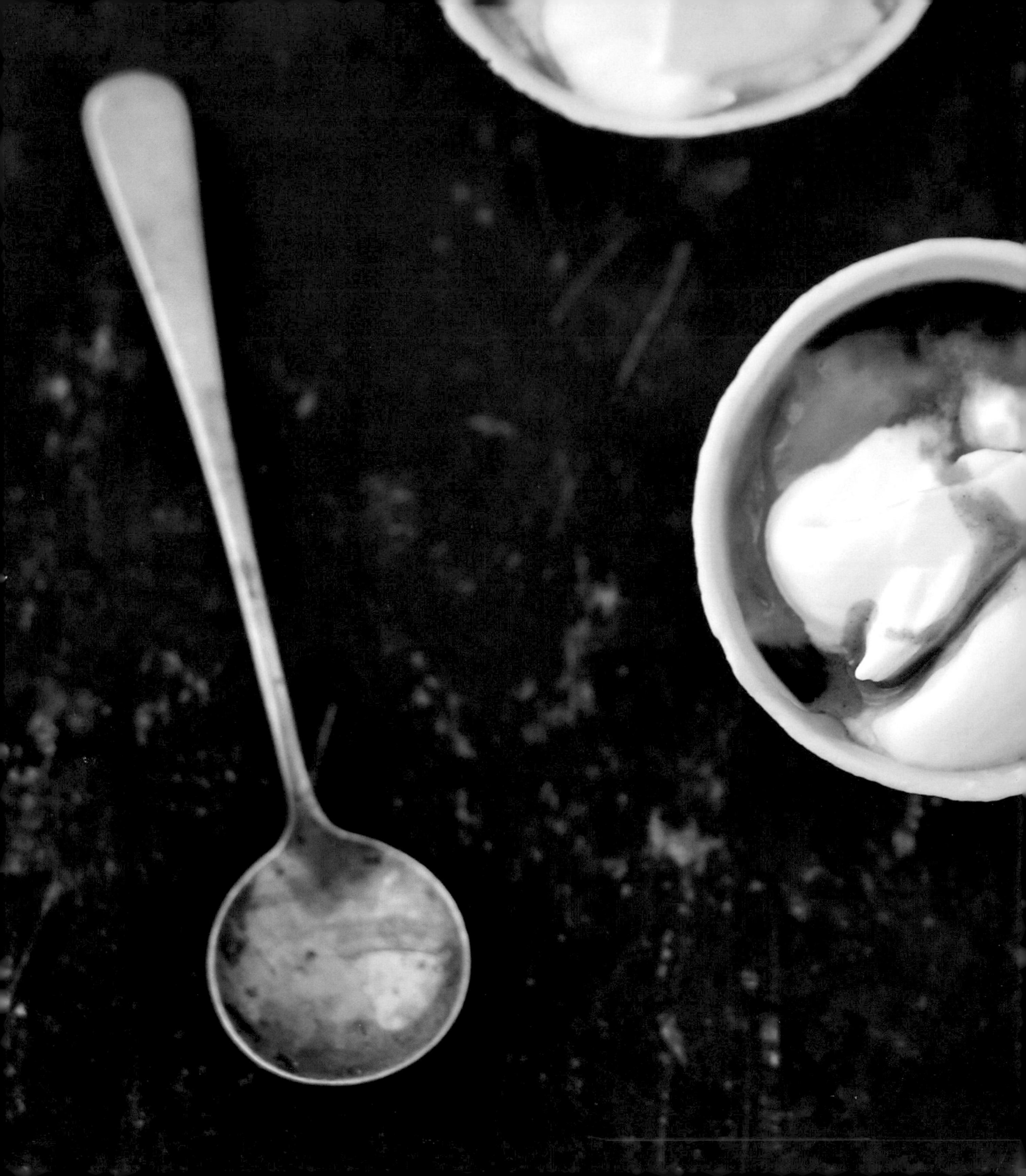

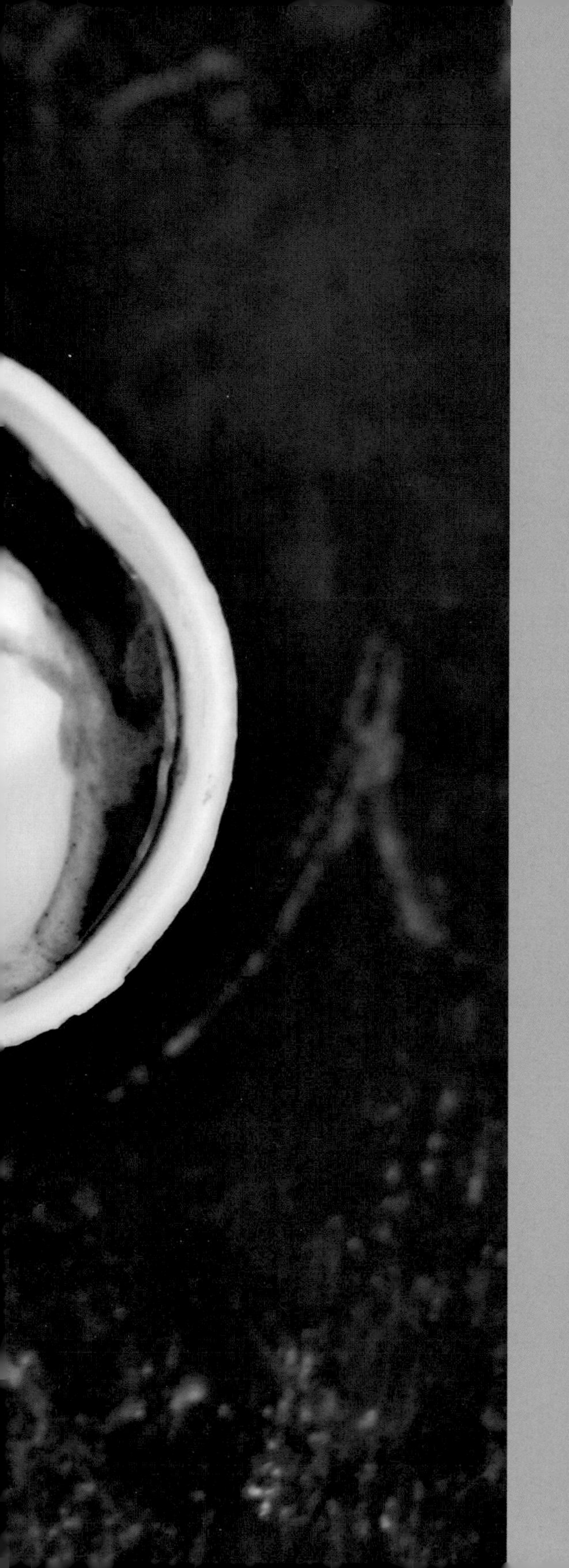

DESSERTS

ALMOST AS GOOD-LOOKING AS ROBERT REDFORD

Feeds 12

Look, there's no way I could resist a dessert with a name like this. I suppose if this dessert suddenly became popular now, instead of in the 1970s, it would be Almost as Good-Looking as Ryan Gosling. Eh, this one's better. It's also known as Better Than Sex in some circles, but that's just a sad name to me. I mean, this is a scrumptious dessert when you make it from scratch: a walnut-butter crust, chocolate pudding, dolloped with sweetened whipped cream cheese–coconut cream. It's fantastic. Better Than Sex? I hope not. Almost as Good-Looking as Robert Redford it is.

FOR THE CRUST

140 grams All-Purpose Gluten-Free Flour Blend (page 17)

8 tablespoons (115 grams) cold unsalted butter, cut into 1-inch cubes

1 cup (100 grams) finely chopped walnuts

FOR THE WHIPPED TOPPING LAYER

12 ounces cream cheese, softened

2 cups coconut cream (see Note)

1½ cups (185 grams) powdered sugar

FOR THE PUDDING

⅔ cup (140 grams) organic cane sugar

½ cup (60 grams) unsweetened cocoa powder

¼ cup (32 grams) arrowroot flour

¼ teaspoon fine sea salt

2¼ cups coconut milk

4 large egg yolks

2 tablespoons (29 grams) cold unsalted butter, cut into cubes

1 teaspoon vanilla extract

Prepare to bake. Preheat the oven to 350°F.

Make the crust. Put the flour blend and butter into a large bowl. Rub the butter into the flour with your fingers until the flour looks like sandy crumbs. Add the nuts and stir. Press the mixture into a 9 x 13-inch baking dish and bake until the crust feels firm to the touch, about 10 minutes. Take the dish out of the oven and allow the crust to cool completely.

Make the whipped topping. In the bowl of a stand mixer with the paddle attachment, whip the cream cheese and coconut cream

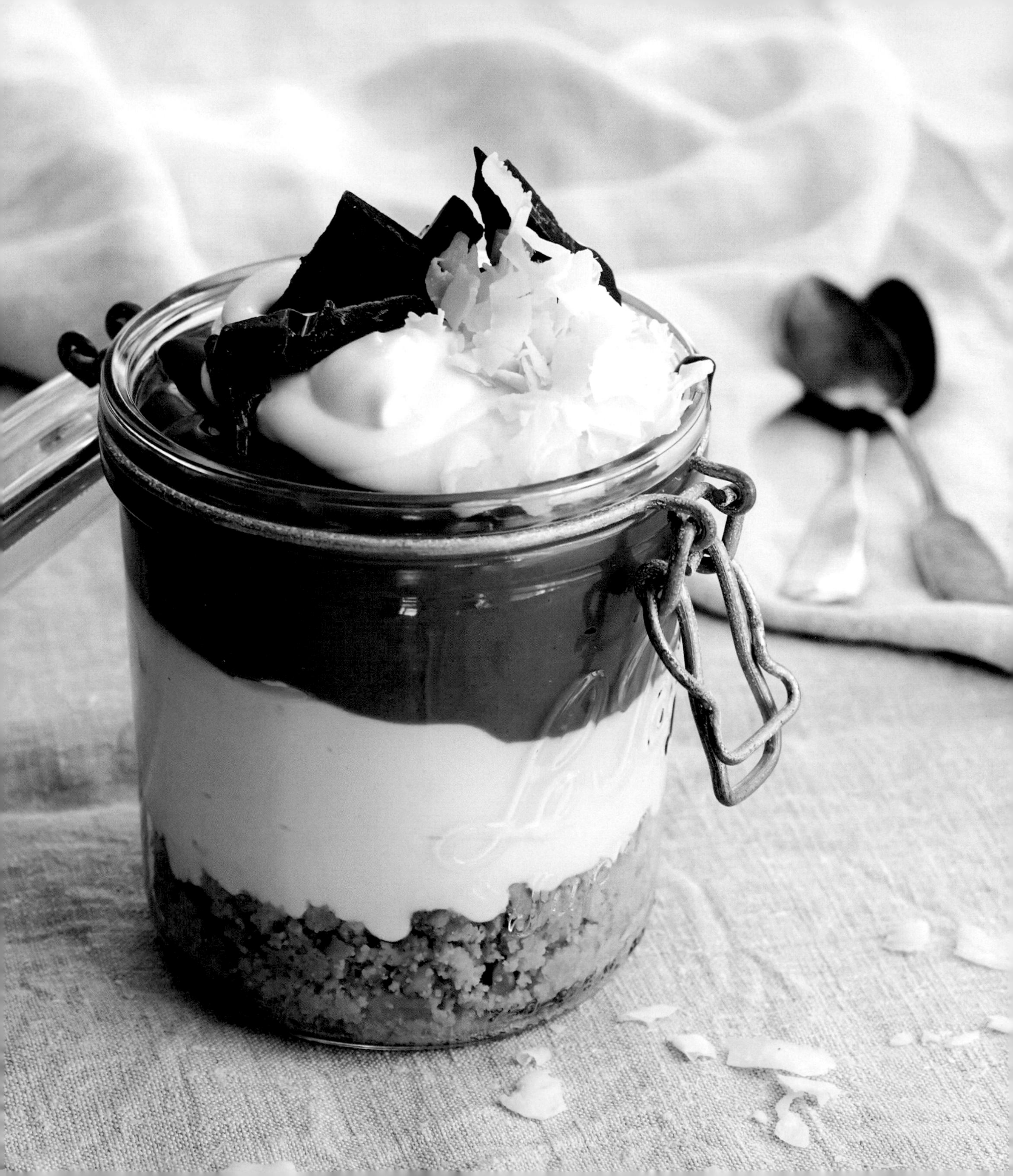

together. Sift in the powdered sugar with the mixer running on low. When they are well combined, put the bowl in the refrigerator to chill.

Make the pudding. In a large pot, whisk together the sugar, cocoa powder, arrowroot, and salt. A few drops at a time, whisk in the coconut milk, making sure that the arrowroot does not clump up. Continue pouring and whisking the milk until it has all been added. Whisk in the egg yolks.

Set the pot over medium heat. Whisk the pudding as it comes to heat. When the pudding starts to boil, turn the heat down to low and whisk vigorously for 1 full minute. Take the pudding off the heat. Add the butter and vanilla and whisk them in. Pour the pudding into a large bowl, cover it with plastic wrap, and refrigerate it for 4 hours.

Assemble the dessert. Spread half the whipped topping over the crust in the pan. Dollop the chilled chocolate pudding on top and spread it to the edges. Top with the remaining whipped topping. Refrigerate until chilled and you are ready to serve.

Note: To make coconut cream, put a couple of cans of full-fat coconut milk in the refrigerator overnight. Open the cans and scoop out the thick part of the coconut milk, which will have all gathered at the top of the can, into a bowl. There's your coconut cream.

Feel like playing?

We really prefer coconut cream to whipped cream for taste and texture, as well as coconut milk in the chocolate pudding over cow's milk. That makes this dessert almost dairy-free. To make it completely dairy-free, use a nondairy cream cheese for the topping and coconut oil to make the crust and finish the pudding.

Traditionally, this dessert is made in a 9 x 13-inch pan, which works with this recipe as well. But making it in individual jars makes it even sexier.

BROWNIES

Makes about 2 dozen brownies

Brownies are the easiest baked good to make and they certainly don't require gluten to make them good. If you want a brownie with a crackling crust on top that disappears into a fudgy center, with crisp edges and an intense chocolate taste, this is your brownie. Teff has a faint taste of chocolate and hazelnuts, so if you add both to the brownies, the entire flavor jumps for joy.

Fat for greasing the pan

8 tablespoons (115 grams) unsalted butter

2 ounces bittersweet chocolate, chopped

1 cup (210 grams) organic cane sugar

2 large eggs, at room temperature

1 teaspoon vanilla extract

100 grams teff flour

2 handfuls (100 grams) chopped hazelnuts

½ cup (85 grams) semisweet chocolate chips

Prepare to bake. Preheat the oven to 350°F. Line an 8-inch square baking pan with two pieces of parchment paper going opposite ways, leaving enough paper to hang over the edges. Grease the parchment with butter or oil.

Melt the butter and chocolate. Put the butter and chocolate in a microwave-safe bowl. Run the microwave for 1 minute. Whisk together the melted butter and chocolate. If there are any remaining chunks of chocolate, microwave for 30 more seconds. Stir well. (You can also melt the chocolate over a double boiler.)

Make the batter. Let the butter-chocolate combination cool until you can touch it. Add the sugar and stir until it is dissolved. Add the eggs, one at a time, stirring in between. Pour in the vanilla and stir. Add the teff flour and stir the batter thoroughly, with a rubber spatula, for at least 1 minute. Toss in the hazelnuts and chocolate chips and stir until just combined.

Bake the brownies. Pour the batter into the prepared pan and spread it evenly into the corners. Bake until the edges have begun to pull away from the pan and the center is just starting to set, 20 to 25 minutes. Remove the brownies from the oven. Cool for at least 15 minutes. Lift both pieces of parchment paper and the brownies out of the pan and cool on a wire rack. Dig in.

Feel like playing?

I like adding cacao nibs to brownies at times. Any nuts will do here, of course. And if you hate nuts in your brownies, just add two more handfuls of chocolate chips here instead. Also, coconut oil works really well as a replacement for the butter, if you have to be dairy-free.

NOODLE KUGEL

Feeds 8

This Ashkenazi Jewish recipe, typically a Shabbat dish, is the ultimate comfort food: slippery egg noodles baked with full-fat dairy and sugar and eggs, all tumbled together to make a warm, sweet pudding. Our friend Katie Workman told us in New York on our potluck tour that after the horror of September 11th, she and her young son put together a dish of noodle kugel the first time she cooked after the tragedy. She now associates this dish with that time, the trying to come alive again by cooking with her kid. This is food that helps to comfort and heal.

16 tablespoons (230 grams) unsalted butter, melted

1 pound gluten-free tagliatelle

8 large eggs, at room temperature

1½ cups (315 grams) organic cane sugar

1½ pounds full-fat cottage cheese

2 teaspoons vanilla extract

¼ teaspoon freshly grated nutmeg

Pinch kosher salt

Prepare to bake. Preheat the oven to 350°F. Grease a 9 x 13-inch baking dish with a bit of the butter.

Cook the pasta. Set a large pot of salted water over high heat. When the water comes to a boil, add the pasta. Stir continuously for the first minute, then cook without stirring until the pasta is just starting to soften, about 5 minutes. Drain the noodles.

Make the kugel. In the bowl of a stand mixer with the paddle attachment, beat the eggs until they are frothy. Slowly, with the mixer running, add the sugar and beat until the eggs and sugar are fluffy, then add the remaining butter, cottage cheese, vanilla, nutmeg, and salt. Turn off the mixer and stir in the noodles with a rubber spatula. Pour it all into the prepared pan.

Bake the kugel. Bake the kugel until the kugel is set and the tops of the noodles are browning and crisp, about 1½ hours. Serve immediately.

Feel like playing?

Is there such a thing as nondairy cottage cheese? If you know a good substitute for that here, please use it. I have a feeling this dish is probably rooted in the tradition of these foods. But that doesn't mean you can't reinvent it!

CHOCOLATE-BANANA BREAD PUDDING

Feeds 8

Although the South has a special affection for bread pudding, this is a dish loved across the United States. It's a great way to make stale bread into something extraordinary. With a bit of milk (we like coconut milk here), some spices, eggs, bananas, and chocolate chips, you have something great to make out of those bread slices going stale in your kitchen. Danny and I had a chocolate-banana cake at our wedding, so we have a fondness for this flavor combination with bread pudding as well.

2 cups full-fat coconut milk

¼ cup (52 grams) coconut oil, melted

2 large eggs, beaten

½ cup (105 grams) organic cane sugar

½ teaspoon fine sea salt

½ teaspoon ground cinnamon

½ teaspoon ground ginger

6 cups gluten-free bread cubes

3 ripe bananas, cut into thick slices

1 cup (70 grams) semisweet chocolate chips (we like Guittard)

Prepare to bake. Preheat the oven to 325°F.

Heat the milk. Set a large pot over medium-high heat. Pour in the coconut milk and coconut oil. Cook, stirring, until the mixture is fully heated and beginning to simmer.

Make the bread pudding. In a large bowl, mix together the eggs, sugar, salt, cinnamon, and ginger. Stir in the bread cubes. Add the bananas and chocolate chips and toss everything together to coat. Pour in the milk mixture and stir everything together.

Bake the bread pudding. Pour the bread pudding into a 9 x 13-inch baking dish. Bake, uncovered, until a knife inserted in the center come out clean, about 45 minutes. Let the bread pudding cool for 15 minutes, then serve.

Feel like playing?

You can easily take out the chocolate and bananas here and use whatever flavorings you want: apples and walnuts; maple and bacon; apricots and hazelnuts; coffee syrup and pumpkin custard. You can make up what works best in your kitchen.

BOSTON CREAM PIE

Feeds 4 to 6

A Boston cream pie is a cake, not a pie. Our version of the recipe contains coconut milk, not cream. But at least this dessert was truly invented in Boston. However, the first person to make it was an Armenian-French chef, not an American. We learned how to make this gorgeous dessert of sponge cake, creamy filling, and chocolate glaze from one of Boston's preeminent pastry chefs, Joanne Chang of Flour Bakery. Chef Chang is gracious and fiercely talented. First a chemistry major at Harvard, she realized she really wanted to make pastries instead. Her meticulous scientific mind creates spectacular recipes that always work. We're honored to know her, and we recommend her cookbook Flour, *in which the original recipe for her Boston cream pie is printed. I think she'd like this version too.*

FOR THE PASTRY CREAM

1¼ cups coconut milk

½ cup (100 grams) organic cane sugar

¼ cup (32 grams) arrowroot flour

½ teaspoon fine sea salt

4 large egg yolks

1 teaspoon vanilla extract

FOR THE SPONGE CAKE

4 large eggs, separated, plus 3 large egg whites

1 cup (210 grams) organic cane sugar

2 tablespoons freshly squeezed lemon juice

105 grams All-Purpose Gluten-Free Flour Blend (page 17)

Pinch fine sea salt

⅓ cup coffee syrup (page 309)

FOR THE CHOCOLATE GANACHE

One 14-ounce can full-fat coconut milk

½ teaspoon vanilla extract

12 ounces semisweet chocolate, chopped as small as possible

Prepare to bake. Preheat the oven to 350°F. Line a baking sheet with parchment paper.

Make the pastry cream. Set a large pot over medium-high heat. Pour in the coconut milk. Cook, stirring, until the milk comes to a low simmer. Simmer for 10 minutes, stirring frequently. Turn off the heat. In a bowl, combine the sugar, arrowroot, and salt. Beat the egg yolks and add to the mixture. Slowly, whisk the warm milk mixture into the mixture, a little at a time, until everything is well combined. Pour the pastry cream back into the pot and turn the heat back to medium-high. Whisk the pastry cream continuously until it starts to thicken, about 3 minutes. Do not let the pastry cream boil for longer than 10 seconds. If it starts to boil for too long, pull it off the heat. Stir in the vanilla. Allow the pastry cream to cool to room temperature, then cover it with plastic wrap and chill it in the refrigerator.

Beat the egg yolks and sugar. In the bowl of a stand mixer with the paddle attachment, beat the egg yolks, 1⁄4 cup of the sugar, and the lemon juice on high speed for 6 to 8 minutes, until they have doubled in volume and have thickened. Transfer the egg yolk mixture to a large bowl.

Beat the egg whites. Clean the bowl of the stand mixer thoroughly and dry it well. With the whisk attachment, beat all of the egg whites to stiff peaks. Add the remaining 3⁄4 cup of the sugar, 1 tablespoon at a time, until stiff, shiny peaks form.

Finish the batter. Fold one-third of the egg whites into the yolks, then fold in the remaining egg whites. Sprinkle the flour blend and salt over the top of the eggs and gently fold them in too.

Bake the sponge cake. Spread the cake batter evenly over the parchment-lined baking sheet with a rubber spatula. Bake for 9 minutes, then rotate the baking sheet 180 degrees in the oven. Bake the sponge cake until a toothpick inserted into the center comes out clean, another 9 to 14 minutes. Take the cake out of the oven and let it sit for 5 minutes.

Cool the cake. Set a piece of parchment paper on a wire rack. Run a sharp knife around the sides of the cake. Quickly, invert it onto the parchment paper. Peel off the top layer of parchment paper and cool the cake completely.

Cut the cake. Using a sharp knife, cut the cake in half lengthwise, then again crosswise. This should give you 4 equal-size pieces. Brush each of the pieces with the coffee syrup.

Assemble the cake. Put the first layer of cake on a flat platter, syrup side up. Spread one-quarter of the pastry cream over the cake, spreading to the edges a little thicker. Put the second layer of cake on top of the pastry cream and repeat the process. Repeat this until you have used all the cake pieces and pastry cream. Press down gently to make sure that the cake is flat. Cover the cake with plastic wrap, loosely, and put the cake in the freezer. Freeze overnight. You want the cake frozen solid.

CONTINUED

Prepare to serve the dessert. Three hours before you intend to serve the cake, pull it out of the freezer.

Make the ganache. Set a medium pot over medium-high heat. Pour in the coconut milk and vanilla. Bring the milk to a boil, stirring frequently. As soon as the milk boils, pour it over the chopped chocolate in a bowl and stir it up as quickly as you can. When the chocolate is fully melted and incorporated into the milk, it should be smooth. You have ganache.

Finish the cream pie. Pour the warm ganache over the top of the cake. Using an offset spatula, work quickly to spread the ganache evenly over the surface. Some of the ganache will drip down the sides. Believe me, you want that. Let the pie thaw to room temperature, and serve.

Feel like playing?

You can use the sponge cake for a number of other recipes, including jelly rolls. Pour this batter into a tube pan and you have angel food cake. Chocolate ganache is good on almost everything, especially dribbled onto homemade ice cream.

CHURROS

Feeds 8

This much-loved fried pastry from the Southwest is much simpler to make than it seems. It involves pâte à choux, *a French pastry term that might terrify just by the fact that it sounds French. Don't worry. It's a simple butter, flour, sugar, and eggs combination, made airy by heat and constant whisking. I love that a French culinary technique traveled to Mexico to help make these treats, which then made their way to New Mexico and Arizona. And now, they're gluten-free, via a kitchen on an island in the Pacific Northwest. That seems very American to me.*

1 cup water

5 tablespoons (75 grams) cold unsalted butter

2 tablespoons plus ¼ cup (60 grams) organic cane sugar

½ teaspoon fine sea salt

140 grams All-Purpose Gluten-Free Flour Blend (page 17)

1 teaspoon psyllium husks

2 large eggs, at room temperature

½ teaspoon vanilla extract

3 cups fat or oil of your choice for frying (we use rice bran oil)

1 teaspoon ground cinnamon

Feel like playing?

If you can't eat butter, coconut oil makes a great nondairy substitute here.

Cook the flour and sugar. Set a large pot over medium-high heat. Add the water, butter, 2 tablespoons of the sugar, and salt to the pot. When they come to a boil, whisk continuously to avoid burning. Add the flour blend and psyllium husks and whisk until everything is well combined and starting to bubble.

Make the churro batter. Add the mixture to the bowl of a stand mixer with the paddle attachment. With the mixer running, add the eggs, one at a time, making sure each is fully incorporated before adding another. Finish by adding the vanilla.

Heat the oil. Set a large wok over medium-high heat. Add the oil. Heat it to 375°F. Combine the remaining ¼ cup of sugar and the cinnamon on a plate.

Pipe the churros. Pour the churro batter into a pastry bag with a star tip. Pipe out 3 to 4 inches of batter directly into the hot oil, taking care to not burn yourself. (You can use a paring knife to release the end of the churro from the pastry bag.) Pipe no more than 3 churros in the oil at a time to avoid overcrowding. Fry until the churros are golden brown and crisp, 4 to 5 minutes. Remove the churros from the oil with a Chinese spider or slotted spoon and place on a paper towel–lined plate.

Toss the hot churros onto the plate of cinnamon sugar and coat them well. Fry the remaining batter the same way.

Eat immediately.

PERSIMMON PUDDING

Feeds 6 to 8

I can't say that I had ever heard of persimmon pudding before we began the research for this book. However, folks from Indiana made it clear they wanted to eat this much-loved dessert without gluten. I'm glad they insisted. This dessert is a lovely mishmash of fruit and sugar, part pudding and part cake. This recipe is adapted from one in Saveur, *which used the recipe of "Eva Powell, a former elementary-school librarian in Mitchell, Indiana, who has won the town's pudding contest five times with her recipe for persimmon pudding." That's good enough for us!*

4 tablespoons (58 grams) unsalted butter, melted

210 grams All-Purpose Gluten-Free Flour Blend (page 17)

1 teaspoon baking powder

½ teaspoon ground cinnamon

½ teaspoon fine sea salt

2 cups persimmon pulp (about 5 persimmons, peeled and pulped)

2 cups (420 grams) organic cane sugar

2 large eggs, beaten

1½ cups low-fat buttermilk

1 teaspoon baking soda

¼ cup coconut milk

Prepare to bake. Preheat the oven to 350°F. Grease a 9 x 13-inch baking dish with 2 tablespoons of the butter.

Combine the dry ingredients. In a bowl, whisk together the flour blend, baking powder, cinnamon, and salt. Set aside.

Make the batter. In the bowl of a stand mixer with the paddle attachment, mix together the persimmon pulp and sugar. Add the eggs and combine well. In a separate bowl, stir together the buttermilk and baking soda (watch it fizz!). With the mixer running on low, add the buttermilk to the pulp. Add the flour mixture, a bit at a time, making sure that all the flour is incorporated before adding more. Scrape down the sides of the bowl with a rubber spatula. Pour in the coconut milk and the remaining 2 tablespoons of butter. Mix until everything is thoroughly combined.

Bake the persimmon pudding. Pour the batter into the prepared dish. Bake until the edges are starting to crisp, the top is dark brown, and a toothpick inserted into the center comes out clean, about 1 hour. Allow the pudding to cool to room temperature.

Serve with whipped coconut cream, if you wish. Berries are also lovely. (These are optional.)

Feel like playing?

Mango pulp would work well here, as would mashed berries. Simply sub in 2 cups of the fruit you wish for the persimmons.

INDIAN PUDDING

Feeds 8

We stood on the green grass of the Common Ground Country Fair, surveying the scene. It was September, turning a bit chilly after a warm day filled with fun, Maine organic farmers' style: horse and wagon rides, wood whittling stations for the kids, milking demonstrations and apple cider making and wheat grinding (we skipped that one). The kids had participated in an organic garden parade; Lucy had been dressed as a pea in a pod. We were there with our friends Tara Barker and Josh Hixon, who run an incredible restaurant in Rockland called 3Crow. Tara is a gluten-free pastry chef and one of my favorite people in the world. After years of talking online, we finally knew each other in person. It was such a good day.

At the beginning of the evening, as the air grew cooler, Tara treated me to Indian pudding. A woman pulled a scoop of the least pretty dessert I've ever seen out of a slow cooker. One bite and I stopped caring about pretty. Deeply sweetened with molasses and ginger, mingled with cornmeal and milk, this pudding tasted of the place it was made. While this is a naturally gluten-free recipe, we offer it here because most of us outside New England have not eaten it. Besides, it's based on the British hasty pudding, which requires boiling wheat flour. Settlers in New England substituted the cornmeal they learned to use from the Native Americans. This is a resilient pudding, very much American, made gluten-free from necessity and even more delicious for it.

5 tablespoons (79 grams) unsalted butter

3½ cups coconut milk

¼ cup molasses

¼ cup (35 grams) cornmeal (make sure it's gluten-free)

1 large egg, at room temperature

½ cup (105 grams) organic cane sugar

½ teaspoon fine sea salt

½ teaspoon ground ginger

½ teaspoon ground cinnamon

Prepare to bake. Preheat the oven to 325°F. Grease a 9 x 13-inch baking dish with 2 tablespoons of the butter.

Thicken the milk. Put a small pot over medium-high heat. Pour in 3 cups of the coconut milk. Bring the milk to a low boil. Immediately whisk in the molasses and cornmeal. Cook, stirring frequently, until the coconut milk has thickened to the consistency of pudding, about 10 minutes.

Finish the batter. In a large bowl, whisk together the egg, sugar, salt, ginger, and cinnamon. Slowly, whisk in the hot milk mixture until everything is thoroughly combined. Pour the pudding into the prepared pan.

CONTINUED

Bake the pudding. Bake the pudding for 30 minutes, then add the remaining ½ cup of coconut milk and remaining 3 tablespoons of butter. Stir vigorously to incorporate, then continue baking until the pudding is firm, about 1 hour. Allow the pudding to cool before serving.

Feel like playing?

We make this with coconut milk to allow dairy-free folks the chance to make it. (If you are dairy-free, you can substitute coconut oil for the butter here.) We also like the way that milk thickens and flavors the pudding. If you would prefer, however, you can use cow's milk instead.

COFFEE MILK CUSTARDS

Feeds 6

Rhode Island has a more specific food culture than any small state we have ever visited. The folks in Providence who came to our potluck were kind, enthusiastic good cooks who had very definite opinions on every dish we mentioned. When someone talked about coffee milk, Danny and I both looked puzzled. "Wait, you haven't tried coffee milk?!" someone said, and then the entire room seemed to roar. It turns out that coffee milk—like chocolate milk made with sweetened coffee syrup instead of chocolate syrup—is the state drink of Rhode Island. After we made some for ourselves, I saw why. Most folks buy their coffee syrup (Autocrat being the dominant brand in Rhode Island, with Dave's Coffee supplying a syrup without high-fructose corn syrup), but we found it so easy to make our own that we had to stop making it for fear of drinking it all the time. Instead, we put it into these coconut milk custards. Coffee milk indeed!

FOR THE COFFEE SYRUP

1 cup water

1 cup strong brewed coffee (you could even try espresso)

1 cup (210 grams) organic cane sugar

FOR THE CUSTARDS

1½ cups coconut milk

½ cup (105 grams) organic cane sugar

3 tablespoons whole coffee beans

1 teaspoon vanilla bean paste (or 1½ teaspoons vanilla extract)

4 large egg yolks

3 tablespoons arrowroot flour

½ cup cold coconut cream

Make the coffee syrup. Set a large pot over medium-high heat. Pour the water, coffee, and sugar into the pot. Stirring constantly, heat until the liquid starts to come to a boil. Turn the heat down to low and simmer the liquid, stirring frequently, until the sugar dissolves and the liquid starts to thicken into a syrup, 5 to 6 minutes. Use a pastry brush to wipe down the sides of the pot once in a while. Keep the heat low, because boiling the syrup will turn it bitter. Take the pot off the heat and pour the syrup into a thick glass or mug.

Simmer the milk. Clean out the pot in which you simmered the syrup and set it over medium-high heat again. Pour in the coconut milk, sugar, coffee beans, and vanilla bean paste (or extract). Bring the milk to a simmer and then turn the heat down to low. Stir occasionally until the sugar has entirely dissolved. Turn off the heat.

Make the custard base. In a large bowl, whisk the egg yolks, ¼ cup of the coffee syrup, and the arrowroot. Slowly, whisking continuously, add the warm milk mixture until it has all become fully incorporated. Return the mixture to the pot and turn the heat to medium-high. Whisk continuously until the custard starts to thicken, about 3 minutes. Turn off the heat. Strain the custard base through a fine-mesh sieve into a large bowl. Let the custard base cool to room temperature, then pour it into 6 ramekins. Cover the ramekins loosely with plastic wrap and refrigerate for at least 2 hours to chill entirely.

Serve with coconut whipped cream and a drizzle of the coffee syrup.

Feel like playing?

I think cinnamon would be delicious in this. Use the coffee syrup for cold drinks (we prefer fizzy water to milk, ourselves) and other desserts. Watch out: it's pretty addictive, that coffee syrup.

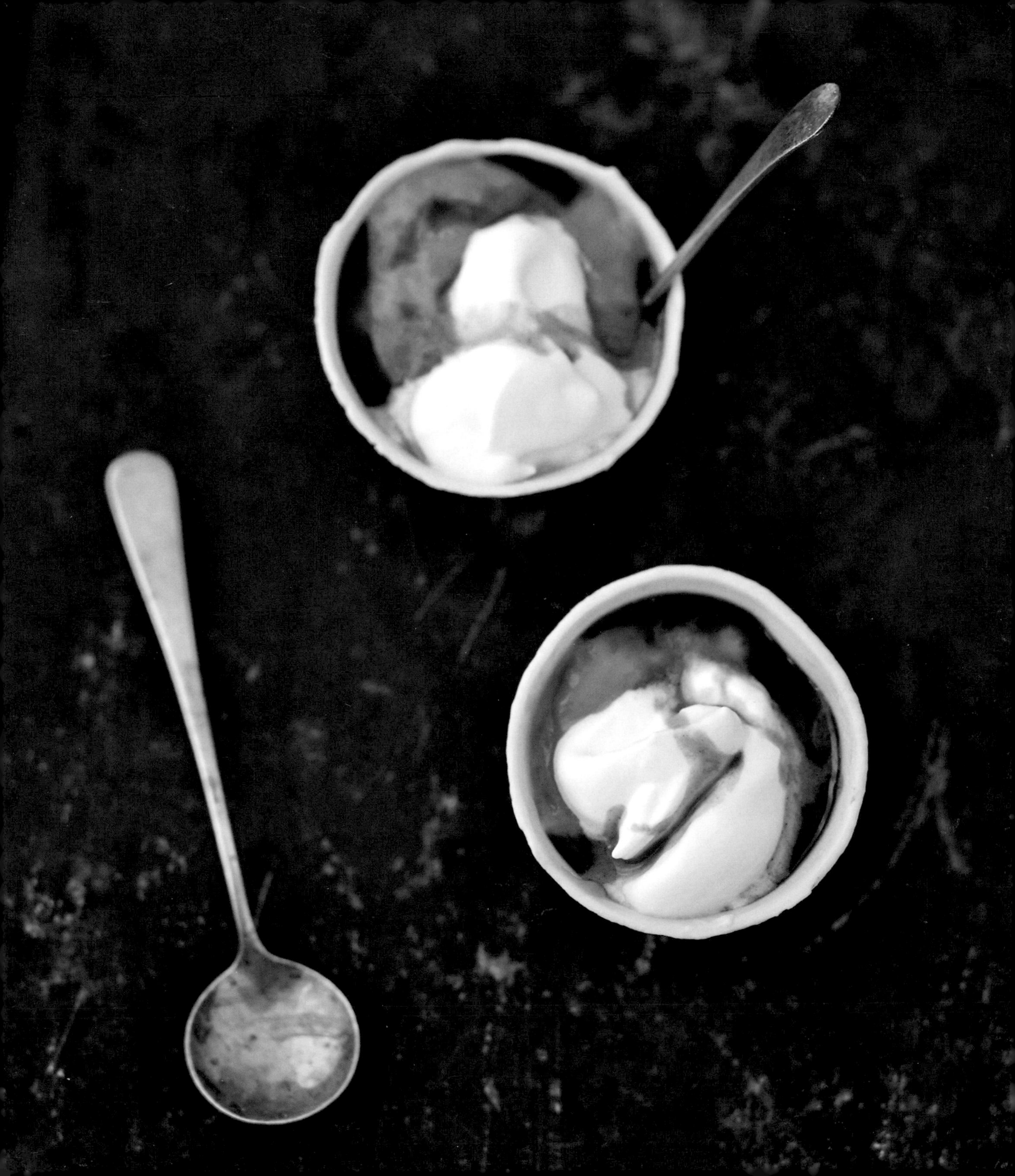

Index

C

D

E

F

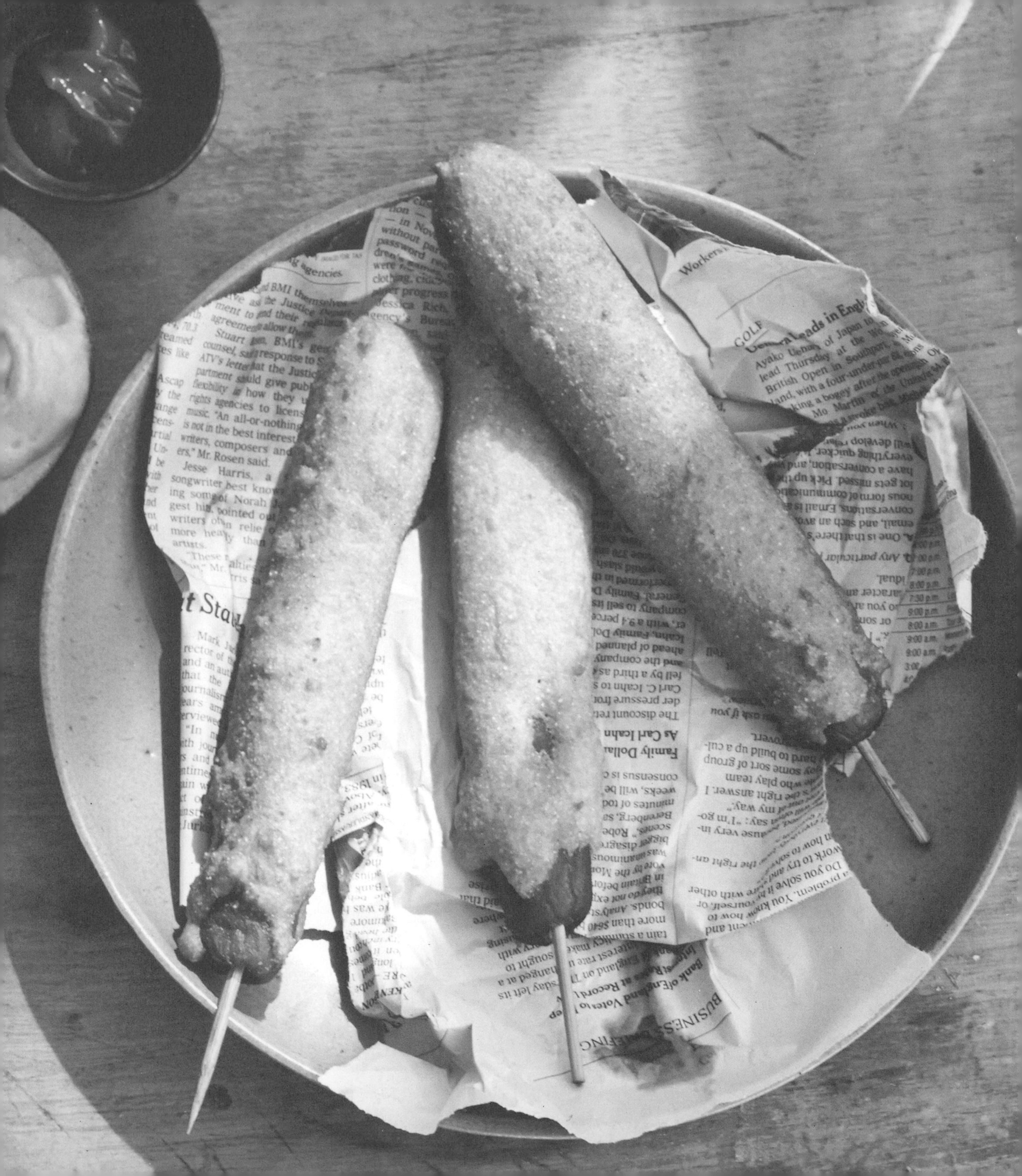

is not in the best interest
writers, composers and
ers," Mr. Rosen said.
Jesse Harris, a
songwriter best know
GOLF